The Complete Idiot's Reference Card

Basic Weight-Lifting Exercises

Legs:
Leg extensions
Leg curls
Leg presses
Standing toe raises

Back:
Lat pull downs
Cable rows
Upright rows

Triceps:
Triceps pushdown
Triceps kickback

Abs:
Crunches
Reverse crunches
Oblique crunches

Chest:
Bench presses
Incline presses
Dips
Pec deck

Shoulders:
Military presses
Lateral raises
Front raises

Biceps:
Seated biceps curl
Concentration curl

Ten Commandments of the Weight Room

1. Lift to improve your strength, not to show off your strength.
2. Progress from larger muscles to smaller muscles.
3. Work out two or three nonconsecutive days per week.
4. Always use a spotter for freeweight exercises such as the bench press, squat, and military press.
5. Never hold your breath when lifting.
6. Use slow, controlled movements—don't swing or bounce the weights.
7. Always use collars on barbells.
8. Warm up and stretch before lifting—loose, warm muscles are less prone to injury.
9. Never sacrifice form to lift more weight.
10. As you get stronger, increase the weight by 5 to 10 percent.

Cardiovascular Exercises

➤ Exercise three to six days per week.
➤ Work out 20-plus minutes per day.
➤ Train in your target heart rate zone—60 to 85 percent maximum heart rate.
➤ Always warm up before and cool down after your workout.

alpha
books

Stretching Exercises

- ➤ Warm up before you stretch—cold muscles are more prone to injury.
- ➤ Stretch all major muscle groups.
- ➤ Hold stretches 20 to 30 seconds.
- ➤ Never bounce or stretch to the point of pain.
- ➤ Don't hold your breath while stretching.

Nutrition

- ➤ Drink at least 80 ounces of water per day—more when you exercise.
- ➤ Don't skip meals.
- ➤ Avoid high-fat foods and empty calories.
- ➤ Limit fat intake to 20 to 25 percent of your daily intake.
- ➤ Carbohydrates are your most efficient and effective source of energy.

Advanced Techniques

- ➤ **Supersets:** Perform two consecutive exercises with no rest between. Use approximately 25 percent less weight than normal for the second exercise.
- ➤ **Negatives:** Allow a spotter to lift the weight for you, but slowly lower the weight by yourself. Use up to 40 percent more weight than usual for negatives.
- ➤ **Breakdowns:** After you end your set, decrease the weight by about 20 percent and try to do an additional three or four reps.
- ➤ **Assisted reps:** Once you reach fatigue, continue to work as hard as possible and allow a spotter to help you complete three or four more reps.
- ➤ **SuperSlow:** Slow your reps down to a ten-second positive, five-second negative pace.

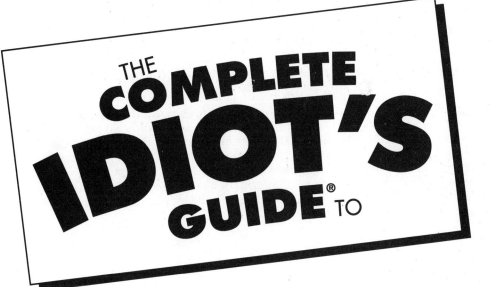

THE **COMPLETE IDIOT'S GUIDE**® TO

Weight Training

by Deidre Johnson-Cane, Jonathan Cane, and Joe Glickman

alpha books

201 West 103rd Street
Indianapolis, IN 46290

A Pearson Education Company

To our families—who gave us the passion to lift and chutzpah to write.
—Deidre, Jonathan, and Joe

International Standard Book Number: 0-02-863197-8
Library of Congress Catalog Card Number: Available from the Library of Congress.

02   01   8   7   6   5   4   3

Interpretation of the printing code: the rightmost number of the first series of numbers is the year of the book's printing; the rightmost number of the second series of numbers is the number of the book's printing. For example, a printing code of 00-1 shows that the first printing occurred in 2000.

Printed in the United States of America

Note: This publication contains the opinions and ideas of its authors. It is intended to provide helpful and informative material on the subject matter covered. It is sold with the understanding that the author and publisher are not engaged in rendering professional services in the book. If the reader requires personal assistance or advice, a competent professional should be consulted.

The authors and publisher specifically disclaim any responsibility for any liability, loss or risk, personal or otherwise, which is incurred as a consequence, directly or indirectly, of the use and application of any of the contents of this book.

Publisher
Marie Butler-Knight

Editorial Director
Gary M. Krebs

Product Manager
Phil Kitchel

Associate Managing Editor
Cari Luna

Acquisitions Editor
Amy Zavatto

Development Editors
Nancy D. Warner
Suzanne LeVert

Production Editor
Michael Thomas

Copy Editor
Faren Bachelis

Illustrator
Jody P. Schaeffer

Cover Designers
Mike Freeland
Kevin Spear

Book Designers
Scott Cook and Amy Adams of DesignLab

Photographer
Peter Baiamonte

Indexer
Angie Bess

Layout/Proofreading
Terri Edwards
John Etchison
Mary Hunt
Gloria Schurick

Contents at a Glance

Contents

33 What's Up, Doc?   397

Appendixes

A Glossary   409

B Resources   415

Index   421

Introduction

We've all seen the infomercials on TV where some model using the "Superduper Tummy Tuck" machine has achieved his statuesque body by supposedly using this gizmo for 20 minutes every other day. Never mind that that body-beautiful model is an out-of-work actor who has spent three hours a day working out for the last 10 years. The selling point behind virtually all of these "quick-and-easy" fitness devices is that honing your body into a figure Michelangelo would be eager to sculpt is basically effortless. This, of course, isn't the case.

Getting into peak physical shape takes time and effort. That's the bad news. The good news is that you have plenty of time to realize the strong and supple physique that you've always wanted. Why? Getting into and then staying in shape is a life-long process and not something that you do in frenetic preparation for your twentieth high school reunion or to look good at the beach. Done properly, strength training is an important piece in a process where you learn how to restore your body's natural gifts, gifts that are often stymied by our busy, modern lives.

While we can't guarantee that reading this book will turn you into the next Arnold Schwarzenegger, we feel quite confident that if you follow our advice and implement it correctly you will look and feel better than you've ever felt before—it just might take longer than 20 minutes.

What You'll Find in This Book

This book is a complete guide to strength training, but it is also a primer on getting and staying in shape on a more comprehensive basis. While we concentrate on lifting weights, we hope to impress on you the importance of proper nutrition, posture, stretching, and cardiovascular exercise. Strength training will get you strong; implementing these other aspects will get you fit. We'll present you with everything the beginner needs to know to make his or her introduction to weight lifting as painless (literally and figuratively) as possible. You'll learn about everything from shopping for a gym to setting up your first exercise program to pushing through plateaus as you progress. We've divided the book into several major parts.

Part 1, "Priming the Pump." In this first section, we'll fill you in on everything you need to know before you begin a weight-lifting program, including some important advise about how you really can't afford *not* to work out. Many people want to work out but feel intimidated by the newness of this foreign place with sweaty strangers and loud music. In fact, a gym is a social place where you're likely to make good friends. We'll familiarize you with the nuances of the gym so that those first days are largely anxiety-free.

Part 2, "Gearing Up." This section is a complete primer on everything you'll need to know before you actually get to a gym. In addition, we'll discuss the importance (or lack thereof) of looking good in your exercise threads. In other words—what to wear and why. We don't necessarily agree with Andre "Image is Everything" Agassi, but we don't want you to walk around in hip waders and boxer shorts.

Part 3, "Ready to Roll." Now the fun starts. We'll take you through a guided tour of the gym—from soup to nuts, or rather machines to shower stalls. To the uninitiated, gyms can be confusing institutions of higher fitness; we'll familiarize you with the basics you'll need to know before you get started. Understanding the way most gyms organize their equipment is an excellent way to learn the lay of the land.

Part 4, "The Workout." It's funny how many people who start lifting have little or no idea what muscles they're working. "I want to work these things," they say, pointing to their deltoids. You'll find a complete list of weight-lifting exercises for your entire body. Each exercise is accompanied by photos and a thorough explanation of what to do. Why is it important to hold your elbows here or your knees there? This section, which tells you how and why, is your own personal trainer guiding you in print.

Part 5, "Leaner and Meaner." Now that you've learned the nuances of the equipment, the exercises, and the philosophy behind working out, we're going to show you how to put it all together. We'll give you guidelines on which exercises to include in your routine depending on your goals and time constraints, and what to do if things aren't working out the way you expected.

Part 6, "When in Rome." In this section, we'll address special health issues that may be important to some of you. We'll talk about strength-training issues specific to women; the importance and viability of strength training for seniors; overcoming obstacles; guidelines for a safe and effective workout for youngsters; and working out with injuries and illness. The bottom line that unites all of these disparate categories is passion, common sense, and desire.

Extras

To make the learning experience as easy and as fun as possible, we've highlighted lots of tips and facts along the way. Look for the following elements in the book to guide you along.

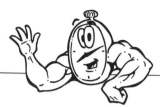

Weight a Minute

The Weight a Minute sidebars will highlight safety issues that are important to your health and welfare. The gym can be a dangerous and intimidating place if you don't know what to expect. Read these cautions carefully to ensure that your workout is pain-free.

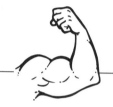

Flex Facts

Flex Facts are interesting tidbits and anecdotes. They're not essential for you to have a safe or effective workout, but you should find them informative and sometimes amusing.

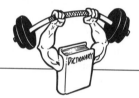

Bar Talk

Bar Talk sidebars provide you with definitions of new terms that are introduced in the text. By adding them to your gymspeak vocabulary, you might not lift any better, but you will be better informed.

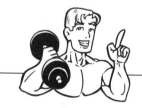

Spot Me

Spot Me's are tips and pointers to help make your lifting more effective. Think of them as having a personal trainer giving you help throughout your workout. They highlight little things that might otherwise go unnoticed.

Acknowledgments

Writing a book is a little like building a beautiful body: It's a great idea with many rich rewards, but man, it boils down to plain old hard work. The three of us—friends when we started, better friends when we finished—enjoyed working on this project, but there were plenty of times when we would rather have been doing something else. Of course, writing this book would have been far more difficult without the invaluable input of quite a few people. In no particular order, we'd like to thank: Ralph Anastasio, of Printing House Fitness Center in New York City, for the use of his great facility. Special thanks to our models, Sejal "Big Dog" Vyas, Barrie "Sheba" Lifton, David Duhan, Aristides Maisonave, Chris Zogopoulos, and Melissa Silver (and baby Ethan) for their friendship, good looks, and good cheer. We couldn't have done this without Nancy Warner and Suzanne LeVert, who tolerated endless questions and e-mails from Jonathan.

Special thanks from Deidre to her father and sister for their endless faith in her and to Laura Giovanella for her patience and support.

Jonathan would like to thank a few of his teachers—Bob Otto, John Wygand, Bob Perez, and Ralph Carpinelli, without whom this book would contain far fewer big words and sophisticated ideas. In addition, he'd like to give a big high five to his friends, cycling teammates, and most of all his family, for their support and patience.

Last, but not least, Joe wishes to thank his lovely, literate wife, Beth, and darling daughter, Willa, who at age three can already type her name. Most of all, he'd like to thank his coauthors, Jonathan, a terrible mountain biker but great fitness trainer, and "D," a beautiful woman who gets downright ugly when she wins World Powerlifting Championships. Without their wit and wisdom, he would be wandering lost in the fitness forest.

Special Thanks to the Technical Reviewer

The Complete Idiot's Guide to Weight Training was reviewed by an expert who double-checked the accuracy of what you'll learn here to help us ensure that this book gives you everything you need to know about weight training. Special thanks are extended to Dr. Bob Otto.

Dr. Robert M. Otto is Professor and Director of the Human Performance Laboratory at Adelphi University, Garden City, NY. He currently serves on the Board of Trustees of the American College of Sports Medicine. He has published and presented more than 200 papers on the role of exercise in health, disease, and functional performance. He is an avid triathlete and runner who has completed more than 80 triathlons and a dozen marathons.

Trademarks

All terms mentioned in this book that are known to be or are suspected of being trademarks or service marks have been appropriately capitalized. Alpha Books and Pearson Education cannot attest to the accuracy of this information. Use of a term in this book should not be regarded as affecting the validity of any trademark or service mark.

Part 1

Priming the Pump

In this first section, we'll fill you in on everything you need to know before you begin a weight-training program, including some important advice about how you really can't afford not to work out. Many people want to work out but feel intimated by the newness of this foreign place with sweaty strangers and loud music. We'll familiarize you with the nuances of the gym so that those first days are largely anxiety-free.

Chapter 1 is loaded with compelling reasons why you should lift weights—to feel and look good, to lose weight, to improve your serve, as well as to make friends—and more.

Once we've convinced you that you should lift, in Chapter 2 we'll give you some tips on how to find the time in your busy schedule. Working out may seem totally impractical until you realize how to do it efficiently. In Chapter 3, we'll explain what exactly happens to your muscles when you lift and discuss the pros and cons of lifting in the gym or at home. (Hint: we're biased to heading to a gym.)

Chapters 4 and 5 tell you all you need to know about choosing the right gym. And we also give you the lowdown on how to equip your home gym if that's the route you choose to take.

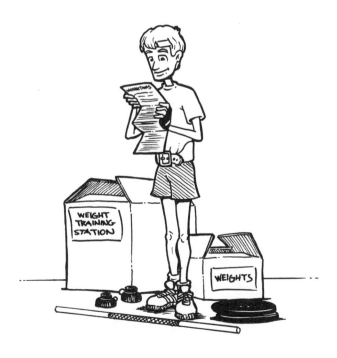

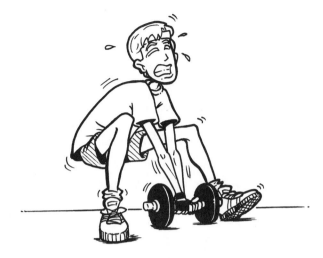

Let's Get Physical!

In This Chapter

➤ Choosing to stay healthy and fit

➤ Understanding how weight training burns fat

➤ How to get the winning edge—safely

➤ Anyone, even you, can weight train!

There's a scene in an episode of *Seinfeld* in which a brassy, no-talent comedian tells Jerry that he's gotten so big from lifting weights that his suits no longer fit him. "I'm huge!" he brags. "You really oughta lift," he instructs the slender Seinfeld. Jerry replies: "Why?" This basic bit of logic throws the "pumped" lifter for a loop. "Don't know," he says quizzically.

Actually, there are more good reasons to lift weights than there are good sitcoms on television. In this chapter, we'll show you what those reasons are and how they might apply to your own life and fitness goals. Read on!

Some Good Reasons Why

Here are eight:

1. It will improve your overall health and sense of well-being.

2. It will make you stronger and help prevent injuries on the playing field—virtually a must if you're a competitive athlete or weekend warrior.

3. It's great for the ego: It's an excellent way to turn a soft body hard and a trim body into one that turns heads. People will be saying to you, "Wow, you look much younger!" Trust us.

4. Weight training can help a self-conscious teenager develop more confidence. (Poor body image is often a source of anxiety for high school–age kids.)

5. A regular gym routine is a perfect way to release stress for office types who rarely lift anything heavier than a telephone. (Many of the gym regulars we know are teachers and cops who maintain their sanity by working out.)

6. It's the perfect way for a new mother to regain her prepregnancy figure.

7. Research has shown that the best way for senior citizens to retard muscle loss and reduced bone density is strength training.

8. Your social life is apt to improve, both because you're going to look and feel better—and thus be more attractive—and because you'll probably meet some people just by working out, either in the gym or around the neighborhood.

And we could go on! But here's the good news/bad news wrinkle. The upside of strength training is that the health benefits are unquestionable, and just about anyone between the ages of 15 and 105 can reap huge benefits from pumping iron. The downside is that there's a lot of misinformation floating around in the fitness world, and worse, scores of personal trainers who do more harm than good. Sounds odd, but it's true.

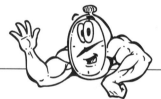

Weight a Minute

Don't assume that the impressive-looking trainer with the great body knows what he or she is talking about. There is no degree or national certification requirement for fitness instructors or exercise physiologists; anyone can call himself or herself a personal trainer, fitness instructor, or exercise physiologist. However, academic credentials in exercise science or certification from an organization such as the American College of Sports Medicine (ACSM) provides recognition of minimal competence.

Collectively, the authors of this book have lifted for more years than we care to admit. Deidre became a physical therapist, and Jonathan earned a master's degree in Exercise Physiology, so we've learned a little about the science behind lifting as well.

We've made dozens of mistakes: from overtraining to neglecting certain exercises that are essential to building core strength. We've learned a lot though trial, error, and study, and along the way, Deidre became a world-champion athlete; Joe became a nationally ranked kayak paddler; and Jonathan transformed from an inactive musician to a competitive cyclist. While we can't guarantee that reading this book will transform you from a 98-pound weakling into a muscular Charles Atlas look-alike (genetics, diet, and years of hard work determine that), we'll provide more than enough information to teach you what works and what doesn't. We'll help you weed through many of the myths and pieces of misinformation that clutter the path to a healthier and stronger body, and in between offer enough training techniques to help you look and feel like a thoroughbred.

"Why lift?" you ask. The truth is, you really can't afford *not* to.

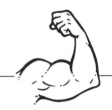

Flex Facts

There are approximately 58 million Americans between the ages of 20 and 74 who are considered overweight. That's about one-third of the country's population whose health would benefit from a decrease in body fat.

Slim Fast

Odd as it may seem in a culture so obsessed with appearance, we Americans are the most obese nation in the world. (All right, there might be an island in the South Pacific with a higher percentage of heavyweights, but you get the point.) We might have more gyms than any other country, but apparently not enough people are using them. The number of books, videos, and "miraculous" medical procedures designed to beautify you in no time could fill an auditorium large enough for a Richard Simmons dance-a-thon. As P. T. Barnum might have said, "Beware of snake oil salesmen and infomercials guaranteeing you'll 'lose ugly pounds in as little as 10 minutes a day'."

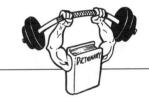

Bar Talk

Hypertrophy is the growth of the individual fibers that make up a muscle. This growth usually occurs as a result of a stimulus to the muscle provided by an external stimulus like weight lifting.

Interestingly, until recently little focus has been placed on how effective weight lifting can be in the battle of the bulge. How does building muscle help you lose fat? The average American adult loses half a pound of muscle each year. Done properly, strength training will maintain or increase your muscle mass, a phenomenon physiology students and fitness geeks refer to as *hypertrophy*. In other words, because each pound of muscle burns up to 30-40 calories a day (the exact figure is debatable), someone who lifts regularly will burn more calories than someone who doesn't.

Here's the beautiful byproduct of weight training: By adding muscle, you may increase your daily caloric expenditure even when you're sitting at a desk, watching the tube, or sleeping. (Now there's an outrageous advertising claim: "Get slim while you sleep.")

There is, of course, a catch. Lifting weights alone won't make you slim. We all know people who come to the gym faithfully for years yet never seem to loose those unwanted pounds. We've even seen some who get fatter—no easy feat. And as any football fan knows, the gridiron is littered with turbo-powerful no-neck muscleheads who are as rotund as prize-winning heifers. In other words, just because you're strong or diligent about working out doesn't mean you'll be slim, nor does it mean you're actually fit. Weight training alone does not expend a lot of calories (only 8-12 calories/minute during the actual muscular contractions).

The bulk of this book is devoted to showing you proper weight-lifting techniques and principles; however, showing you how to merge strength and fitness—health and wellness, if you will—is a large part of what we're eager to teach you. We'll show you how to become strong and lean, as well as how to look your best. But we also want you to feel good—an aspect of fitness that is often underemphasized.

Here's something to keep in mind: There is no quick fix, no pill, sweat suit, or tummy-tuck that will turn fat to muscle. Getting and staying lean is about making intelligent decisions: how and when to exercise, how and what to eat. Put simply, lifting weights should be an important element of anyone's fitness regime.

In Chapter 7, "Food for Thought," we'll cover all you need to know about diet. In Chapter 11, "Safety First," we'll show you how to stretch—a woefully neglected part of overall fitness. And in Chapter 25, "Lift Well, Play Hard," we'll give you enough information about aerobic exercise to prepare you for the Ironman Triathlon. For now, know this: Pumping iron is a strong ally in your efforts to prune unwanted pounds from your physique.

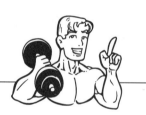

Spot Me

If you want to improve your game—no matter what game you play—try weight training. Dr. Wayne Westcott, research director at the South Shore YMCA in Quincy, Massachusetts, found significant improvements in golfers' club head speed and drive distance with just eight weeks of strength training. The good news is that increased strength can help almost any athlete's game.

The Winning Edge

It seems so obvious now since virtually every professional athlete lifts weights, but it wasn't long ago that many athletes thought that weight training would make them "muscle-bound" and impair their athletic ability. In fact, until Evander Holyfield, the "built up" heavyweight champion, hired a strength coach and showed the boxing world what weights could do for one's prowess in the ring, few fighters ever touched a barbell. (If you want to see a near-perfect back, check out "Real Deal" Holyfield.)

Here's a random sampling of athletes who've benefited from time in the gym:

➤ Martina Navratilova, who dominated women's tennis in the 1980s, says weight training transformed her from a "pudgy player" to the strongest woman in the sport. (Chris Evert, her chief rival, was convinced she couldn't compete with Navratilova unless she weight trained herself. Once she did, she began beating Martina again.)

➤ Would Mark McGwire have hit 70 homers in 1998 without the added oomph he gained from the weight room?

➤ Even Tiger Woods—a golfer!—proved the benefits of lifting. Had he not pumped iron, it's doubtful he could drive the ball a country mile.

➤ Six-time NBA champion Michael Jordan lifted like a fiend even during the season—though it didn't help his golf or baseball any.

And the list goes on and on.

No matter what sport you play—whether you're a jockey, gymnast, rock climber, surfer, swimmer, skier, softball player, tennis player—weight lifting will help improve your game. If, for example, you're a golfer, strengthening the muscles in your shoulders, arms, hips, and abdomen will help you add distance to your drive (assuming you practice). Perhaps more important, staying strong and limber will cut down on the number of injuries you incur, which means you'll be able to play more rounds.

Of course, don't assume that Kryptonian strength will make a professional star out of mere mortals, but you're likely to be amazed at how much weight training can help your performance in your game of choice.

Buffer Bod

Call us mavericks for going so far out on a limb with this statement, but muscles look good. And to many people, especially men, bigger is better.

Not convinced? Arnold Schwarzenegger, a six-time Mr. Universe before he turned to the silver screen, banked on an anatomically perfect (albeit inflated) body, not his acting ability.

Visit Rodin's *The Thinker* and Michelangelo's *David*, two sculpted hunks depicted sans clothes, and the transfixed gazes on admiring spectators highlights our inherent fascination with the male ideal. (Having seen them, we can tell you that both statues have bigger biceps than Arnold.)

Flex Facts

Arnold Schwarzenegger is one of the world's most popular movie stars. The Austrian-born ex-bodybuilder has gone from Mr. Olympia to Conan the Barbarian to a stint as the chairman of the President's Council on Physical Fitness. Today, Arnold is one of the 10 wealthiest entertainers in America, worth an estimated $50 million.

While excessive vanity is a turnoff—Narcissus, where art thou?—properly controlled, it's a positive force since it's the primary reason most people come to the gym. How many times have you heard people make this springtime resolve: "Got to get in shape for the beach." (As if it's okay with them to be grossly out of shape the other 10 months of the year.)

One of the amazing, even addicting, aspects of weight lifting is seeing how quickly your untoned muscles respond to the task at hand. The body is an amazing machine, adaptable, responsive, capable of more than you probably ever thought possible—but it needs to be challenged to reach its potential.

After just a few weeks of steady working out you're likely to be amazed by the changes that occur. Not only does adding muscle burn more calories, but adding mass to your upper body will change your proportions and make your waist look smaller. (Women often try and create this illusion by wearing shoulder pads—a poor fashion choice if you're wearing a bathing suit.)

Strain to Avoid Pain

Preventing injuries may not be the most glamorous aspect of strength training, but it may be the most important. Here's a predictable pattern we've seen time and again.

1. Highly motivated man lifts like a fiend.

2. Sees significant results.

3. Piles on more and more weight until he suffers an injury (shoulder or elbow typically) that sends him to the sidelines for weeks.

4. Slowly, steadily he works himself back into shape until he gets strong enough to make the same mistakes that led to the injury in the first place.

Welcome to the "More isn't better, don't listen to your body" syndrome (better known to certain experts as The MIBDLTYB Syndrome).

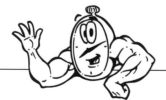

Weight a Minute

One of the main causes of injury in the gym is working with too much weight or going for that extra repetition on your own. Never let your ego get in the way of proper form and safety.

Here's a basic lesson in physiology: One of the primary functions of muscles—besides allowing you to move—is providing protection for your joints. Strong, supple muscles absorb more impact than weak, tight ones and reduce stress on your ankles, knees, hips, and vertebrae. As a result, increasing muscular strength and endurance will not only make everyday activities—from walking and running to mowing the lawn, carrying your kids, schlepping suitcases through the airport—easier for you, but will also reduce your risk of back injuries and other problems. After all, the time you spend in the gym each day pales in comparison to the physical challenges that await you in the "regular" world. Which is why it's ironic that some people will huff and puff for an hour on a Stairmaster, but will refuse to walk up a few flights of stairs. As fitness expert Steve Ilg says, "Take your gym everywhere."

Good Back

Millions of us suffer from back pain. In fact, the complaint Deidre hears most often in her physical therapy practice is: "My lower back hurts!" Why? As a people we sit more than we do just about anything else. We slouch in our car to and from work. Most of us sit in an office chair for eight or more hours a day (usually in front of a computer that isn't designed with the human anatomy in mind). Then we slouch on the couch at home for hours in front of the tube. We are, after all, a people who will wait in line at the drive-through window even when there's no one waiting inside.) No wonder our backs ache—we're assaulting them with poor posture which weakens our muscles by putting them in an habitually stretched position.

In Chapter 31, "Tots and Teens," we'll give you some help if your back is aching. In the meantime, while it won't help Deidre's business any, know this: Done properly, strengthening the muscles in your lower back and abdominal region, coupled with a good stretching regimen, will turn all but the most persistent lower back pain into a thing of the past. The key is maintaining good technique and knowing which exercises to do and when to do them.

Walking on That Tightrope

We've all heard the saying, "Balance in all things!" True enough, but living and playing invariably upsets the proverbial apple cart. Unless you take special care to stay aligned, muscle imbalances occur when repetitive activities are done consistently without regard to the opposite musculature. Huh?

For example, swimmers are prone to anterior (front) shoulder (deltoid) problems because their *pectorals* (chest muscles) and posterior (rear) *deltoids* are far more developed than their counterparts. In other words, the front is stronger than the back, and that screws everything up. By strengthening the weaker muscles in the upper back and rear shoulder, a swimmer's muscular balance is restored and the chance of injury minimized.

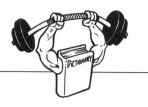

Bar Talk

Pectorals (commonly referred to as "pecs") are the chest muscles responsible for the pushup motion. **Deltoids** (often called "delts") are the muscles that cover your shoulder and are responsible for lifting your arm.

The same is true for runners, kayakers, cyclists, and any other athlete who calls on one particular set or sets of muscles—the other muscles of the body may need some help. The key, of course, is knowing which muscles to work and how to work them. Read on, and we'll show you how.

Over and Over and ...

The most common overuse injuries that Deidre treats are golfer's elbow (don't try to say this if you're not warmed up: *medial epicondylitis*) and tennis elbow (*lateral epicondylitis*). These tongue-twister syndromes afflict not only recreational athletes, but also a sizeable cross-section of folks who do a repetitive activity that requires using joints of the lower arm.

For example: One of Deidre's patients, who hadn't played tennis in 20 years, came to her with a bad case of tennis elbow. Apparently, the elbow became inflamed after he chopped onions for several hours for a dinner party he was hosting. To make matters worse, the condition worsened to the point that just turning his key in his front door and opening a jar of pickles was painful.

The point of this example, which happens more than you think, is that athletes are not the only ones to suffer overuse injures that weight training can help. Whether you're using a set of muscles too much or too little, pumping iron purposefully should have you chopping pain free—onions, pickles, even your house keys if you so desire.

Head Strong

The classic image of passionate weight lifters—no-neck goons pumping colossal amounts of iron on Venice Beach, for example—does not usually conjure men of prodigious intellectual prowess. "Uh, well, am I doing back and chest today? Or is it arms and chest?" While this stereotype has largely gone the way of the hula hoop, most people don't think of working out in a gym as a real heady way to spend time. This is both true and extremely false.

Here's why.

Grunt and Chill

First off, working out correctly requires concentration—on your technique, breathing, and the task at hand. It's important when you're performing any exercise—especially risky ones like squats—to concentrate on the exercise completely. In other words, you don't want to just mindlessly pick up the weight, count to 10, set it down, and move on. We'll go into this in far greater detail later, but suffice it to say for now, being mindful while you work out produces far greater results.

Second, we can't even count the number of times we've headed to the gym feeling as lifeless as an old sock and an hour or two later hit the streets as revitalized Homo sapiens. While we've experienced this Jekyll-to-Hyde switch a thousand times, the process still seems astounding. We'll talk about this more later, but you should know that the chemical effect of working out is rather heady stuff. And in fact, the natural high that comes with exercising can be quite addictive.

The Barbell Blues

Other than the beach, you're not likely to see more uncovered surface area of your fellow man than at the gym. Big deal? Well, yeah! If you want to see and be seen by your local fitness brethren, the gym is the joint to frequent. We know one guy who takes the yoga class offered at his club not because he's interested in this ancient and subtle art, but because the class consists primarily of women. His strategy hasn't netted him any hot dates, but his flexibility has greatly improved.

Gyms obviously are for working out, but the social component (which varies from gym to gym) is always a factor. We'll talk more about this in Chapter 4, "Look Before You Lift," but it's clear that some folks do more schmoozing than lifting. (They might not get fitter, but they're conversationally quite strong.) Some do a bit of both. No matter. Whether you're training for the Decathlon or for a coed badminton outing, the ability to socialize with a variety of people is one of the most enjoyable sides of becoming a gym regular.

The wide variety of people in our gym in Brooklyn produces some conversational classics. Joe often finds himself in the locker room sandwiched between Dick, the Ivy League historian, and Richie, a chatty Brooklyn sanitation worker with a proclivity for the inane and profane. "Hey Joey," he asked one memorable time, interrupting Joe's conversation about the publication of Dick's latest book on the Korean War. "Have you noticed that blankin' baby food tastes different these days?"

Such interchanges are not likely to motivate you to run to the nearest YMCA, but it is worth noting that that's where the three authors of this book met. In fact, it's where husband and wife—Jonathan and Deidre—met. (For the record, their eyes met over the leg extension machine at the Hunter College Gym.)

The Diverse Population of Weight Lifters

While the weight room has long been the province of young males, anyone with a clean bill of health—young, old, male, female—can benefit from weight lifting. There are hard-core "muscle" gyms where large men grunt like wildebeests in heat. There are all-female gyms for women who prefer a more genteel atmosphere. Our experience, however, is that most gyms are equal-opportunity employers: If you show up regularly, learn the basics, and act relatively civilized, you'll be fine.

I Am Woman

It wasn't long ago that women and muscles mixed about as well as oatmeal and sushi. Strong, muscular women were considered "unlady-like" or worse, "butch." This, of course, reeked of sexism, but it was just part of the raw deal women had to endure. Now that strength and muscles are chic on Madison Avenue—thanks in part to women like Carla Dunlap, Madonna, Gabrielle Reece, and scores more—women have come to see that weight lifting burns unwanted calories as well as enhances their appearance, self-esteem, and performance on the playing field.

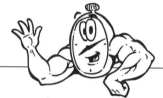

Weight a Minute

Weight-bearing exercise alone will not delay the onset of osteoporosis, but it does help. However, many nutritionists also recommend that women especially need as much as 1,500 milligrams of calcium per day to help preserve their bone density.

From a medical point of view, there's good reason for women to lift weights. Osteoporosis, a serious health risk related to decreased bone density, is a major concern for women as early as the age of 40. Lifting weights regularly can help prevent or delay the onset of the conditions and can often strengthen brittle bones. Furthermore, exercise also has a tendency to reduce cramping during menstruation. And there's ample research that shows that lifting combined with aerobic exercise is extremely good for pregnant women since having strong supple muscles helps during delivery, and strength training after labor will get them back to their prepregnancy weight more quickly.

Seasoned Citizens

In many ways, "act your age" is one of the most damaging sayings we have in our culture. For some reason, there seems to be a societal expectation that once you reach the age of 50 or so, you're "middle aged" and supposed to sit around and take it easy.

Actually, staying in shape is far more crucial as we crack the half-century mark. So while too few senior citizens frequent the gym, they really should do so.

Why? Because most inactive seniors have lost significant amounts of muscle mass. This muscle loss or *atrophy* isn't due to age but rather to sloth. The bottom line is that the muscles of older adults will respond to weight lifting the same way that younger people's do. In fact, if you compete in marathons, triathlons, and other assorted acts of masochism as we do, you'd see that there are 50-, 60-, and 70-year-old competitors with physiques that look 10 to 20 years younger—and they're kicking butt.

Around mile 22 of the 1986 Honolulu Marathon, Joe fell into a conversation with a wizened runner who sidled up next to him. Just before the gent ran off ahead, Joe learned the chipper runner was 72. On the back of his T-shirt, he'd inscribed: "Smile, you've just been passed by an Old Coot!" Now there's a guy "acting his age."

In Chapter 29, "With Age Comes Wisdom," we'll outline the specifics of a safe, effective program for old coots eager to outrun "kids" half their age.

May I See Your ID?

Perhaps it's true that "youth is wasted on the young," since we're baffled when we see so few teens working out. It's almost as if kids are too consumed with being kids to realize how much they'd benefit from even a modest gym routine. Not only is it a wonderful outlet for youthful enthusiasm, it's certainly time well spent away from video games and/or TV. (We certainly wish we'd lifted regularly during our own teen years.)

Physically, teens who lift will be planting the seeds for a strong and healthy body that will only improve as they reach their twenties and beyond; psychologically, lifting fosters discipline, self-knowledge, and a whole host of good qualities that are better experienced than described. In Chapter 30, "Physically Challenged," we'll lay out the details of an appropriate plan for teens.

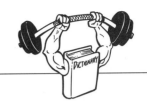

Bar Talk

Atrophy is the opposite of hypertrophy and refers to the loss of muscle mass. Atrophy is not an inevitable result of aging—it's caused by inactivity.

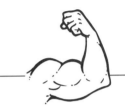

Flex Facts

Jack LaLanne is credited with opening the nation's first modern health club, on the third floor of an old office building in Oakland, California. LaLanne is also well-known for performing mind-boggling physical feats. On his 70th birthday in 1984, he successfully swam in Long Beach Harbor in hand- and leg-cuffs while towing 70 boats carrying 70 people. LaLanne, who is still going strong today, has said, "I can't die. It would ruin my image."

No Worries

So far we've listed a dozen reasons why you should lift weights—and we haven't even tossed in the exaggerated claims that lifting will immediately improve your personality, bolster your performance at work, and help lower the gross national product. However, after all that you may still have reservations about heading to the gym. After all, there are plenty of myths floating around. We hope the words that follow will put your mind at ease.

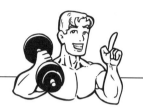

Spot Me

Don't be discouraged by people who spend all day in the gym. A weight-lifting workout that takes more than 30 to 45 minutes is a sure sign of a lifter with an inefficient routine or a tendency to talk more than lift.

It Won't Take All Day

Some people assume that in order to build a physique they can be proud of, they need to spend three hours a day in the gym, every day. Not even close! Unless you plan to become a Greco-Roman wrestler, there is no need to lift for more than 30 to 45 minutes a day, three or four times a week. In fact, if you're spending two or more hours at a stretch with the barbells, you're probably doing too much or spending too much time yakking between sets.

One of the huge factors is how intensely you train, not how long. Throughout the book, we'll give you lots of tips on how to make the most of your time in the gym and how to fit lifting into your busy schedule.

It Won't Make You "Too Big"

Ironically, one of the reasons people say they don't want to lift weights is that they don't want to "bulk up" and look like an American Gladiator. This is a particular concern for women. Don't worry! While women can reap all the positive effects we've discussed, very few have the genetic make-up to produce the same increase in muscle size that their male counterparts do.

Even Deidre, a former two-time world powerlifting champion who was able to squat nearly three times her body weight, looks exquisitely feminine. Very fit? Yes. Masculine? Not even close. In other words, lift to your heart's content. You probably couldn't "bulk up" if you tried. We'll show you how to "customize" your workout to the particulars you desire, but to a large extent genetics determine how much each of us can change and how quickly these changes will occur.

In other words, don't fret that lifting will have your neighbors whispering that you look like the Incredible Hulk. Even if you were to follow Lou Ferrigno's routine religiously, you wouldn't look like him. You'll get very muscular, sure, but his enormous mass, perfect proportions, and green hue can be attributed to Mother Nature—or at least to his mother and father (and the makeup people).

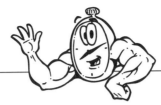

Weight a Minute

Don't be fooled into following someone else's lifting routine. Just because something works for an elite athlete, or for your pal from the gym, doesn't mean that it will work for you—in fact, it might be a perfect recipe for an injury.

It Won't Make You Walk Funny

Another common concern we often hear is that weight lifting will make you "muscle-bound" or inflexible. (Again, this is why boxers rarely lifted weights before Evander Holyfield showed pugilists how important it could be.)

In fact, as long as you use proper form, there's no reason why lifting will compromise your flexibility. Conversely, lifting won't help improve it either, which is why we've included a series of stretches in Chapter 11. Combining the two will leave you armed, dangerous, and rather lithe.

Finally, don't worry about all the tales of woe about people being injured in the weight room. Yes, people suffer aches and pains while weight training. And no, it's not as safe as reclining in front of the evening news, but as long as you learn the basics (outlined in Chapter 9, "Getting a Clean Bill of Health"), there's no reason for anyone to get hurt pumping iron. In fact, as we've mentioned, it can actually help you avoid injures. Come to think of it, perhaps lifting *is* safer than sitting around doing nothing!

The Least You Need to Know

➤ Combined with cardiovascular exercise and a sensible diet, strength training will have you looking lean and strong.

➤ Whether you're a weekend warrior or Mark McGwire, training in the gym will help you on the playing field.

➤ One of the least discussed but most beneficial aspects of weight training is injury prevention.

➤ Whether you're young or old, male or female, weight training can help you reach your physical potential.

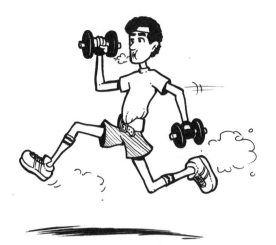

Chapter 2

Hurry Up and Weight

In This Chapter

➤ Getting rid of the excuses

➤ Making the time

➤ Planning is the key

➤ The social side of working out

Okay, let's assume you've read our persuasive prose in Chapter 1 and agree (unlike that recalcitrant Seinfeld character) that there are sound reasons why you *should* lift; the concern you might have now is that you're not sure if you *can.* Fret not! The old saying, "Where there's a will, there's a way" is especially true when it comes to exercise. In this chapter, we'll help you rid yourself of all the usual excuses so that you can get on the road to fitness.

It's Easier Than You Think

First off, working out effectively (and efficiently) is easier and far less time-consuming than you may think—if you know what you're doing. In Chapter 13, "Gluteus What?" we'll script several sample workouts that you can complete in 30-45 minutes. Sound skimpy? Do each set to failure (to the point that you can't do one more) and you'll leave the gym so exhausted (and well-trained) that you'll be unable to lift anything heavier than a tofu sandwich for a while.

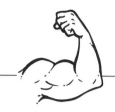

Flex Facts

Ashrita "Mr. Guinness" Furman, who has set more Guinness book fitness records than anyone else, once pogo-sticked up all 1967 stairs in Toronto's CN Tower, the tallest building in the world. This isn't the fastest way to the top (it took him just under an hour), but keep it in mind the next time you're waiting for the elevator.

Like we said, if time is an issue and you're unable to work out as often as you'd like, you need not despair. There are ways to fit working out into your lifestyle. For instance, if you live a reasonable distance from your place of business, you can walk to work instead of driving. (Just for the record, 70-year-old former running great Ted Corbett walks 11 miles from his home in the Bronx to work in Manhattan each day.) Similarly, if you work in an office building, you can motor up the steps instead of using the elevator. Not only will you be stretching your legs and improving your cardiovascular fitness, but you're likely to earn a reputation as "the fitness nut."

The main point to keep in mind is that nothing has power over your training unless you give it power. In other words, take stock of the excuses you manufacture, and gently toss them where they belong: the garbage heap. While we all do it, the ability to generate excuses—the "my piranha ate my gym shorts" kind of thing—has more to do with fear, sloth, or some other mental block than it does with an insurmountable obstacle. Surrounded by terrorists? Nice try. See Chapter 3, "What Goes Where and Why," for ways to work out at home.

Just for fun, let's look at the "Top 10 Lame Excuses Not to Exercise" that we've heard:

1. "I forgot my socks."

2. "My dog ate my membership card."

3. "I'm having a bad hair day."

4. "My tattoo is drying."

5. "I just did my nails."

6. "My outfit doesn't match."

7. "I'm premenstrual."

8. "My allergies are acting up."

9. "I don't have time; happy hour will be over soon."

10. "I'm hungover."

A few of the honorable mentions include: "I had a fight with my girlfriend/boyfriend," "My cat died," and "I got some Ben Gay in my eye." While those feeble lines are easy to debunk, let's take a quick look at the top five excuses that carry a bit more weight.

1. *I'm too busy.* Good solid excuse. However, consider the triathlete Joe often trains with, a 50-year-old architect we'll call Frank L. Wright. Mr. Wright works at his job at least 40 to 60 hours a week, yet has qualified for three Hawaii Ironman triathlons, run more than 25 marathons, and trains as many as 30 hours a week, including three weight-lifting sessions a week. Okay, so he's a training freak. The point is that if he can work and exercise that much, you can manage to work out two to four hours a week. It's all a question of desire and time management.

2. *I'm too tired.* Not bad! But, ironically (or not), most of the time exercising will revive you, turning a groggy, cranky human into a more delightful version of your prestressed self. Being flexible helps. If you're feeling weary, you can just lighten the load and lift less strenuously. Sometimes a good warm-up will turn you around. If not, just breathing deeply for the time you lift will do wonders for you.

3. *Gyms are too expensive.* We'll get into this one in more depth later, but for now, remember that a gym doesn't have to be expensive at all: There are a wide variety of fees and even many ways to work out without a gym.

4. *My back, neck, wrist, shoulder, knee hurt.* Stressing an injured body part is plain stupid; however, there are many ways to work out with your injury and as many exercises to help injured body parts mend faster. An example of the former occurred when Joe broke his wrist while training for the Boston Marathon. Not only did he continue to run (no problem there), he continued doing strength-training exercises on his noninjured side. (Studies show that exercising the uninjured or contralateral (opposite) side speeds recovery.)

5. *It takes too long.* Sorry! As we've said, not only can you make biking, walking, skating, or running part of your daily transportation, you can make terrific strength-training gains by spending as little as 90 minutes to 2 hours a week lifting weights at home or at the gym.

Now that we've got the excuses out of the way, read on and we'll discuss the options available to even the busiest multitaskers.

Working Out Before Work

This spring, Joe took a Navy SEAL training course for two weeks as research for an article he was writing for *The New York Times*. A notorious slow starter in the morning, he grimaced at the thought of exercising at 5 A.M. in Manhattan's Central Park. What he realized, other than the fact that homeless men do their most productive collecting between 4 and 6 A.M., is that working out early gets the day off to a flying start and affords an expansiveness that is likely to leave you feeling downright giddy. In fact, Joe felt so virtuous that when he'd finished at 6:45 A.M., he shouted "slaggards" at the joggers and cyclists circling the park in the cool of the morning for getting such a "late" start.

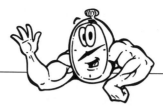

Weight a Minute

If you're planning to go for a run or bike ride at dawn, make sure you've chosen a safe route. And in the darker winter months, it's a good idea to wear a reflective vest.

Clearly, getting out of bed early in order to get to the gym or park requires some good solid willpower; however, once you make it a part of your daily routine you'll start to get cranky if you're unable to start your day with an endorphin rush. To quote that old adage: "One hour in the morning is worth three in the afternoon." (Just for the record: It typically takes about eight weeks to establish a routine as a habit.)

Getting an early start requires some organizational skills. One of the guys in Joe's Navy SEAL class, a Wall Street trader who had to go from Central Park to his office, ran through the park schlepping a garment bag over his shoulder. While he looked like a complete goof, we have to admire his dedication.

While that particular exercise predicament may not occur to you, some people are resistant to the morning workout simply because they don't know what to do with their gear—sweaty clothes, towels, beauty aids—when they go from the gym straight to work. If that's the case, invest in a rental locker at the gym where you can store your accoutrements. (As we'll discuss in Chapter 3, the difference between gyms has to do with more than the type of equipment they feature.)

For years, Deidre was an early-morning training monster. Here's how she managed these early workouts when she was competing as a powerlifter.

On the days that she went to the gym at 6 A.M., the night before she:

➤ Prepared her coffee.

➤ Set out her workout clothes.

➤ Picked out what she was going to wear to work so as not to disturb Jonathan, her slumbering husband tucked neatly in the fetal position.

On the days she rode the stationary bike (in her living room) at 5:45 A.M., she:

➤ Prepared her coffee. (Do you see a pattern developing?)

➤ Had her work clothes set out so as not to disturb her sleeping husband.

On Saturdays when she woke up at 4:45 A.M. to work out with her training partner who lived upstate, she:

➤ Packed her powerlifting suits, knee and wrist wraps, weight belt, and lifting shoes.

➤ Set out her pre- and post-lifting clothes.

➤ Set out her shower gear for her postworkout shower.

➤ Made sure she had enough money for a round-trip train ticket, subway tokens, news-paper, and French vanilla coffee and cranberry muffin.

➤ Before leaving, tried to wake her snoozing husband, who refused to wake up and pay homage to her dogged efforts.

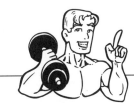

Spot Me

The more prepared you are the night before, the more likely it is that you will work out the next morning. Preparation is like a promise to yourself that you'll feel bad about breaking.

The Lunch Break Plan

If, however, waking at the crack of dawn is as ap-pealing as getting pecked to death by ducks, con-sider working out during lunch. For this strategy to be effective, your gym needs to be within shouting distance of your workplace. If you have to travel far to get there, you'll end up frittering away much of your exercise time.

Unless you live in a country that recognizes a daily siesta, don't plan on going hog wild at lunch. Re-member, you've got to change into your workout gear, pump iron, shower, and change back into your Calvins—so plan your routine accordingly so that it won't have you rushing through your work-out like a bike messenger through Manhattan. Working out under duress can turn a stress-buster into a stress-inducer, and often leads to injury because you're more focused on finishing than being mindful about using proper form.

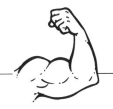

Flex Facts

Americans spend 2,300 hours in front of the television set every year; researchers report that the average family member now spends more than seven hours a day watching television and 14 minutes a day talking to other family members. We're asking you to devote 75 to 100 hours a year to lifting.

"But it's lunchtime," you say. What about that deli around the corner that whispers your name? Well, call us austere, but here's a good way to approach the midday meal: First, eat a large, healthful breakfast (a mixture of protein and carbs to avoid that coffee-and-donut, late-morning crash), then snack on a piece of fruit and/or some nuts an hour or two

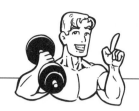

Spot Me

Before you go to the gym, eat yogurt, a piece of fruit, or some nuts, which will provide you with some preworkout energy. After lunch, try a turkey, lettuce, and tomato sandwich with mustard on whole wheat bread. The combination of carbohydrates and protein will prevent fatigue; the mustard is less fattening than mayo; and whole wheat bread is more nutritious than the white stuff.

before noon. This way, by the time lunchtime rolls around, you've kept your blood-sugar level elevated and won't be ready to gnaw on the pencil sharpener. (Having a low sugar level is the reason we become hungry.) After your workout, eat a sandwich, a piece of fruit, or a yogurt at your desk. This combination of protein, carbs, and fat should fill you up without the threat of you curling up for a nap under your desk.

Finally, working out during the day may give you more energy and incentive to work a bit harder and more effectively at your job. This increased productivity may even get you a raise. But beware—a promotion may lead to more responsibility, and that could crimp your midday power workout!

Work Out Postwork

The most popular time to work out is after work. While scores of your cronies saunter up to the corner bar, you'll be loading iron onto another kind of bar—one that will leave you without a headache or a cash deficit.

Let's look at the pluses of working out after work:

➤ You'll have more time to do a thorough workout.

➤ It's a fine time to schmooze with the workout set.

➤ You'll head home feeling refreshed after a long day at the office.

➤ You're less likely to kick the dog or quarrel with your mate.

That's the good news; the bad news about an after-work workout includes the following:

➤ A crowded gym can be a tough place to get a good workout. Unless your facility is spacious and well-equipped, you might have to wait for a particular apparatus (bad for the flow) and/or be rushed off the station you're using. (We'll give you some strategies for how to deal with this later.)

➤ Too much chatting. It's one thing to be social and another to try to work out at a cocktail party. If you're trying to work out efficiently, it can be disconcerting when someone is telling you the latest "good news/bad news" joke. Sure, your repertoire of bad jokes may increase, but you may find yourself barely breaking a sweat.

The fact is, the hardest part of working out is getting to the gym. The "just take the day off" devil sitting on your shoulder is a loud and divisive force, especially if you've had a hard day of work.

That's why location should become an important consideration when you're choosing a gym. We'll talk more about this in a later chapter, but to ensure that you get the most out of your gym, choose one that's near your home or job. We all know people who chose a fine gym with a reasonable membership fee but who are unable to take advantage of it because it's such a pain to get to. If you have to take a train, bus, or rickshaw to get there, you're more likely to blow it off, promising yourself that you'll "work out harder and longer tomorrow."

Clearly it's important to listen to the rhythms and whims of your body—exercise is, after all, supposed to enhance your life, not turn you into a guilt-ridden mess. (Always remember: A fitness regimen is not punishment for a flawed body, but a way to enhance your natural gifts.)

Keep in mind that the fatigue you're feeling is usually all in your head. After a few minutes of working out, you're likely to get your second wind. Once this happens, you'll be glad you exercised your willpower as well as your body. As fitness expert Steve Ilg writes, "You are developing inner strength in addition to outer strength." Put another way, Shakespeare said: "Our bodies are our gardens, to which our wills are gardeners."

Just to show you what's possible if you're really motivated, consider Joe's Ironman architect friend who typically runs before work, swims at lunch, and cycles after work. While he might not have the world's most exciting social life, he does shower more than a supermodel and gets to consume more calories than your average circus elephant.

Let's Get Ready for the Weekend!

Working out is generally easier on the weekends than during the week, for the simple reason that most of us have more free time on those precious two days. How-ever, it's also far too easy to fritter away your workout time when you have the whole day stretching out in front of you. That's why it's a good idea to "schedule" your exercise for an hour or two the day before so that you have a plan—and then stick to it.

If family responsibilities present a conflict, do what we've suggested in the preceding text. Either get up early and squeeze in a workout while the toddler is napping (you'll need someone to watch the snoozer of course), or time your exercise for late in the afternoon just before you plan to paint the town red. We know a lot of city dwellers who follow this weekend ritual: A late afternoon nap, work out at the gym, light dinner, and then it's party time.

Depending on the location of your gym, the weekend workout can get tricky. If you both work and live near your institution of higher fitness, you're fine. If you have to travel very far from home to the gym, on the other hand, you might want to make the trip more utilitarian by running errands en route. If the weather is good and you're not pressed for time, cycling to the gym is a great way to warm up and burn some extra calories. Regardless, keep the gym's distance from home as well as from your workplace in mind when you purchase your gym membership. If it's possible to find one located relatively equidistant from both, that's the way to go. Another approach is to consider joining a gym that's part of a chain so that you can work out at any of its affiliated gyms. That way, at home, at work, or even on the road, you've got your endorphins covered.

You Brush Your Teeth, Don't You?

There's a great quote by a woman named Lady Mary Wortley Montagu who said: "The trick is to die young as late as possible." Working out is a time-honored way to accomplish this noble aim.

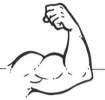

Flex Facts

Dr. Urho M. Kajala of the University of Helsinki tracked 16,000 healthy sets of twins for an average of 19 years. Those twins who exercised regularly—taking half-hour walks just twice a week—cut their risk of death by 44 percent. Even occasional exercisers were 30 percent less likely to die young than were their control group (sedentary) twins.

By now we hope we've convinced you that not only *should* you work out, you *need* to work out. Most civilized people find the time every day to eat, bathe, and brush their teeth. Similarly, working out should become a standard part of your daily (or almost-daily) health maintenance program.

Weight training may not make you live longer, but it will help ensure that you live better. Your muscles, connective tissue, and bones will get stronger; you'll have more energy, coordination, agility, and savoir faire. (Okay, the last one is debatable, but it sounds good and French lifters claim this as an added benefit.)

For all these reasons, and more, thinking about working out not as a negotiable option but as something that is necessary for your general health and well-being should help get you off your duff and into action.

Sweat Socially

The gym is a great equalizer: status, wealth, and social airs are generally tossed out the window since the assembled crowd—corporate bigwigs, bus drivers, unemployed actors, teachers—sweats under one roof in shorts, spandex, and T-shirts. (It's hard to take even a dignified CEO seriously when he's walking around with a sweaty crotch.)

Sure, there are the muscleheads flexing in the mirror and beauty queens sashaying around the room, but just about everyone in attendance is there for similar reasons that serve to unite us.

Although each gym is different, in general the social dynamics in a gym are amusing: a curious combination of neighborhood watering hole, soap-opera set, and endorphin commune. You'll be able to discuss the big game, mourn the stock market losses, hear about the latest movie, and dish the dating gossip. But, unlike a bar or party where there's a premium placed on "making a connection," the gym is a lower-pressure conversation zone—the best of both worlds. You can chat if you like or remain mum and pump iron with a purpose.

We've worked out next to people for years and never done more than bat an eye in their direction; other gym rats become fast and lasting friends. And we've peacefully coexisted silently next to familiar faces only to find out one day that they are excellent company. That's part of the fun about hanging out in a place filled with aspiration.

As we mentioned in Chapter 1, "Let's Get Physical," Deidre and Jonathan met at Hunter College gym. And Joe and Deidre met at their gym in Brooklyn. The three of us are quite serious about working out—heck, Deidre can *deadlift* a compact car and has won two World Powerlifting titles—but when you encounter a smiling face you just can't help but schmooze. Before you know it, you're part of a healthy subculture—a fitness cult!

It's interesting to note that more and more businesses are finding that a healthy and relaxed employee is a more productive employee, and an employee who is less likely to take sick days. That's why corporate fitness centers are appearing all over the country. If your company provides an on-site gym (or has a contract with one nearby), run, don't walk there ASAP. Many are free (or modestly priced) and often offer payroll deductions so that you never have to think about paying your gym bill. Furthermore, these facilities tend to be spiffy—stocked with all the amenities to leave you looking and smelling like a rose.

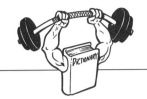

Bar Talk

The **deadlift** is a powerlifting maneuver; the weighted bar is on the floor and the lifter bends his or her knees and hips to reach the bar. Once ahold of the bar, the lifter stands up, pulling the bar to midthigh. See Chapter 16, "Flip Side," for a complete description.

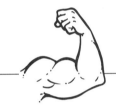

Flex Facts

Six months after the start of a fitness program for Dallas police officers, officer commendations jumped 39 percent, while the amount of sick leave taken by exercising officers dropped 29 percent. Such statistics only confirm the integral relationship between mind, body, and spirit. If this sounds like New Age mumbo-jumbo, ask the Dallas cops about their regimen. Better yet, work out and see for yourself.

If, even after reading this chapter, you still find yourself saying, "Well, yeah, working out is cool, but being around all those sweaty apes isn't my cup of tea," turn to Chapter 3 where we'll discuss the pros and cons of working out at home. We'll familiarize you with some of the better home equipment and show you how to get a safe and efficient workout under your own roof.

The Least You Need to Know

➤ It's important to try not to fall prey to excuses that will keep you from meeting your fitness goals.

➤ Choose your workout time with care, but you have plenty of options: before work, at lunch, after work, and on weekends.

➤ View working out not as an option or a hardship, but instead as a joyous and necessary part of life's journey.

➤ Joining a gym just might expand your social life—if you want.

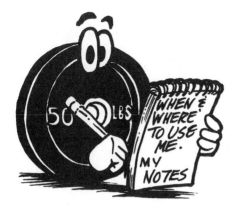

Chapter 3

What Goes Where and Why

In This Chapter

➤ Learning how your muscles work

➤ Deciding if home or the gym is right for you

➤ Weighing the risks and benefits of solo training

Get in your car, press the gas pedal, and it moves. Go to the gym, lift enough weight, your muscles get bigger and stronger. Although that's all you really need to know in order to get someplace in an automobile, some people like to have a greater appreciation for the inner workings of things. Just as understanding how your car works can help you keep it in tip-top condition, developing a basic appreciation of how muscles work can give you a better awareness of how and why they get stronger. That's what we'll do in this chapter: show you how your muscles work and how you can make them stronger and thereby make yourself more fit. We'll also help you decide where—in your gym or in your home—you might be best suited to begin working out. Let's get started.

The Basics About Muscles

First of all, let's get one thing clear: This book is about getting in better shape by building your muscles, which will make your muscles stronger and change the shape of your body at the same time. Weight lifting is different than cardiovascular exercise. As its name implies, cardiovascular exercise (like running, biking, stair climbing, dancing) primarily works the heart, making it pump faster and harder, thereby making it stronger (it's a muscle, after all), as well as making you breathe harder and faster, and getting your blood flowing through your vessels more efficiently.

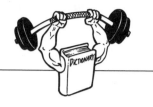

Bar Talk

Each muscle consists of millions of **myofibrils**. Myofibrils are muscle fibers that work to contract the muscles of the body. They are what you're trying to build when you lift weights.

We'll talk more about including some sort of cardio-vascular exercise into your fitness routine in later chapters. For now, we want to explain a little about muscles, the parts of the anatomy you're working on when you lift your barbells or press those machines.

There are more than 600 muscles in your body, and collectively they make up about 40 to 50 percent of your body weight. While our focus is on skeletal muscle (whose primary function is voluntary body movements), we also have visceral muscles that are located in internal organs and act involuntarily, and cardiac muscles, which, as the name implies, are found in the heart.

Muscles are made of numerous muscle fibers, which are made of small, threadlike strands called *myofibrils*. Myofibrils are made of two different types of contractile proteins: actin and myosin, which act together to create muscle contraction, the process in which a muscle is activated and generates force.

The Art of the Contraction

For a muscle to contract, it must receive a signal from the brain that tells it what to do. These signals come from nerve cells called neurons. A neuron and the muscle fibers it controls are collectively known as a motor unit. Muscle fibers and motor units are generally classified into two types, slow twitch (type I) and fast twitch (type II), with fast twitch further divided into type IIa and type IIb. Slow-twitch motor units are used when low force production is required, and they can work for extended periods of time, whereas fast-twitch motor units are capable of greater force production than slow-twitch, but require greater stimulation before they will work, and fatigue much more rapidly. Think of slow-twitch fibers as cheap labor that will work all day but never produce quickly, while fast-twitch fibers need more money before they'll come to work, and they won't stay long but they'll get a lot of work done while they're there.

A key point to understand is that motor units are always recruited in size order, from smallest to largest (or slow twitch first, then fast twitch), regardless of the speed of the movement. Fast-twitch motor units are never used unless the slow-twitch fibers have been recruited first. This phenomenon is known as the size principle. If the force requirements of an activity are low, you will use slow-twitch fibers only, even if it's a quick movement like swatting a fly. If the force requirements are high, as in a maximal effort like trying to push a car (or lift heavy weights), you will use your fast-twitch fibers in addition to your slow-twitch fibers, even if you're moving very slowly.

Positive, Negative, and In-Between

There are three types of muscle "contractions": positive (sometimes referred to as concentric), negative (or eccentric), and static (also called isometric). In a positive contraction, the muscle's force overcomes the resistance posed by the weight and shortens to lift the weight. This is also known as the positive phase of the lift.

In the case of a negative contraction, the muscle is still exerting force, but it's not enough to overcome the resistance, so the weight is lowered as the muscle lengthens. This is the negative phase of a lift.

A static contraction occurs when there is no movement of the resistance or change in the joint angle. This can occur when you try to move an immovable object, such as pushing against a wall, or when the force exerted by the muscle is equal to the weight.

Gotta Grow

When a muscle experiences a great enough work-load, it adapts by gaining strength. This increased strength comes from improved communication between the brain and the muscles as well as an increase in the size of the muscles. That's how you can get stronger without any significant changes in muscle size. As we'll show you in future chapters, various types of strength training are all capable of increasing both muscle size and strength. There are two mechanisms by which muscle size may increase. The first is hypertrophy, in which the individual muscle fibers that make up the muscle grow wider not longer. Hypertrophy is caused by an increase in the size and number of myofibrils within the fiber, which takes place in both slow-twitch and fast-twitch fibers, although fast-twitch fibers have greater potential for growth.

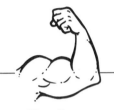

Flex Facts

Hyperplasia does not occur in humans except in certain muscular dystrophy–type conditions where there is growth of the muscle without any strength benefit. In such cases, hyperplasia may take place. When a human's muscles grow, it's from hypertrophy—not hyperplasia.

The second is hyperplasia, a phenomenon in which individual muscle fibers split, creating an increase in the total number of fibers. This method of muscle building appears to occur primarily in cats and other mammals, but there is little evidence that it takes place in healthy humans.

So now we know that fast twitch fibers have the most potential for growth, but they're also the hardest ones to recruit. Since they'll only work when the slow twitch fibers can't handle the job, one of the keys to a successful strength-training program is ensuring that we get those stubborn fast twitch fibers involved. How to do that safely and efficiently is the question. If you've already thumbed through this book, you've see that there are no exercises demonstrated until Chapter 14, "Now What?" That's because in many ways, the exercises themselves aren't as important as how you do them. Indeed, proper technique is the key to success.

When beginners first get started on a lifting program, they invariably get stronger almost right away, usually much stronger within just a month or so. While it's not unreasonable to expect some muscle growth in that time frame, hypertrophy can't explain all the strength gains. During that initial learning phase, most of the increase in strength is caused by your brain and not your brawn.

What does that mean? Well, when you learn a new exercise, your brain adapts and gets used to the new movement. As it learns the movement, you become much more efficient due to the neurological adaptations that take place. And it's only after you've become proficient at the movement that you really work your muscles. This is a significant concept for you to grasp, because it dictates how you'll start your lifting program. The most important thing to keep in mind as you get started is to pay attention to proper form and to focus on every exercise. Once you have established a foundation based on good habits and proper form, we can build from there. After you have learned the exercises, the only way to continue to improve is by intensifying the physical challenge.

So what do you do to get stronger? In the gym, you'll encounter a variety of different contraptions, all designed to help make you stronger. Some will be good old-fashioned "freeweights": barbells and dumbbells that use gravity as resistance. Others will be newfangled machines that use a variety of means to create resistance. Some use air pressure, some use magnetic braking, and most use a stack of weights attached to the machine by a cable. Ultimately, what all of them do is make your muscles work hard.

Here are a few things you need to know about how to get your muscles stronger:

➤ *Give them enough stimulation.* As a muscle and its individual fibers become stronger, a greater stimulus is required to elicit further strength gains. If all the variables (including weight, repetitions, sets, rest periods, and speed of movement, all of which we'll discuss later) remain the same, there will be no stimulus to cause further adaptations. Manipulation of any of these variables can create increased stimulus and lead to greater muscle recruitment and strength. If you constantly do the same thing over and over again in the weight room, you'll maintain your strength, but you won't get any stronger.

➤ *Give them enough rest between workouts.* When you lift weights, your muscles fatigue. It's during the time between workouts that your muscles get stronger. Matt Brzycki, coordinator of strength and conditioning programs at Princeton University and author of *A Practical Approach to Strength Training* (Masters Press), compares recovery between lifting sessions to allowing a wound to heal. "If you had a scab and picked at it every day you would delay the healing process, but if you left it alone you would permit the damaged tissue to heal."

➤ *Work them through a full range of motion.* When you lift a weight, you should start with your muscle in a stretched position and move to a fully contracted position before returning to the starting position. By working a muscle from its longest length to its shortest length, you have worked it through its full *range of motion*. Since muscular strength gains are specific to the angle at which you train, a full range of motion is necessary to ensure maximum strength gains. In her physical therapy practice, Deidre sometimes has reason to have a patient work through a limited range of motion, and for certain exercises such as the squat, safety concerns dictate that the range of motion be limited. We'll give you full explanations of the appropriate range of motion for all the exercises we describe.

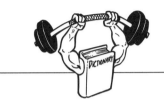

Bar Talk

A full **range of motion (ROM)** refers to the movement of a joint from its fully extended (straight) position to its completely bent (flexed) position.

So by now, we hope we've convinced you that you should lift, shown you how you can find time to lift, and told you what happens when you lift. Now let's figure out *where* you should lift.

Where Oh Where Do I Train?

Before we explain the pros and cons of working out at home, let's get one thing out of the way: We prefer training at the gym. Why? Well, being city dwellers where space is precious, we hardly have room to store our bicycles and running shoes, let alone a separate place to house all the equipment a solid gym has to offer. (Just for the record: Joe, who hasn't thrown out a pair of running shoes in years, is the Imelda Marcos of athletic footwear. And Jonathan, who's raced bicycles for years, has more spare wheels and gear cogs than most bike shops.) That, of course, doesn't mean you can't create a great home setup. You can. And you'll be able to do so without the hassle of rubbing elbows with the rest of humanity. In this chapter, we'll help you figure out what will work best for you—working out at a gym, or creating a great gym at home.

As we've discussed, one of the key factors in maintaining a workout regimen is convenience. Unless you follow the credo of the U.S. Postal Service (neither rain, sleet, nor snow ...), you're not likely to stick with a workout regimen if getting to your gym is an ordeal, no matter how well-intentioned you are. If you happen to live a stone's throw away from a good gym, your decision is basically made for you: Sign on the dotted line and have at it. If, however, you have the space and would prefer to work out at home, then you may want to create a gym for yourself there. After all, what could be more convenient?

Well, hold on. Before you rush out to become one of the millions of people who buy home exercise equipment that ends up unused in the basement, here's where you need to do a bit of self-evaluation. Some people can work out on their own; some people can't. We each know athletes who will wake up at an ungodly hour to train with a partner, but when left on their own will roll over in bed and blow it off. On the other hand, there are those who will head out alone at twilight into a raging snowstorm to complete a workout. In other words, if you need the company and motivation supplied by others, joining a gym is the best way to fly. On the other hand, if you're a self-starter and find you are more focused and intense on your own, a home gym is your best bet.

Of course, to borrow a basketball phrase, you may be a "tweener"—someone who may prefer working out at a regular gym but just doesn't have the time to make it work. You might be someone like Joe's kayak-racing friend, Nels Akerlund. A freelance photographer who works irregular hours, Nels set up a variety of equipment in his basement (including an indoor climbing wall). No matter the hour, 6 A.M. or midnight, he heads downstairs, cranks the tunes, and lifts to his heart's content (although he is sometimes inconvenienced by his wife's tendency to hang laundry on his bench).

Weighing the Pros and Cons

As that old baseball philosopher Yogi Berra might have said: "Like anything, there's pros and cons to everything." We have no idea if Yogi lifts at home or on the road, but here are a few of the pluses of working out at home:

➤ *Convenience.* You certainly don't have a membership card you can forget!

➤ *Efficiency.* You'll cut *way* down on travel time if you work out at home—unless, of course, you live directly above a gym!

➤ *You choose the tunes.* One of the constant complaints we hear at the gym is, "This station sucks!" Or, "Make it louder!" and so on. In fact, persistent music gripes is why many gym regulars wear Walkmans. (FYI: Watching workout partners communicate through hand signals when each is wearing headphones is always amusing.)

➤ *No waiting for machines.* One of the most familiar phrases in a gym is, "Can I work in with you?" Meaning, when you're done with your set, can I squeeze one in? Without fail, all but the rudest bench hogs will gladly agree. Nevertheless, waiting for a machine can prolong your workout and/or interrupt your rhythm.

➤ *You'll work out more often.* This is probably the biggest reason to set up a home gym: the "use it or lose it" syndrome. When your equipment is a whopping 10 seconds from where you sit, there are precious few excuses that can keep you from using it.

➤ *Long-term cost savings.* Belonging to a gym is like renting an apartment: You have no equity in it. While setting up a home gym can get a bit pricey, it's far cheaper over the long haul.

➤ *No intimidation factor.* To gym regulars, it seems a bit silly, but until it becomes familiar, the gym scene can intimidate many beginners since it's not uncommon to find large men with bulging eyes shouting like—well, like weightlifters. In the privacy of your own home, you too can bellow like an opera singer.

So there are some very good reasons to exercise at home and you may, in fact, get a lot out of choosing to do so. On the other hand, there are some negatives attached, some of which we mention here:

➤ *Loss of living space.* Basements, spare bed- rooms, garages, and so on will be consumed by a good home gym. If you have plenty of room (and/or live by yourself), this may not be a concern, but if space is tight, you may not want to choose the home gym option. This is especially true if you have a significant other whose response to the idea is, "You'll bring that thing into my house over my dead body!"

➤ *Less external motivation.* As we've already men- tioned, some folks are driven on their own to work out; others need the stimulation of like- minded people. Know thyself and you may spare your home a piece of equipment that soon turns into a very expensive clothes rack.

> **Spot Me**
>
> If you work out at home and you're unable to let the answer- ing machine pick up, turn off the ringer. It's also a good idea to treat your home workout like you would a honeymoon in a hotel—tell your family and friends not to disturb you when you're working out.

➤ *More distractions.* As a freelance writer who works at home, Joe can speak vol- umes about the distractions of working in his apartment: phones, refrigera- tors, doorbells, e-mail, and deadliest of all, the reclining chair where drowsy would-be lifters go to drift off into a dreamlike state faster than you can spell Schwarzenegger. That's why it's important that you're able to treat your workout at home as if you were performing it in an actual gym. (In fact, you are.) We'll give you some tips on how to accomplish that later, but for now, if you don't think you'll be able to turn your home "off" while you're working out, a gym is probably the place for you.

➤ *Less diversity.* One of the best things about a well-equipped gym is the different machines that allow you to vary your workout. Not only will they keep the boredom factor at bay, but you can also work the same body part in a variety of ways.

33

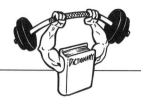

Bar Talk

A **spotter** is someone who stands by to help the lifter if and when he or she can't finish a repetition. While it takes time to learn the nuances of spotting, the most important thing is making sure the lifter doesn't drop the weight on his or her head.

➤ *Fewer partners and* spotters. It's quite typical for gym regulars to pair up on days that they work the same body parts (chest/back, legs, and so on) and train together. Similarly, if you decided to work "heavy" on a particular exercise, there's always someone around to make sure you don't drop the weight on your forehead at the gym. At home, you're far more likely to be working out on your own.

In the end, the question of where you lift is not nearly as important as *if* you lift. In the best of all worlds we prefer the gym, but if it's not practical, there are lots of sensible alternatives to consider. In the next chapter, we'll show you all you need to know about working out in a gym. Then we'll take you back home and show you what you'll need if you decide to work out there.

The Least You Need to Know

➤ Muscles need a challenge to get strong.

➤ Your brain needs to know the exercises before your muscles can do the work.

➤ Working out, both at home and at the gym, offers risks and benefits, pros and cons, that you need to consider carefully before making a decision.

➤ Working out alone means knowing the risks and taking special care, especially if you use freeweights.

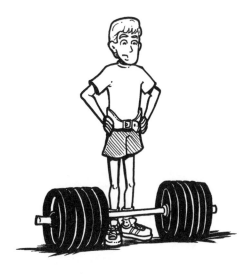

Look Before You Lift

Okay, you've decided after weighing the pros and cons of the "home versus gym" controversy outlined in the last chapter that working out in a gym might be best for you. The good news is that there are more gyms in the United States than there are fake blondes in Los Angeles. In fact, according to the Yellow Pages, there are more than 14,000 health clubs in this great nation of ours. (If you're looking to drop a few other health club facts at your next cocktail party, mention that the health club industry generated $9.6 billion in 1997. The number of health club members: 22.5 million.) With all these choices, how can you find the right gym for you? That's what we'll discuss in this chapter.

Eenie, Meenie, Miney, Mo

Here's an obvious bit of advice that, oddly enough, takes many people by surprise: The more specific your fitness goals, the easier it will be for you to pick a gym that suits your needs. In other words, are you just there to pump iron or are you interested in taking aerobics classes, yoga, swimming, boxing, or playing basketball? Is taking a sauna a big plus or a big ho-hum? Remember, if your gym has these amenities and

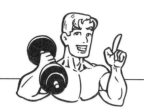

you choose not to use them, then you're likely subsidizing someone else's use of them. (If you're just there to lift and use the cardio machines, you may be able to save money by selecting a "restricted" membership. Restricted memberships also may be available if you're willing and able to work out during "off-peak" hours, which are generally midmorning and midafternoon (not prework, lunch, or postwork hours).

As long as we're on the obvious front: Check to make sure the gym you join has hours that work for you. We know one gym in Brooklyn that sits over a synagogue and hence must close on the Sabbath as well as whenever there's a Jewish holiday. "Closed for the Ninth of Av? Never heard of that one!"

"Gosh," you may be saying, "I just want to find a gym and get in shape, not select a four-year college." Don't worry. In the pages that follow, we'll help you figure out what you should look for in an institution of higher fitness, factoring in everything from your legal rights to your creature comforts.

Neatness—or at Least Cleanliness—Counts!

Surveying a gym is a bit like looking for an apartment, only different. Instead of looking for closet space and listening for street noise, you'll want to focus on the general cleanliness of the gym area and locker rooms as well as the quality of the equipment. When you enter a new gym for inspection, don your white gloves and prepare to judge!

Look for the following in the gym area:

➤ Take a good look at the general condition of the equipment. For example, are the cables that you'll find on many pieces of gym equipment in good repair or are they frayed?

➤ Check out the equipment's manufacturer. If it's Bodymaster, Cybex, or Nautilus, that's a good sign. Stu's, Herb's, or Skip's should send up a warning signal. Other reputable companies to look for are Hammer, Icarian, TK Star, and Paramount.

➤ Is the upholstery covering the equipment worn and/or torn? If the equipment looks like the inside of a honky-tonk, you may consider your alternatives.

➤ Check out the dumbbells—the handheld weights you'll soon become familiar with. Are they the plated variety, which hold up well, or the hexagonal type that tend to bend and rust?

Now get yourself into the locker room and evaluate the following:

➤ Is the locker room clean?

➤ Are the lockers large enough to accommodate your gear? We've been to gyms where fitting your clothes into a skinny locker is like squeezing a thick English muffin into a narrow-slotted toaster. In winter, when you'll be toting even more clothes, this toaster phenomenon gets worse. So buyer beware.

➤ Are there lockers for rent? Renting a locker allows you to leave stuff at the gym like a weight belt, shampoo, deodorant, or hair dryer—a lifesaver if you'll be heading for the office or the movies after your workout.

➤ Are the stalls in the bathroom clean? Or is the place like the restroom at a rest stop on the interstate? Is there toilet paper in the stall?

➤ Ditto for the shower stalls. A nice, hot, re-laxing shower after a workout is supremely satisfying, unless the space is a moldy mess reserved for jungle explorers and cattle rustlers. Also, it's not a bad idea to check the water pressure. The dribbling shower just doesn't get it done.

➤ How about the upkeep of the steam room, sauna, and whirlpool? Again, these are excel-lent features—provided they're fit for human enjoyment.

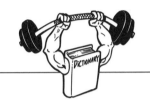

Bar Talk

In gym speak, a **musclehead** is an extremely muscular man or woman, usually a hard-core reg-ular. The inherent suggestion when using the term is that those muscles weren't acquired while attending Harvard—but that's not necessarily the case!

Do You Have X, Y, and Z?

Gyms are a bit like restaurants: The basic product is the same, but the pomp and cir-cumstance surrounding the workout/meal varies widely. To some, the only factors that concern them when selecting a gym are 1) do they have enough equipment? and 2) is the price right? Everything else is window dressing.

Consider a *musclehead* gym we know in Brooklyn called The Fifth Avenue Gym that's so austere and grungy it's almost cool. Inside, large, animated men with biceps the size of cantaloupes hoist prodigious amounts of free weights around like NFL linemen tossing back spare ribs. The grunting and groaning is so intense you'd almost think you were listening to natural childbirth. Shampoo and conditioner in the shower stalls? Get real! Patrons are lucky there's water in the water fountain. Nevertheless, the gym has nine million pounds of free weights and the annual membership is about the cost of dinner for nine at McDonald's. For some, that's just what the doctor ordered.

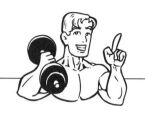

Spot Me

When you decide to check out a health club, try to bring the gym bag you'll be using and see if it will fit into the locker. If it's summer when you join, keep in mind you'll be jamming it with more stuff during the winter months.

On the other hand, if you prefer a prettier setting, or if the sight of a spider in the bathroom sends you scurrying for a vaccination, you may want to consider a classier establishment.

Let's look at the amenities you may want to consider, realizing ahead of time that the more you get, the more you'll pay!

Towel, Please

Belonging to a gym that provides towels to its paying customers is a major plus, especially if you work out nearly every day. First off, stuffing a towel in your gym bag or backpack takes up a lot of room, and washing and drying the things takes time and energy you might spend better elsewhere. Health clubs with juice bars, massage therapists, and stores with workout gear generally dispense towels as you enter, the way Carnegie Hall provides mints at a concert, but that's because they charge a much higher membership than their "no frills" counterparts. Less-refined establishments like the Brooklyn gym Deidre and Joe be-long to charge patrons a buck for the use of a towel—and they aren't the fluffy face savers you'll find in Bloomingdale's. Essentially, if you travel this daily towel route you'll add about $50 to $100 per year to your annual membership.

Scrubbing Bubbles

With few exceptions, if the gym you choose offers a "free" towel service, you'll also find plenty of soap, shampoo, and conditioner in the showers. If you have to pay for your towel, you're likely on your own in the cleansing department. At Joe and Deidre's gym, it's BYO. For people like Deidre (a classy massage therapist who needs to interact with human beings after her workout), remembering to bring her own is more important than it is for Joe, the freelance writer who works alone at home with his grouchy cat. By way of contrast, when Joe had occasion to work out at a classy establishment in Manhattan, he lathered up so heavy with the sundry free potions that he left smelling like a rose!

Ambience

Although you rarely hear the word *ambience* used to describe a gym, each establishment has its own feel, its own character and mood. How do you feel when you enter a club? Are you comfortable there or do you feel like racing out like a prisoner pardoned from jail? It's probably a good practice to trust your initial impression, since very often your gut-level feeling is what will determine whether you stick with the place or not.

After working out in her neighborhood gym for many years, Deidre decided to join a gym that was closer to her job. Deidre appreciates the finer things in life, but cares little if her gym has soft hankies in the ladies' room. However, the new club she joined had old, run-down equipment, a decrepit locker room, and played awful music really *loud!* Even for a tough gym-rat like her, the squalid scene detracted from the quality of her workouts. Before too long she was back in her bare-bones gym, which suddenly seemed much more pristine.

Know this: Very few gyms will let you tour their facility on your own. Usually, you'll be chaperoned by a salesperson whose job it is to get you to join. Keep this in mind and don't let them rush you through a suspect area of the gym. In addition, don't let them hurry you into signing a contract on the spot if you're on the fence about whether to join or not. The salesperson will tell you that the club is running a "special" sale, but more often than not this select opportunity happens as frequently as a full moon— like every month! In other words, if you're not ready to buy, we assure you there will be another promotional deal sooner rather than later.

Curiously (or not), the same gym has a different feel depending on when you visit. Why? Gym regulars cycle through in predictable shifts: There's the prework crowd, the midmorning and afternoon lull set, the postwork rush, and the late-night revelers. That's why it's best to check out the gym you're examining at the hour you'll be working out. There's no sense in looking at a mellow, half-empty gym at noon if you're going to be rubbing elbows during peak evening hours with dozens of other patrons jockeying for the equipment.

If the place is too trendy or too low-rent; too loud or eerily silent for your tastes; or if the price is right but the neighborhood is wrong, remember that you've got options. Make sure you check out one of the other 14,000-plus gyms out there. You're no doubt bound to find one that feels right for you.

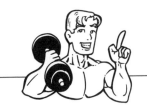

Spot Me

When health club shopping, try to go with a friend who is interested as well. You can discuss what you liked and didn't like, and, if you decide to join, ask for a discounted rate for signing up at the same time. Sometimes, you can even get a "two-for-one" deal.

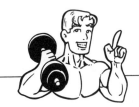

Spot Me

For you Web surfers, a great resource when shopping for a gym is www.healthclubs.com. Narrow your search by telling them your zip code and what type of facilities you're looking for and they'll instantly supply you with a list of gyms that fit your needs.

Bond or Bust

Here's a situation you may not have considered: On Monday you go to the gym to work your chest and back; on Wednesday you're back to do arms and shoulders when you learn that the gym is going belly up. Out of business. Chapter 11. Gone. Goodbye.

If the gym you join is bonded, you're guaranteed at least a partial refund. A bond is a contract between the state and the gym that provides that, should the facility go out of business before the the consumer's membership expires, the member will have some financial recourse. Roughly half of the states in the country require that a fitness center carry a bond of at least $50,000. If a bond is required in your state, the gym must have proof that it has one should you ask. Again, if a bonded gym bites the dust, this doesn't mean you'll get a full refund, but it's insurance that you'll get at least some money back. If your gym is not bonded, there's not much you can do.

You might think that calling your state's chamber of commerce or Better Business Bureau to see if your gym has a bond might seem like overkill, but gyms go out of business all the time, and sometimes under shady circumstances. Deidre once worked as a massage therapist at a health club that one day just closed its doors as suddenly as a three-card monte dealer folds his cardboard table. Even worse, in the days preceding this unannounced event, the owners offered tremendous deals on multiyear memberships. Obviously, these guys were trying to rake in as much cash as possible before closing up shop. (The only recourse any member had was to break in and hock the furniture. Try selling a used leg extension machine on the street—it's not a pretty sight.)

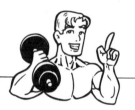

Spot Me

Always read your health club contract. Clarify confusing points before you sign anything. If you have special needs or considerations, say so and have them included in the contract via a rider.

Your Escape Clause

You've got another good reason to read your gym contract carefully before you sign. Most states provide some sort of "buyer's remorse" clause in the contract that gives you anywhere from 24 to 72 hours to cancel your membership without being penalized. Similarly, there may be a clause in the contract to cover you if you move out of the area or are injured before your contract runs out. Some gyms allow members to "freeze" their memberships for certain periods—after having a baby, after being in-jured, in order to take a long vacation, and so on. And often if you move a significant distance from your gym (usually 25 miles), you'll be entitled to a prorated refund.

We realize you didn't buy this book to read about contracts, but know this: You can often have riders added to your contract. Remember that smiling salespeople often have more flexibility in what they can offer than they let on. You might be able to negotiate a family membership deal or a group discount if you recruit new members. If the gym doesn't offer discounts, you may be able to add another month on your membership or have a personal training session tossed in the mix. Remember, if you don't ask, you'll never know what accommodations you may be able to obtain.

For example, if you regularly travel out of town for weeks or months at a time, you can probably have the contract amended to account for this. Alternatively, your club might be affiliated with a national chain or organization (IHRSA, the International Health, Racquet and Sportsclub Association is the largest and most reputable) that allows you to work out at another gym while you're on the road—usually free or at a discounted rate.

Just How Much Is This Going to Cost?

Pick a number between $99 and $9,999 and you've narrowed the price of joining a gym. (Needless to say, the latter figure would indeed include shampoo and towels!) In other words, the cost of a health club membership can vary widely, even within the same gym, since there are peak and off-peak memberships, month-to-month or annual contracts, and several options in between.

What's this about a month-to-month contract, you ask? Well, many clubs offer them, and they have several advantages over an annual contract:

➤ You won't have to lay out a lot of cash when you join.

➤ If you're not comfortable with the gym, just finish out the month, and you won't feel a financial pinch.

➤ Ditto if you move, travel a lot, get injured, or are abducted by aliens.

But there's always another side of the coin, isn't there? Here are some of the disadvantages of having a month-to-month contract:

➤ If you continue to work out, it will end up costing you more at the end of the year.

➤ There's usually an "initiation fee" associated with month-to-month memberships that is often waived or nonexistent with annuals.

Give Me Exercise or Give Me Death

Okay, we said we were done talking about your gym contract, but there are a few more things we think you should know. Here's an incident that illustrates a bogus practice employed by a gym in Brooklyn. This particular club allows you to pay on a monthly basis by automatically deducting the fee from your checking account. However, when a patron we know wanted to quit, she had to mail a certified letter.

Then the gym could charge her another monthly fee until 30 days after it received the letter. In short, they made getting out of the contract as easy as settling a debt with the Mafia. Familiarize yourself with the club's policy on cancellations in order to protect yourself. Many of them require 30 to 60 days' written notice.

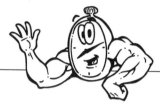

Weight a Minute

Beware of multiple-year contracts; few clubs offer them, and those that do may not be on sturdy business ground. Not only that, but you don't know where your own life will take you in terms of physical distance from the gym or from your personal preferences about where and when to work out.

As a consumer, you have rights when you purchase a membership from a health club. (Remember that the contract not only spells out your commitment to the gym, but it also protects you against fraudulent acts by the owners.) In fact, most states have specific statutes that spell out consumers' rights when it comes to health clubs.

Below are highlights from the New York Health Club Statute. Check for specifics in your state.

➤ You can pay in installments or in one lump sum. Paying in full in advance may seem cheaper, that it may involve taking a financial risk you don't want to incur.

➤ A contract becomes void if the club fails to provide the services it offers in the contract within one year from the day the contract is signed.

➤ A contract should provide you the option to cancel within three business days after signing your name on the dotted line. Your notice of cancellation should be sent by certified or registered U.S. mail at the address specified in the contract.

➤ The buyer (that's you) may cancel the contract if you move more than 25 miles away from the health club.

That said, we don't mean to imply that every gym—or even most gyms—is out to rook you. Far from it. Most gyms are legitimate businesses that make a profit by providing good service. But, as in all things, when it comes to signing on the dotted line and handing over a check—buyer beware!

Now that you've had a chance to evaluate the idea of making a gym a part of your life, let's take a look at another viable option: creating a home gym that works for you.

Evaluating the Trainers

Trainers present yet another one of those good news/bad news deals. The well-trained, knowledgeable, concerned fitness expert is an invaluable asset in the gym. They can help motivate you, offer advice on everything from nutrition to stretching, and they'll help guide you through your workout. If you've got the will—and sometimes even if you don't—a good trainer has the way. The bad news, however, is that the staff at many fitness centers isn't always well-trained, informed, or concerned.

Depending on a trainer's qualifications, reputation, and demand, expect to pay anywhere from $25 to $100 an hour for a training session. (Introductory sessions are often available to new members.) Some trainers will trim the price if you work with a partner.

School of Hard Knocks

As we mentioned in Chapter 1, "Let's Get Physical," anyone who walks and talks can call himself a "personal trainer," "exercise physiologist," or "fitness instructor." Scary as it sounds, in most states you need a license to cut hair, but not to be a personal trainer.

The better establishments will be staffed with trainers with graduate degrees in exercise physiology, biomechanics, or other health sciences. In others, the instructors may have no laurels to rest on other than their beefy pectoral muscles. In-house certifications offered by some of the big national chains are as tough to pass as basket weaving. Essentially, their requirements are minimal, and the certification is just a way to let the gym tell folks that its staff is certified.

It's a good idea to check with the salespeople about the staff's qualifications. There are scores of alphabet-soup certifications out there. The most respected is the American College of Sports Medicine (ACSM). Jonathan was certified as a Health and Fitness Instructor by ACSM before getting his master's degree in Exercise Physiology. He recalls the difficult ACSM exam with the same warm feelings that his broken collarbone evokes. ACSM has various levels of certification, but each requires passing both a written exam and a practical exam, and you can be sure that an ACSM-certified trainer knows his or her stuff.

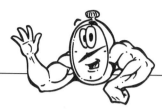

Weight a Minute

Don't be impressed just because a trainer is "certified." Clubs often have their own certifications—usually just a gimmick to pump up the appearance of the staff's credentials.

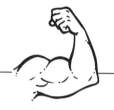

Flex Facts

Jonathan, who once dreaded taking the challenging ACSM Health/Fitness Instructor exam, now serves as an examiner for ACSM, administering the practical exam to a new generation of terrified subjects. After completing a three-hour written exam, they're looking at Jonathan's smiling face for the next hour.

In addition to the ACSM, there are other reputable organizations that offer certification for personal trainers. They include:

➤ The National Strength and Conditioning Association (NSCA). This organization offers two levels of certification: Personal Trainer and Certified Strength and Conditioning Specialist. The difference isn't worth noting here; suffice it to say that each is geared toward strength training. While the NSCA has gained nationwide prominence over the past few years—many strength and conditioning coaches at the college and pro level are NSCA-certified—some of the techniques it advocates are too severe for the beginner. In fact, some authorities (including us!) question the use of these explosive movements even for seasoned athletes. While we'll get into plyometrics later in the book, you can be sure that an NSCA graduate is more than qualified to help you.

➤ The American Council on Exercise (ACE), the Aerobics and Fitness Association of America (AFAA), the National Academy of Sports Medicine (NASM), and the National Sports Performance Association (NSPA) have also spawned a healthy number of trainers out there. The requirements of each of these are far less stringent than those of either the ACSM or NSCA. While most of the trainers who study with those groups lack formal education in health sciences, these four organizations do ensure a basic level of competence.

Insure Me

If you do opt to work with a trainer, even for a few sessions to help you get started, make sure that your trainer is not only qualified but insured as well. While we sincerely hope it never happens, if you are injured due to a trainer's neglect you'll want your trainer to have liability insurance.

Okay, so there's all you need to know about gym basics, at least for now. Does gym life sound right for you, or are you beginning to think that working out at home may be your best bet? If so, read on: Chapter 5, "There's No Place Like Home," brings it all home to you.

The Least You Need to Know

➤ If you know what you want to do and when you want to do it, you'll find the health club that's best for you.

➤ Not all trainers are created equal. Learn which degrees are worth more than the paper they're printed on.

➤ A good gym is the sum total of its parts. Know what to look for, and you won't regret your choice.

➤ Before you sign on the dotted line, read the contract with care.

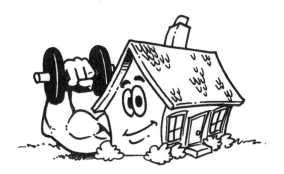

Chapter 5

There's No Place Like Home

In This Chapter

➤ Choosing home exercise equipment wisely

➤ Understanding all-in-one machines

➤ The ABC's of freeweights

Okay, let's say that you're starting to think that working out at home is the way to go for you. What now? Well, now you've got to look into the future a bit and anticipate some of the challenges you may face. Don't worry, we'll walk you through it! As we mentioned in Chapter 3, "What Goes Where and Why," one important disadvantage of working out at home is that you have no spotter, a kind soul who will make sure you don't drop a weight on your head. While most home gym equipment is designed to minimize (and/or eliminate) this problem, the potential still exists. Let's take a look.

Recognizing and Avoiding Home Gym Pitfalls

It sounds perfect, doesn't it? If you have gym equipment at home, you can work out in privacy on your own schedule. What could be better? Well, before you assume home is where the exercise is, consider a few built-in pitfalls. Perhaps the most important one concerns safety—an issue we'll return to again and again throughout this text. If you're working out at home, you're almost always also working out alone, and that can be dangerous.

For instance, one day many moons ago, Joe came home and found his father stuck upside down like a bat hanging helplessly in a pair of inversion boots (an odd but once-popular piece of home gym equipment). One can only imagine what his poor old man would have done had no one come along to extricate him from his perilous predicament. Another time, Mr. Glickman was benching a modest amount of weight and was unable to press the bar from his chest. Stuck like a mouse in a trap, he slowly, painfully, rolled the weight toward his knees until he was able to squeeze out from below. Atlhough these examples are humorous, each year 5 to 12 deaths are reported from weight training. Usually the cause of death is suffocation from dropping the bar across the neck during the bench press. These kinds of stories are virtually nonexistent in a gym, where patrons and trainers typically rush to your assistance.

Needless to say, since you are alone you need to take extra care to read the instructions that come with your home unit. If there's anything that you don't understand, don't hesitate to call the manufacturer. Many units come with a video. Take the time to watch it—it could spare you an injury.

What You'll Need, and What It'll Cost

Assuming you're like us and plan on working out until you're put out to pasture, setting up a home gym is more economical over the long term. (Actually, working out in a pasture is rather appealing as well!) Of course, if your shiny high-tech piece of equipment becomes the featured item in a garage sale, you've been penny-wise and weight-foolish.

First of all, if you decide on the home gym route, expect to pay from about a couple of hundred dollars a year for a special at the YMCA to thousands at a "see-and-be-seen establishment," like the Vertical Club on Manhattan's trendy East Side. You might find less expensive deals where you're from, and always be on the lookout for two-for-one deals or other specials.

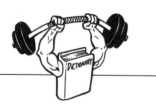

Bar Talk

Cardiovascular exercise is any activity that elevates your heart rate over a sustained period of time. Your body's cardiovascular system includes your heart and lungs.

Now, let's compare that to the cost of a complete home gym. We'll start with the equipment, which should include these three components:

➤ *Cardiovascular equipment.* You'll need some type of machine—stationary bike, rowing machine, or treadmill—that gets your ticker ticking.

➤ *Resistive equipment.* This apparatus will help you build muscle.

➤ *An exercise mat.* We'll discuss stretching at length in Chapter 12, "Revving the Engine," but for right now know that working on your flexibility should be an integral part of any fitness regimen. Without a mat, you're even less likely to follow our advice.

Cardio Action

What type of cardio machine should you buy? And how much can you expect to spend? Let's do a little imaginary shopping.

A stationary bike with bells and whistles like the Lifecycle can cost as much as $2,000, or you can spend as little as $300 for a basic stationary model. Here's the Catch-22. If you're not sure that you'll use it, it's best to start with the cheaper model. If, however, you're planning to become the next Greg LeMond, the sturdier machine is preferable. Years ago, one of Jonathan's teammates on the Stephen Roche Cycling Team, a guy who hadn't cycled or exercised in years, started riding on a low-rent stationary bike he bought for a song. Before long, he rode it so often he ground it into pencil shavings. Afterward, he started riding on the road and went on to become one of the better riders in the state. If you already have a bicycle, a fine way to work out indoors is to buy a contraption that allows you to remove the front wheel and ride your bike indoors. Usually, such an apparatus goes for between $100 and $200.

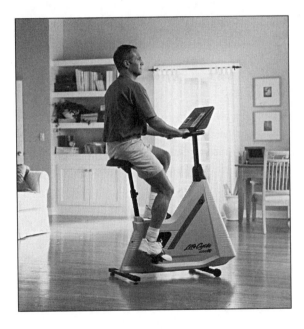

The Lifecycle stationary bike is a staple in homes and gyms.

(Photo courtesy LifeFitness)

If biking isn't your thing, let your feet do the walking and buy a treadmill. As is true for the stationary bike, there's a whole range of options for the treadmill, ranging in price from $500 to $5,000. Again, if you're going to use it regularly it's far better to drop four figures on a solid machine. Three brands we endorse are Star Trac, Quinton, and Trotter.

Treadmills can give you a great cardiovascular workout.

(Photo courtesy Star Trac)

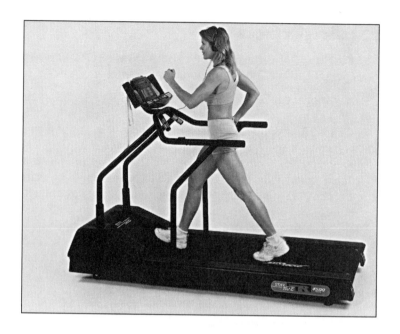

Don't like to run or bike? There are a variety of other machines that will help get your heart pumping. Our favorites include:

➤ *The Concept II rowing machine.* This calorie-burning contraption used by all the elite-level rowers in the off-season works the entire body from the ankles to the elbows. For $850, you get a state-of-the-art machine that represents maybe the most efficient bang for your buck. It's very low-maintenance and easy to learn.

The Concept II rowing ergometer. A terrific work-out that uses both your upper and lower body.

(Photo courtesy Concept II)

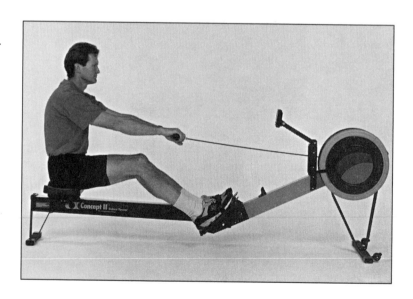

➤ *The VersaClimber.* Imagine climbing a ladder where the rungs are moving—Jack and the Bean Stalk meets Jack LaLanne—and you've got the general idea of this all-body workout. It sells for about $1,500 and doesn't take up much room. This is one of the best cardiovascular devices on the market, though it takes a bit of coordination to get started.

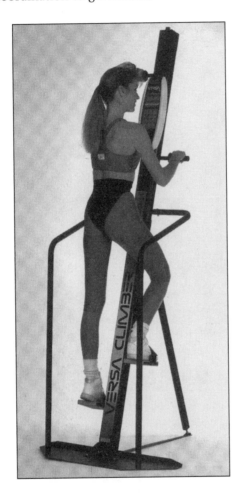

The VersaClimber provides a challenging cardio workout.

(Photo courtesy Heart Rate, Inc.)

➤ *Cross-country ski machine.* Cross-country skiers are always at the top of the list of athletes with the highest VO_2 *max,* or cardiovascular fitness. This machine won't help you carve turns on the trail, but it will help you get lean. Like the preceding two machines, we like this one since it works both your arms and your legs at the same time. At first the Nordic Track can be a little awkward, but once you get it, you'll enjoy one of the most efficient indoor workouts available. Nordic Track makes a variety of ski simulators ranging in price from $500 to $2,000.

➤ *Stairclimber.* This might be the most popular piece of indoor equipment at most gyms. While it's a terrific cardio workout that works the quads and gluts, unlike the three mentioned above it doesn't work the upper body. Stairmaster was the innovator in the market, but LifeFitness, Star Trac, and ClimbMax are among the many companies that have now given them some competition. Prices range from $1,000 to $2,000.

The Stairmaster is the original stair climbing machine.

(Photo courtesy Stairmaster)

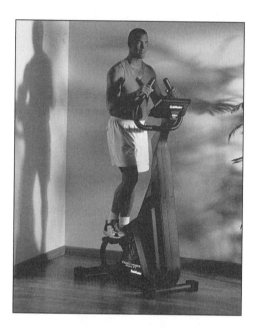

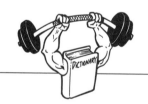

Bar Talk

VO$_2$ max refers to an individual's capacity for aerobic work. It is generally considered to be one of the most important factors in predicting an athlete's ability to perform in activities of more than three to five minutes.

The Weight Stuff

Now that we've explored the world of cardio equipment, it's time to discuss the meat and potatoes (or better yet, the fish and rice, but we'll get to the diet stuff later in the book!) of the home gym: resistance equipment.

Here's what you should look for in an "all-in-one" unit:

➤ *A variety of exercises.* No matter how effective the exercise, a continuing routine of the same few exercises will leave you feeling bored.

➤ *Ease of movement from one exercise to another.* If transitioning from one exercise is difficult or time-consuming, you're not likely to use the machine. Or if you do use it, you're not likely to get a good workout.

➤ *Enough resistance to grow with you as you get stronger.* Right now, the lightest weight on the machine may be just a little too heavy for you to lift, but—as hard as it may be to imagine now—you won't be in that position for long. You'll get stronger and stronger, and you'll want a machine that will help you do just that. If you have to do 38 repetitions of an exercise to tax yourself, you need to increase the weight.

➤ *An objective measure of your progress.* In other words, you need a way to tell how strong you're getting from one week to the next. Progress is inspirational. If you see that you're able to do 10 more repetitions of a particular exercise, you're more likely to keep at it.

There are quite a few multifunction strength-training machines on the market that are versatile, sturdy, and safe. Of course, each has its advantages and disadvantages. As a relative guide to our subjective rating of this equipment, we offer a barbell rating system from one to five—one being poor and five being the bee's knees. Let's look at some of the best options.

Total Gym (Cost: $795 plus shipping)

Featuring celebrities like Christie Brinkley, the manufacturers of the Total Gym have spent a small fortune popularizing their machine, making ambitious claims in their infomercial about how the Total Gym led these celebrities to superstardom—and how it can do the same for you. Well not quite, but once you get past the hyperbole, you'll find a well-designed machine. Unlike other machines, this one uses your own body weight, instead of metal plates or bands, at a variety of angles to provide resistance.

As with all the other pieces of equipment we've discussed so far, the Total Gym has its pros and cons. First, the pros:

➤ It offers a wide variety of exercises.

➤ It's compact, easy to store, and weighs only 95 pounds.

➤ It's safe. No worries about dropping weight on your toes or getting stuck under a bar.

➤ It's a well-made machine with fewer "bells and whistles" than most, and so requires relatively little maintenance.

➤ It provides resistance through a full *range of motion,* a key to a good workout.

➤ The manufacturers offer a lifetime warranty on the frame and a five-year warranty on parts.

And here's the downside of the Total Gym:

➤ Resistance is limited to 65 percent of your body weight—not enough for everybody.

➤ Since there are just six levels of resistance, this means that there are large jumps from one setting to another, as opposed to the ability to increase resistance gradually.

➤ The machines offer some relatively unconventional exercises, which means that it will be hard for you to translate exercises you might have learned at the gym.

Five-barbell rating: 3 barbells

Overall, the Total Gym is a fine piece of equipment but not well suited to someone who is already really strong or for someone who wants to duplicate the same types of exercises he or she has performed in a gym.

Soloflex (Cost: $1,195, plus shipping)

Thanks in part to its well-done ad campaign and elegant design, Soloflex has more name recognition than just about any other home gym. Using rubber "weight straps" instead of *freeweights* to provide resistance (though they now offer a freeweight option), Soloflex falls into the good-news, bad-news category.

Once again, we're going to offer you a neat little list of the pros and cons of this particular piece of machinery. Let's start with the pros:

➤ This is a safe and effective machine.

➤ It doesn't take up a lot of space.

➤ If a machine can be pretty, this one is pretty!

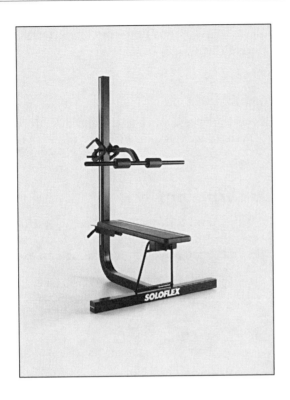

Soloflex uses rubber straps instead of weights for resistance.

(Photo courtesy Soloflex)

➤ It provides both positive and negative resistance for all exercises.

➤ The floating bar feature ensures that you don't favor your dominant side. Some other machines allow you to move the bar evenly, even if you push harder on one side.

➤ It offers a wide variety of exercises.

➤ The manufacturers provide a five-year warranty.

And now for the cons:

➤ The Soloflex offers uneven resistance. Because rubber bands become tighter as they stretch, as you move through the exercise—known as the range of motion (ROM)—it will be either too "easy" at the beginning or too "hard" at the end, especially on longer movements like the squat. To remedy this you can use the freeweights option, but this means spending more money to purchase them as well as taking time to change the weights.

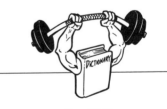

Bar Talk

Freeweights, namely barbells and dumbbells, are freestanding and not part of a machine.

➤ In the infomercial, it looks like a snap to transition from one exercise to the next. In reality, it's a little more difficult.

Five-barbell rating: 2.5 barbells.

Overall, the Soloflex looks good, but the bands present a problem since the beginning part of the exercise doesn't provide as much resistance as the end does. It feels almost like you start the exercise with a 10-pound weight, and increase it to a 20-pounder by the top of the movement.

Bowflex (Cost: $999 plus shipping)

While the Bowflex looks more like a medieval torture device than a piece of exercise equipment, it is an effective and versatile apparatus. Using "Power Rods," which look like arrows in an archer's quiver, the rods bend as you move through an exercise's range of motion.

The Bowflex creates resist-ance using Power Rods.

(Photo courtesy Bowflex)

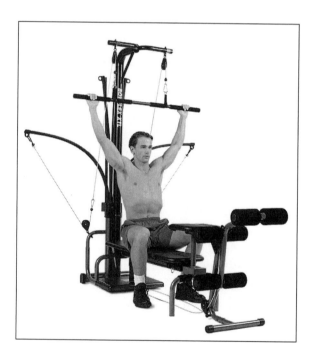

Here are this machine's best qualities:

➤ It's well built and sturdy.

➤ It allows you to increase resistance in low weight increments.

➤ The Bowflex folds and rolls for storage.

➤ The manufacturer offers an unlimited warranty on the Power Rods and a five-year limited warranty on materials and workmanship.

And here, of course, are the cons:

➤ A few of the adjustments between exercises are tedious.

➤ If you need more resistance than the 210 pounds offered by the standard model, you'll need to upgrade.

Five-barbell rating: 4 barbells

Overall, we like it. It works well for both the beginning weight trainer and the grizzled veteran. Our favorite home gym option.

The Power of Freeweights

If newfangled ideas like rubber bands and Power Rods don't do it for you, you can buy an adjustable bench ($300 to $500) and a set of freeweights (price discussed in the next paragraph), and knock yourself out (but not literally!). Although initially this might seem like the simpler, less expensive way to go, the costs quickly add up, and it can become far more expensive that you anticipated. Furthermore, for the novice, the use of freeweights in an unsupervised setting makes us more than a wee bit nervous. Still, a freeweight setup at home can work quite well if you take the time to learn the rules and then follow them.

Now for the cost. Unless you're training to be the next Barry Sanders, you probably don't want or need a full set of dumbbells in your home. A good option is a pair of adjustable dumbbells such as The PowerBlock. Selling for roughly $200, The PowerBlock allows you to easily and quickly adjust the weight of the barbell from 5 to 45 pounds.

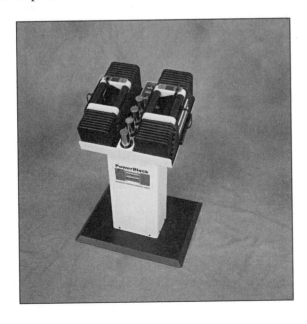

The PowerBlock is a terrific freeweight option, offering versatile, easily adjustable dumbbells.

(Photo courtesy Intellbell)

When shopping for a bar and weights (also known as plates), you have a few options. "Olympic" bars, found in just about every gym, are seven feet long and weigh 45 pounds. (There are shorter, lighter bars available.)

Plates are available in 2.5- through 100-pound increments. Figure on spending about 25¢ per pound, a sum that adds up if you're a budding moose. Throw on a pair of collars (the clips that secure the plates at either end of the bar), and you're good to go for just about any of the exercises we'll describe in future chapters. We say "just about" because there are a few that are unsafe to do without a spotter. We'll note which are the risky ones so you don't end up with an imprint of the barbell on your nose.

As we've already said, unless you're willing to spend a small fortune, you'll never duplicate the wide range of equipment that a good gym can offer (to say nothing of the guidance trainers can provide). However, even the best gym in the solar system does you no good if you don't use it. As we said in Chapter 2, "Hurry Up and Weight," working out in a gym is the fastest way to build a fitter body, but a home gym option is certainly the next best thing.

The Least You Need to Know

➤ Working out alone means knowing the risks and taking special care, especially if you use freeweights.

➤ Setting up a home gym may be more cost effective than paying a gym membership—assuming you use it.

➤ If you decide to purchase equipment for a home gym, be a wise consumer—and that especially goes for freeweights.

Part 2
Gearing Up

This section is a complete primer on everything you'll need to know before you actually get thee to a gym.

In Chapter 6, we discuss the importance (or lack thereof) of looking good in your exercise threads. In other words—what to wear and why. If you've been wondering about some of the subtleties of jog bras, this is the chapter for you.

In Chapters 7 and 8, we get into the basics of a proper diet, and we spend some time talking about the pros and cons of the scores of nutritional supplements out there today.

Chapter 9 will address that dreaded, but often necessary, visit to the doctor. We'll talk about some of the issues that may come up in his or her office and what to do if you're not feeling up to snuff.

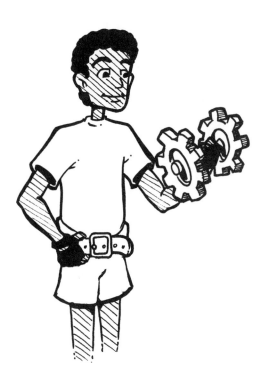

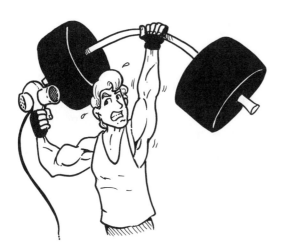

Chapter 6

Strain in Style

In This Chapter

➤ Dress for success in the gym

➤ Threads and treads: do's and don'ts

➤ Sports bras: compression or encapsulation

➤ Accessories: to wrap or not to wrap?

What you wear to the gym is an issue of the utmost importance that really doesn't matter. By that we mean if it's comfortable, allows a full range of motion, and adheres to gym regulations, you could wear a tuxedo with tails or an evening gown and be good to go. While this sounds ridiculous—and it is—there was a terrific runner a few years ago who ran the New York City Marathon in a tuxedo jacket and shorts. (He discarded the black shoes and went with a pair of Nikes.)

So while you could work out effectively in a burlap bag, what you wear is of enormous personal relevance to who you are and what kind of statement you wish to make—if you wish to make any at all. Are you flashy or modest? A lycra proponent or fan of organic cotton? Do you go with the neon lime green bike jersey and large silver hoop earrings or stick with the ripped T-shirt that you wore when you went fishing with your Uncle Sylvester? In this chapter, we'll outline your options and make some recommendations about the workout clothes that might be right for you.

Do Clothes Make the Athlete?

Although we adhere to the philosophy of "to each his own," some people's workout attire can be perplexing. Deidre and Joe frequently find themselves working out next to a hulking guy who can lift a compact car and the kitchen sink. However, no matter how hot it gets he wears an XXL sweatshirt and long baggy pants. Though he has the body of a NFL linebacker, the self-effacing chap refuses to show skin. Another full-bodied woman they know wears Pamela Anderson–type skintight outfits.

Even more confusing is the dignified gent who works out in the same immaculate outfit every time: red tank top, blue shorts, white socks, and white sneakers. While this is a perfectly fine outfit, Joe and Deidre are dying to know if he has two dozen of the same items (and if so why?); and, if he has just one of each, does that mean he's laundering them after every workout? These, dear reader, are some of the questions that can weigh on a petty man's mind.

Simply put, picking an outfit to exercise in at the gym can be purely perfunctory or a fair bit of fun. While we have more than a few biases on the subject that we'll gladly share with you in the following pages, the bottom line is: If the garment fits, wear it. To us, it seems silly (or at least immodest) to have to worry about flashing your goodies to your gym neighbors, adjusting your clothing during each set, and either ignoring or enjoying lascivious looks, but however you're comfortable is fine. We'll assume that the more obvious points of gym attire—wearing socks that match each other, forgoing the evening gown or pj's—are understood. What follows are some common-sense pointers about what to wear and how to wear it. We'll also talk about gym accoutrements like weight belts, gloves, and wrist and knee wraps that you should know about.

The Threads

The best workout clothing consists of any combination of comfortable garments that allow freedom of movement and a modicum of modesty. When Joe began competing in kayak marathons with international paddlers, he was initially surprised to see that the majority of the world-class Australian and South African kayakers he raced against wore baggy T-shirts while the Americans often wore tight tank tops. Why the baggy look? These guys had chiseled upper bodies straight from central casting. It's comfortable, mate! In other words, if you got the goods why compromise comfort for vanity? Before you could say rip curl, many of the Americans started wearing extra-large as well.

Here's a basic list of acceptable gym threads:

➤ Sweat pants

➤ Shorts

➤ Leggings

➤ T-shirts

➤ Tank tops

➤ Sports bras

➤ Sweat shirts

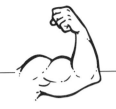

Although some people find wearing a tank top too revealing, keep in mind that it's always a good idea to concentrate on the muscle groups you're working, so if you're concentrating on your upper body, a tank top may be just the thing. Not only is it easier to focus on the task at hand if you can see the muscle actually lengthening and contracting, it can be a good motivational tool to see your muscles grow before you eyes—a phenomenon known as the *pump*.

When working her upper body, Deidre usually wears a sports bra and sweatpants, and she dons a T-shirt and shorts when she works her lower body.

Flex Facts

Lifters often refer to the swelling in a muscle immediately after lifting as the "pump." While it appears that the muscle is growing as you lift, what you see is actually the muscle becoming temporarily engorged with blood—not the same as when the muscles themselves grow.

Joe, who has arguably the largest collection of race T-shirts in North America, tends to modify his attire according to the aerobic activity he's doing that day. If he's going to run and lift he wears jogging shorts and brings along an extra T-shirt (no problem there). If he's going to cycle or use the Concept II rower, he's likely to wear bike shorts, and, you guessed it, a T-shirt. Also, on "leg" day, he prefers bike shorts since they offer better support when he does squats.

Jonathan, the personal trainer who has been known to dine in trendy Manhattan restaurants in a black warm-up suit (arguing that, strictly speaking, it is a suit), doesn't really care what he's wearing as long as he's working out. In fact, Jonathan probably would lift in a lobster bib if he forgot to pack one of his nine million T-shirts.

Jocks for Jocks

While the jockstrap may be one of the most ridiculed and ridiculous garments in the clothing kingdom, it certainly has its place on the so-called clothes chain. One very obvious bit of advice (that for some reason is frequently ignored) is that when you're wearing baggy sweats or loose shorts, please (please!) wear a jockstrap or Jockey shorts/briefs. If you don't, your faux pas will be discussed—before or behind your briefless behind. Joe once worked out in a pair of black bike shorts that, unbeknownst to him, sported a dime-sized hole in the right cheek region. His friends told him about it *sotto voce*; others just pointed and laughed hysterically.

If you don't already know, some gym shorts (and virtually all shorts designed for runners) come with a built-in brief for added support and comfort. *Compression shorts,* a specifically designed undergarment that resembles bike shorts, also work well under shorts or sweats.

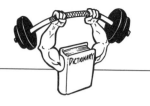

Bar Talk

Compression shorts like the ones favored by NBA players are form-fitting shorts made of nylon and spandex designed to be worn under loose-fitting shorts.

We all know members of both sexes who favor shorts so small that little (if anything) is left to the imagination. Some people can pull this off; others fall into the "shouldn't have tried" category. Again, diversity is the spice of life, and if you don't mind looking like Charo or one of the Village People, fine by us. However, remember that form usually follows function; if the garment is stretched to its limit, it's probably not the best thing to wear. Again, make like Joe's kayak-racing cronies and get comfortable before you get vain.

Women's Wear

Since the 1980s, more and more women have begun flocking to the gym. In the early days, it seemed as if women were wary of "looking like men" and overemphasized their femininity in their dress instead of focusing on the fact that they were athletes working out. This may (or may not) explain the popularity of the thong that scores of women wore to the gym.

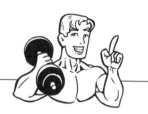

Spot Me

Leggings often become nearly transparent when stretched; if you wear them in the gym be sure to wear something underneath to protect your privacy.

In case you missed it, the thong was (and is) a one-piece leotard cut extremely high on the hips with a thin strip of cloth wedged uncomfortably between the buttocks. In gym parlance it was known as "butt floss." While many women looked downright sexy in the thing, it had to be one of the cruelest fashion hoaxes this side of platform shoes, since essentially you were walking around with a self-imposed wedgie.

Luckily, these days the thong is mostly a collector's item packed neatly beside your collection of *Jane Fonda's Greatest Aerobic Hits*. Today, most women who exercise regularly wear a sports bra or T-shirt with sweats, leggings, or shorts.

If you do go the sports bra route and are amply endowed, make sure you can jog and/or take an aerobics class without doing yourself bodily harm. Similarly, causing a traffic accident might be good for your ego, but it could be bad for your conscience.

The Treads

If you hadn't already noticed, a trip to a well-equipped sporting goods store will reveal just how specialized workout gear has become. This is especially true in the footwear realm. In fact, never-throw-out-a-pair-of-running-shoes jocks like Jonathan and Joe each have at least 44 pairs. (Okay, maybe more, but we don't have the time to tally them all.) Think we're exaggerating? Here's a basic outline of the footwear you could find in our collective closets:

➤ Running shoes for the road (lots of them!).

➤ Trail running shoes.

➤ Cycling shoes for biking on the road.

➤ Cycling shoes for mountain biking and touring.

➤ Basketball shoes.

➤ Tennis shoes.

➤ Cross-training shoes, which are hybrid sneakers designed to do a bit of everything.

➤ Water shoes, which are slipperlike footwear designed for kayakers.

➤ Approach shoes designed for easy hiking.

➤ Sports sandals.

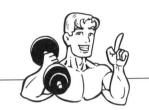

Spot Me

When buying a new pair of shoes, it's a good idea to try them on in the evening, since your feet tend to swell toward the end of the day. What feels good at 9 A.M. might be a wee bit snug at dinnertime.

With the obvious exception of cycling shoes that feature protruding cleats that leave you walking like a petrified tree, most of the above are fine for just lifting weights. Remember that there have been many Olympic-level marathon runners who ran like the wind barefoot. So while the sport specificity in footwear does have its place, you can wear just about anything as long as it fits and gives you adequate support.

Herein lies the rub. Ideally, your footwear should provide you with ample arch support as well as proper medial (inside aspect of the foot) and lateral (outside) support. If you've ever had any foot pain, your best bet is to go to a store known for its sneaker savvy. Be specific with the salesperson about what you'll be doing in these sneakers. If you know that you're *flat-footed* (have no arch), *pronate* (walk on the inner portion of your foot) or *supinate* (walk on the outer portion), inform the salesperson; if he knows what he's doing he should recommend shoes designed for those specific conditions.

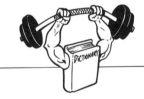

Bar Talk

To **pronate,** as it relates to walking, is to bear most of your weight on the inner portion of your foot. You can often tell by looking at the wear pattern on the sole of your shoes whether you pronate or **supinate,** which means to bear weight on the outer portion of your foot as you walk. To have a **flat foot** (pes planus) means to be without arches.

If you don't understand pronation, buy whatever feels best and, over time, monitor where the majority of the wear and tear on your footwear occurs. (If you're a runner this will quickly become obvious.) Generally speaking, when you're weight lifting, a cross-training shoe would be your best bet for appropriate support.

Don't Mention It

If ever there were a perfect place to discuss the ins and outs of sports bras, here it is. The three things to remember are proper fit, comfort, and structure.

➤ **Fit.** When shopping for a sports bra, always try it on before you get to the gym. Once you've got it on, clap your hands overhead; if the plastic band moves up your chest, it's too tight. You don't want to start working out and discover you're wearing an iron corset that doesn't allow you to breathe. And you don't want to fret about peekaboo bosom while you're lying in the middle of a bench or performing another cleavage-revealing exercise.

➤ **Comfort.** To continue on our sartorial theme: Looking good doesn't equal feeling good. Besides, the better you feel when you work out, the more apt you are to keep training!

➤ **Structure.** Basically, there are two types of sports bras to choose from: compression and encapsulation. While neither sounds terribly forgiving, the latter tends to be the most comfortable. True to its name, the compression bra presses (read squishes) the breasts against the chest in a single mass. This style is more appropriate for small- to medium-breasted women. Like a brassiere, the encapsulation type is built to hold each breast in a cup. This works better for full-figured women.

Wrap It Up

One of the neat things about strength training is that you can do it in a sophisticated gym with high-tech equipment or in a bare-bones basement with a bench, a few hand-held weights, and plenty of desire. In either setting, however, you can bring nothing more than what you're wearing or an assortment of goodies that may (or may not) help you get stronger.

We're talking about weight belts, wrist and knee wraps, and gloves. Is this stuff necessary? Not really. Can the mere sight of this equipment get you psyched to go to the gym? Could be. Let's talk a bit about each one, and you can decide for yourself.

Buckle Up!

To belt or not to belt, that's a question that has generated a fair bit of debate among fitness devotees. The good news is that wearing a *weight belt* reminds you to maintain erect posture while you lift. The bad news is twofold. The belt offers support to the muscles in your lower back and abdomen that you're trying to strengthen. Secondly, wearing one can give you a false sense of security that may have you trying to lift more weight than is safe or necessary. Of course, if you have a weak lower back, a belt may be necessary to work out pain-free until we can help strengthen your abdominal and lower back muscles.

In many ways, wearing a belt offers more psychological comfort than actual aid. If you suffer from low-level chronic back pain, wearing one can be comforting—it's like a heating pad without the heat, if you will. Furthermore, it's like an athlete who rubs the head of the trusty old trainer before taking the field. As they approach an imposing bar loaded with weight, many lifters cinch the buckle one notch tighter, a gesture that gets them psyched for the challenge more than anything else.

During her powerlifting days, Deidre wore a belt. But remember, her sport was about demonstrating strength; your goal in the gym is to gain strength. In other words, her goal was to lift the heaviest weight she possibly could, so wearing a belt while she squatted or deadlifted helped to up her totals. Again, we're concerned about what your muscles can do, not what your gear can do. Unless you feel you need to wear a belt, we recommend you don't.

For a belt to offer any significant support, it has to be pulled so tight you'd barely be able to whistle. By comparison, the corsets worn by female French nobility were as comfy as housedresses. In fact, before Deidre would approach a *squat* or dead lift it would take two strong people to yank on her belt to get it tight enough to give her sufficient support. Hauling a marlin into a fishing boat wasn't as much of a struggle.

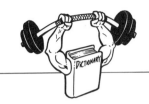

Bar Talk

A **weight belt** is made from thick, dense leather and is roughly six inches wide. It's buckled securely around your waist just above your hips.

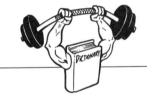

Bar Talk

The **squat** is a great full-body exercise that involves performing a deep knee-bend with a barbell across your back. Sounds intimidating, but fret not; we will take you through the proper execution of this movement in Chapter 18, "The World on Your Shoulders."

It's a Wrap

There are two kinds of wraps that you can use in the gym: wrist wraps and knee wraps. Wrist wraps are shorter and affixed with Velcro, while the longer knee wraps are cinched by tucking the wrap under itself and pulling.

Remember, for wraps to be effective they have to be pulled pretty tight. There are only a few good reasons to wear wrist wraps. Here they are:

➤ If you've recently suffered a wrist injury and need the support.

➤ If you have a tendency to *hyperextend* your wrists while you perform a bench press, it's a good idea to wrap. Otherwise you could drop the bar.

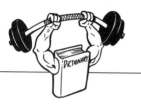

Bar Talk

To **hyperextend** means to bend a body part beyond its normal anatomical or neutral position. For example, if you straighten your arm to lock your elbow, it will end up in a straight line. People who are called "double-jointed" can lock their elbow beyond that straight line position so it looks as though their elbow is bending in the opposite direction. This is called hyperextension of your elbow.

Knee wraps? We're against them. These mummifying wraps are usually worn to support you when you're performing squats or using the leg press or leg extension machine. (For descriptions of these exercises, see Chapter 18.) We don't like knee wraps for the same reason we're generally against weight belts. Unless you're squatting or pressing a ton of weight, a person with healthy knees who wears them is wasting his or her time. Or worse.

The reason one does these exercises in the first place is to strengthen the muscles around the knee joint. When you wrap your knees, you remove a significant amount of the workload from the muscles and transfer it to the wraps. Simply put, wearing knee wraps defeats the purpose of the exercise.

Here's where people get confused. Wearing wraps will help you lift more weight, which should be good, right? Wrong! Being able to lift more weight is only good if it comes as the result of your muscles getting stronger, not because you've fortified yourself with wraps.

This "might makes right" logic highlights an important point: Your lifting should be about getting strong, not seeming strong. This move-as-much-weight-as-possible syndrome, which afflicts men far more than it does women, is counterproductive to health and is as misguided as erecting an ornate roof before you've built a sound foundation.

We can hear the dissenters saying, "If I lift more with the wraps, my leg muscles won't get injured, and I'll get stronger faster." Nice try. Just because your securely wrapped knees can handle an increased load doesn't mean that your back or other body parts can. So ironically, wrapping your knees to protect this complex and vulnerable joint may actually end up jeopardizing your safety rather than ensuring it.

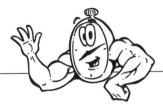

Weight a Minute

We cannot stress how important it is not to be fooled by the use of equipment while lifting in the gym. The potential for harm is extremely high, and we have seen people get seriously hurt in the act of lifting more than they could handle because they were wearing a weight belt or knee wraps.

Finger Wraps

A noncontroversial option in the lifting game is the wearing of gloves. Weight-lifting gloves, which typically cost around $10, have padded palms and cut-off fingers for ventilation and dexterity. Gloves are good if you look at calluses with disdain, and they can come in handy during certain abusive exercises like chin-ups and lat pull downs, which you'll read more about in later chapters.

When Deidre started lifting 10 years ago, she used gloves until she realized that her feel for the weight improved without them. What does "feel for the weight" mean? Many experienced lifters feel that the greater the contact they have with the bar, the easier it is to lift the weight. Try both and see for yourself.

Like Deidre, Jonathan and Joe go gloveless. A kayaker whose hands are usually callused and cracked from gripping a paddle hours a day in salt water, Joe finds that the calluses he's built from lifting help fortify his mitts while paddling.

If you decide to don gloves, try to find a pair that have a grippy texture on the palms, and make sure they fit your hands snugly without restricting your movement.

Pads

Instead of gloves, some folks prefer pads, which are small, flat, neoprene squares that are held in your palms like mini-potholders. Not only do they offer the same comfort and improved grip as gloves, but you also won't have to worry about sweaty-palm syndrome. The downside is that since you have to carry them around, they tend to disappear like socks in a dryer. Jonathan has collected enough pads from his gym's lost and found to tile Madison Square Garden.

Straps

Straps are another common piece of paraphernalia you'll see in the gym. Made of sturdy, nonstretch material, straps are worn around your wrists and then wrapped around the bar that you plan to lift. The purpose of straps is to ease the burden on the gripping muscles in your hands and forearms that often fatigue before the larger working muscles.

Take exercises like deadlifts, pull-ups, and/or cable rows, which we'll explain in depth in Chapter 16, "Flip Side." These exercises all involve movements that tax large muscles and hence require you to lift a fair bit of weight. While overusing straps can prevent those hand and forearm muscles from becoming stronger, they are useful when a weak grip inhibits you from completing the exercise, a common occurrence if you're lifting a lot of weight.

As you may have gathered by now, we're not big proponents of gadgets that will make your exercises easier. Still, after you spend enough time at the gym, you'll see tremendously strong people who lift with a weight belt, wrist and knee straps, and gloves. What's up with that?

People who lift a lot and often have developed their own habits—good and bad—over many years of experimentation. However, when you start out, it's important to establish good habits, to lift with sound technique and with as little interference as possible—just you, the weight, knowledge, and plenty of desire.

The Least You Need to Know

➤ Your workout gear should look good and feel better.

➤ When buying shoes, let fit and function be your guide.

➤ Choose the sports bra that's right for you.

➤ Weight belts, wrist and knee wraps, and gloves can help or hinder you. Use them with care.

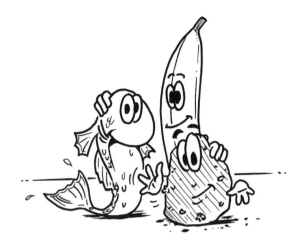

Chapter 7

Food for Thought

In This Chapter

➤ What to eat and when

➤ The pros and cons of protein

➤ Stop dieting and lose weight

Ask any bodybuilder, triathlete, or racehorse trainer and he's likely to say the same thing when it comes to the importance of proper nutrition: You are what you eat.

Sure, lifting can (and should) be an important part of your fitness regimen, but if you neglect proper nutrition, you're likely to sabotage your potential gains in the gym as well as your overall health. While we all know people who seem to flourish while eating a diet of pastrami sandwiches, jelly donuts, and coffee, most people will pay a steep price for such gluttony.

Typically, if you neglect your diet, you're destined to struggle with your weight, feel sluggish during the day, or worse, invite sickness and disease. Even if you exercise regularly and have a washboard stomach, ignoring sound nutrition means you'll probably struggle through your workout. "I just didn't have it today," is a common complaint heard in the gym. It says a great deal about the individual's body chemistry and the lack of the fuel it needs to function.

As you probably know, there are enough myths and misinformation about nutrition floating around out there to confuse even the most knowledgeable doctor. Don't despair. In this chapter, we'll walk you through this dietary quagmire and explain what constitutes a sensible diet. We'll also discuss the changes you may need to make as you improve your fitness level and health. If you have less body fat than Carl Lewis, more energy than Richard Simmons, and eat plenty of fresh vegetables and lean protein, you probably should just skip to the next chapter. If not, grab a pen or pencil and let's get shopping.

How Much Is Just Enough?

Let's start at the beginning—the basics of a sensible diet for the average healthy adult.

According to the U.S. Department of Agriculture, the average healthy male weighs 154 pounds, and his female counterpart tips the scales at 121. The phrase that we often hear—Recommended Dietary Allowances (RDA) or Recommended Daily Intake (RDI)—refers to the levels of protein, vitamin, and mineral intake considered adequate to meet the nutritional needs of these exceedingly normal folks. Of course, if you weigh more than 50 pounds over or under those figures you'll need to adjust accordingly. And similarly, if you're pregnant, lactating, postmenopausal, or a kid, your requirements are different from what the RDA suggests.

That said, here's something to keep in mind: A guideline for dietary intake is laid out in the "Food Guide Pyramid," which breaks down the recommended number of servings for each of the five basic food groups (see the following figure). The groups are:

➤ Bread, cereal, pasta, and rice

➤ Vegetables

➤ Fruit

➤ Milk, yogurt, and cheese

➤ Meat, poultry, fish, dry beans, eggs, and nuts

A sixth group, the one that makes most humans salivate, is pleasing to the palate but high in fat or calories. This group includes fats, oils, and sweets. Sadly, these substances have little (or no) nutritive value and should be eaten sparingly. (One can only imagine the frenzy caused by a study that said the best diet would include copious servings of ice cream, potato chips, mayonnaise, and bacon.)

Here's something else you should know. The six essential nutrients are:

➤ Carbohydrates

➤ Proteins

➤ Fats

➤ Vitamins

➤ Minerals

➤ Water

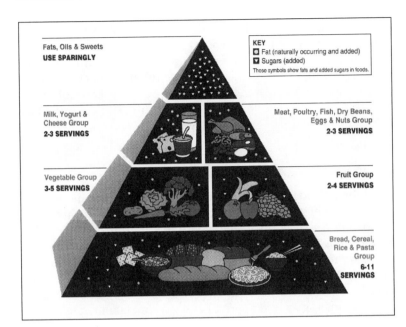

The Food Guide Pyramid is a good visual representation of a healthful diet, emphasizing the need for complex carbohydrates.

Before we get into the nuts and bolts of what and when to eat, let's do a quickie course in basic nutrition.

Carbohydrates (carbs), proteins, and fats are your sources of calories. Carbs supply four calories per gram and are classified as simple or complex. This isn't a psychological profile, but is based on the properties each possesses. Simple carbs, which are quickly converted to energy, are high in sugar and found in treats like cakes, cookies, jams, and soda.

Complex carbohydrates, which provide a more sustained and gradual release of glucose into the bloodstream, are found in pasta, bread, grains, and cereals. Complex carbs should be the mainstay of your diet.

Fats don't provide a lot of vitamins and minerals, but they serve a valuable role in your diet. For example, without ingesting some fat—about two tablespoonfuls a day—your body couldn't process or absorb vitamins A, D, E, or K.

Protein, which forms the structural basis for muscle tissue, supplies energy only when there aren't enough calories available from carbs and fat. Foods high in protein include meat, milk, eggs, and legumes.

That's the basics on what we eat. While many experts disagree on the precise figures, it's our informed opinion that a good diet should consist of 60 to 65 percent carbohydrates, 10 to 12 percent protein, and 20 to 30 percent fat. Here's a helpful key to figure out how much of each type of food you should eat.

First you need to figure out your basal metabolic rate (BMR). Your BMR is the amount of energy (calories) you burn just to keep going if you did nothing but lie in bed staring at the wall. (The ultimate couch potato doesn't even use the remote control.) It's both amusing and informative to figure out the approximate number of calories that your body needs each day to maintain your weight. To figure out your BMR for one day, get your calculator and punch in the following numbers. This estimate should be within 15 percent of your actual BMR.

Men: Body weight (pounds) × 24 ÷ 2.2

Women: Body weight (pounds) × 21 ÷ 2.2

For example: Jonathan weighs 172 pounds. To find out his metabolic rate, he multiplies 172 by 24, which is 4,128, which he divides by 2.2 to get 1,876. So, without exercising, he needs to consume 1,876 calories each day to maintain his body weight, and thus to lose weight, he needs to eat fewer than 1,876 calories. Now Jonathan actually does more than lie prone for the day. In fact, he burns about 1,500 or so calories each day cycling, running, and lifting weights, which means he breaks even at more than 3,300 calories a day. (By way of comparison, the average sumo wrestler consumes 4,600 calories a day.) Being able to approximate your metabolic rate allows you to have an idea of how many calories your body needs each day.

Do You Need More?

As an aspiring body beautiful, you may be wondering if your caloric needs are different than the average. Should you eat some extra protein, and maybe less fat? Good question.

The Truth About Protein

When it comes to strength training and building muscle, the role of protein is perhaps the most misunderstood. First, some facts: The RDA for protein is 0.8 grams per pound. For our prototypical 154-pound friend, that's 56 grams of protein a day, or about one cup of milk (9 grams), 2 eggs (12 grams), and a four-ounce serving of chicken or beef (32 grams). In other words, it's quite easy to meet the RDA requirement.

"Whoa, Nellie!" you may be saying. "You just said that protein helps make up the actual structure of the muscle. If that's true, isn't it best to eat more protein?" At the risk of sounding like a politician on the campaign trail, the answer is "yes and no."

While there is scientific evidence to suggest that some strength and ultra-endurance athletes may benefit from protein intakes of as much as 1.5 to 2.0 times the RDA, this is probably not necessary or helpful for the vast majority of people. The Catch-22 is that you're probably already downing well over the RDA and just don't know it. So before you start doing a Rocky Balboa on us and slurp raw-egg shakes before heading to the gym, know that recent studies show that the average American consumes more than 100 grams of protein per day. So while you may need more than the RDA, you're likely already there.

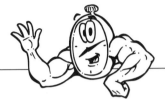

Weight a Minute

Beware of "studies" that claim you should consume more than twice the amount of protein suggested by the RDA. Odds are these are conducted by manufacturers of supplements who have a vested interest in your eating like a lion.

Water, Water, Everywhere

We cannot overstress the importance of proper hydration. Simply put, a human being can go for weeks without eating solid food, but can't survive more than three to seven days without water. A male's body is made up of 60 to 65 percent water; a female's 50 to 60 percent. The human brain is about 75 percent water. Water aids in digestion and eases muscle soreness after a training session. Proper water consumption is crucial to weight loss.

Why, then, are most people, even serious athletes, underhydrated? The two most common answers are: It's a nuisance and maintaining proper hydration means you'll pee a lot. While the first is debatable, the second is not.

In the course of a normal day—no naps in a sauna or foot races in the Gobi Desert—the average adult needs about 80 ounces of water to maintain water balance. Most people probably drink half that, which is why so many of us are sluggish, suffer from headaches, and feel stiff and sore after performing just a moderate amount of exercise.

If you exercise often (especially during the summer), drink a lot of coffee and booze (which act as a diuretic), or take medication, you'll need to drink even more water. Even a slight drop in your body weight lost through perspiration can adversely affect your exercise performance. That means that you should drink about 6 to 8 ounces of fluid every 15 minutes or so when you're exercising. On average, you should be consuming at least 8 ounces roughly eight to 10 times a day. Sound like a lot? Try it for a few days and see how much better you feel.

In short, making a lot of trips to the bathroom is a small price to pay when you consider how much better the human body functions when it's properly lubricated. Although water provides no energy (calories), your body can't use most of the nutrients it needs without water to process them.

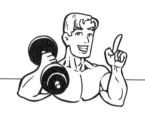

Here are some salient facts about water:

➤ Water is responsible for providing the building materials for cell protoplasm. Don't ask, just trust us: it's important.

➤ Water helps protect the body's tissue and internal organs.

➤ Water helps regulate our body temperature as well as transport other nutrients, hormones, and waste products.

There's more, but we assume you get the point by now: The more water you drink, the better you'll feel.

The Fancy Stuff

Okay, so water is cool, but what about Gatorade, Sportsade, and the scores of other liquid "ades" sprouting up all over the beverage aisle? After all, if it works for Michael Jordan it's got to be good. Right? To which we reply unequivocally, "Maybe."

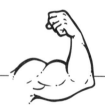

Unless you're running, cycling, or engaging in any cardiovascular activity for at least 45 minutes to an hour a day or working out in a hot, humid gym, sports drinks really aren't necessary. There is no real physiological need for the extra calories or minerals in a sports drink. (You'll replenish everything you need in your next meal.)

However, if you are pounding the pavement with a vengeance, a sports drink may help you speed up the rate at which your body absorbs the fluid. Perhaps the biggest advantage these sporty drinks have over straight water is taste. A cold glass of pure mountain water may be the elixir of life, but after a while your taste buds may be calling out for more. Simply put, the more you like the taste, the more likely you are to drink the stuff.

Here are our top four tips for optimal hydration:

1. Unless a gator is chasing you or you're working out under extreme conditions, cold water is the best bet to keep you running efficiently.

2. Most commercial sports drinks contain a carbohydrate concentration of between 5 and 7 percent. Anything higher than that can cause gastric distress and actually slow fluid absorption. Diluted juice (50 percent juice/50 percent water) with maybe a pinch of salt works just as well.

3. Drink 16 ounces of cold water or diluted sports drink before working out.

4. Drink water every 15 minutes or so to prevent dehydration.

Lose It by the Book

We are a culture obsessed with weight, and for two reasons. First, we have before us the unrealistic standards set by the incredibly thin supermodels and actors who are viewed as "ideal." Second, we are the most overweight culture in the Western world. And oddly enough, despite our nation's keen interest in fitness, the rates of obesity are on the rise.

If you're one of the millions of Americans struggling to lose weight, you're well aware of the countless products and diets promising to help you drop "those ugly pounds" in a matter of minutes. (Okay, days.) Not only are most of these products bogus, dangerous, or worse, even the best of them rarely produce long-term weight loss.

Slow but Steady Wins the Race

Sorry folks, but as much as we'd like to unveil some secret recipe to get you looking like Fabio or Fabia, the simple fact remains: There's no easy way. There is, however, a safe and extremely effective way to reach your ideal playing weight: eat with moderation, variety, and balance.

With few exceptions, low-calorie diets, skipping meals, and fasting are counterproductive. When you make drastic adjustments to your calorie intake, your body's survival instincts sound an alarm and slow its metabolism to a snail's pace. Your goal is to speed up your metabolic rate, not the other way around. When you sit down to your next meal after a fast, your metabolism remains depressed, which actually causes you to gain weight.

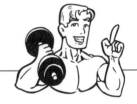

Spot Me

Try weighing yourself before and after a workout. If you're lighter after you train, it means that you've lost more water from sweating than you've replenished in fluids. If that's the case, try drinking more next time. Remember that one pound of body weight is equivalent to 16 ounces of water.

Because most health experts agree that a weight loss of more than two pounds per week is unhealthy, we recommend a weekly goal of one pound. Usually, when you lose more than that per week, you're actually losing muscle as well as fat—a big no-no since not only does muscle look good, but it also helps you to burn calories.

In order to lose a pound a week, you need to burn 500 calories more than you ingest each day. That may seem like a formidable number, but it really isn't if you exercise. If you can manage to burn an extra 250 calories a day—a 2.5-mile jog or 30 minutes on the exercise bike—you're halfway there. As we said in Chapter 2, "Hurry Up and Weight," your body won't know the difference if you get those miles walking to the post office in lieu of running in the park. And keep in mind that as you increase your muscle mass, you'll be burning extra calories. Even as you read this book your muscles are metabolically active. (Reading this book while you walk to the post office is even better.)

Now, here are some handy ways to decrease the number of calories you eat each day:

➤ In the morning eat a piece of whole wheat toast instead of a bagel. Calories saved: 150.

➤ Hold the mayo and use mustard on your turkey sandwich. Calories saved: 100

➤ Use tomato sauce (without sugar) instead of a creamy Alfredo on your pasta. Calories saved: 190.

➤ Use skim or low-fat soy milk in place of whole milk. Calories saved: 60.

➤ Pass on the midday candy bar snack and down a piece of fruit. Calories saved: 180. (If you're still hungry, eat raw nuts.)

➤ Toss that can of Coke and drink water. Calories saved: 150.

➤ Use one instead of two sugars in your coffee. Better yet, use none. Calories saved: 15 to 30.

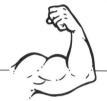

Flex Facts

Men with more than 25 percent body fat and women with more than 30 percent body fat are considered obese. Studies by the National Center of Health Statistics over the last two decades show that today approximately 35 percent of women and 31 percent of men age 20 and older are considered obese. That's an increase of approximately 30 percent and 25 percent, respectively, from 1980.

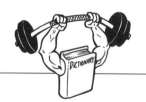

Bar Talk

Glycogen is the form in which a carbohydrate is stored in the body. Glycogen stores are later used by muscles as fuel to perform work. A total of 1,500 to 2,000 calories worth of glycogen is stored in the muscle, liver, and blood.

The Sad Truth About Fad Diets

As P. T. Barnum might have said, "A weight-loss sucker is born every minute." No matter how outrageous or absurd the alternative, many people refuse to apply common sense and sound science to their dietary needs (or their pocketbooks). Recently, we heard a radio spot for a product called "The Fat Assassin" that promised to melt off pounds quicker than you could spell John Wilkes Booth. While the image is clearly preposterous, enough people are apparently buying it to justify the number of ads on the air.

You can learn the hard way or take our word for it right now: Wacky diets like the "Grapefruit Diet" or the "Cabbage Diet" that exclude or severely restrict whole categories of food do more harm than good since they typically exclude important vitamins and minerals.

Take Barry Sears's *The Zone*, a low-carbohydrate diet that in the early 1990s gained more notoriety than Linda Tripp. A few years ago, one of the guys Jonathan trains with raved about how he'd lost seven pounds in just a week by following Sears's 40-30-30 diet (40 grams of carbohydrate, 30 grams of protein, and 30 grams of fat). Basically, the premise of The Zone diet is that eating too many carbs makes you fat.

The ever-curious, always-skeptical Jonathan brought out his magnifying glass and went to work and came away extremely unimpressed. True, this man had lost a whopping seven pounds in seven days; however, when you know that carbs, which are stored in the body as glycogen (energy fuel), hold three times their weight in water, you realize that this suddenly svelte Zone-ite had lost water and sugar, not fat. That's a good way to travel if you're like Deidre trying to make weight for a powerlifting competition, but useless if your aim is to drop fat. Once again, if something seems too good to be true, it probably is.

A Pound of Feathers or a Pound of Rocks

As we've recently noted, the scale doesn't know the difference between a pound of water and a pound of fat. The same can be said about the difference between muscle and fat. Plainly put, "A pound is a pound is a pound" on the scale. However, there is actually quite a huge difference between the way a pound of muscle and a pound of fat looks on the human body.

When clients tell Jonathan that they're frustrated that they haven't lost weight despite their best

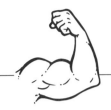

Flex Facts

Marathon runners typically "carbo load" on bread and pasta a day or two before their race in order to "top off" their glycogen stores. Jonathan is encouraged to find that the runners he coaches have gained a few pounds right before the race—a sign that their glycogen levels have increased.

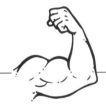

Flex Facts

Elite male marathoners generally carry about 4 to 6 percent body fat. Football linemen can range from 17 to 23%. When Deidre won her first World Powerlifting title she carried 14 percent body fat. This cycling season Jonathan is lugging 7 percent. Essential body fat, the amount necessary for normal physiologic function is approximately 3% in men and 12% in women. These levels may interfere with normal function, and are not necessary for optimal health. Males at 15–18% and females at 19–23% body fat are considered healthy.

efforts, he reminds them that they've dropped a dress size or a belt loop. The bottom line isn't what the scale says but your ratio of fat to lean mass.

Take, for example, two chaps who stand 5 feet 10 inches and tip the scales at 180 pounds. Mr. Stud Muffin has only 10 percent (or 18 pounds) of body fat, while Mr. Potato Latke is schlepping 25 percent of his weight as fat. That means Mr. Latke has more than twice the fat of his counterpart. The scale can't tell them apart, but a measurement of their body fat sure can.

While there are many ways to gauge your percentage of body fat—underwater weighing being the most accurate—most knowledgeable trainers with skin-fold calipers can give you a reasonable assessment. However, the best way to see where you stand is to step in front of a mirror in the buff and look for yourself.

The Least You Need to Know

➤ Sound nutrition starts with sound science.

➤ When it comes to building muscle, protein is the most misunderstood food group.

➤ Proper hydration is crucial, but sports drinks have their place in the diets of serious athletes.

➤ Eschew fad diets and practice the only real way to lose weight: moderation, variety, and balance.

➤ The scale doesn't lie, but it doesn't tell the whole story. Your percentage of body fat is just as important as how much you weigh.

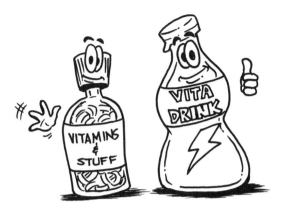

Chapter 8

To Supplement or Not?

In This Chapter

➤ Supplements may do more harm than good

➤ The truth about creatine, DHEA, chromium picolinate, and androstenedione

➤ Using coffee to boost energy and performance

➤ The good stuff about energy bars

No matter the field—computers, architecture, nutrition, you name it—we constantly strive to make improvements, partly because it's in our nature to do so and partly because we're out to make a profit from our innovations. Indeed, these "new and improved" versions are often more cosmetic than substantive because manufacturers are constantly trying to get the public to believe that they've perfected the egg when most of the time they've only come up with a new advertising slogan.

This is especially true when it comes to the wide-open field of nutritional supplements, but that's not to say that there aren't some valuable products on the market that can help you feel and look better. In this chapter, we'll help you decide what supplements will help you meet your fitness goals and which ones may not only fail to help but may actually harm you.

Buyer Beware

First of all, the most common deficiencies are carbohydrates and fluids—neither of which requires a trip to a health food store. Second, vitamin, protein, and mineral deficiency is rare in people with a balanced diet. You should also know that while a shortage of a nutrient can have a negative effect, taking an excess of one particular substance usually does more harm than good. For instance, a protein deficiency can

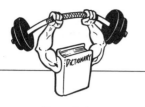

Bar Talk

Amino acids are the structural material or "building blocks" of protein. Of the 20 amino acids, nine are considered "essential." The body is unable to produce essential nutrients, which means that we need to consume them in our diets.

leave you feeling sluggish, but ingesting excess protein can actually cause weight gain and kidney problems.

Of the three of us, Jonathan, who has a master's degree in exercise physiology, is the most knowledgeable on the subject of nutrition. It's also worth noting that one of Jonathan's heroes is the "Amazing Randi," a magician who has made a career out of debunking charlatans like Uri Geller, the performer who claimed that he could bend silverware with his mind. Having a professional skeptic like Jonathan evaluate supplements is good news for you. For a doubting Thomas like him to give a supplement two thumbs up it has to be good.

Before we continue, let's review a few facts to help you understand where we're coming from:

In 1989, the Food and Drug Administration (FDA) defined a dietary supplement as a substance made of essential nutrients such as vitamins, minerals, and *amino acids*. The following year, an act of legislation came down the pike broadening the term *dietary supplements* to include herbs and similar nutritional substances. Then in 1994, another act from the Feds established yet another definition. Here are the rules that allow a company to identify and market a product as a dietary supplement today:

➤ The product must be labeled as a "dietary supplement."

➤ The product must contain one or more of the following ingredients: a vitamin, mineral, herb or other botanical, and amino acids. (There are other criteria, but they're too tedious to mention.)

➤ The product is intended for ingestion in pill, capsule, tablet, or liquid form. In other words, desiccated caterpillars from China fall outside the guidelines.

➤ The product must not be represented as a conventional food or as the sole item of a meal or diet. The Complete One-Pill Breakfast, Lunch, or Dinner ain't cuttin' it right now.

It's worth noting that these regulations require that the statements the manufacturer makes be "truthful and not misleading," but do not establish any standard for the often outrageous claims that supposedly back up such statements. In other words, a single study—even one financed by the manufacturer using shaky statistical methods—is enough even if that one study contradicts scores of other more impartial studies. And you wonder how Jonathan became so jaded.

When you're browsing the aisles in your local health food store, study the fine print on the product's label. If you see "This statement has not been evaluated by the FDA," you should think of the Amazing Randi (read: buyer beware). Claims made on food labels are more strictly regulated than on supplement labels and hence must answer to a higher authority.

Before we get into some of the most popular individual supplements on the market, consider these random facts on dietary supplements:

➤ Supplements include vitamins and minerals as well as herbals and botanicals.

➤ Multivitamins may help some people, but less is known about herbals and botanicals.

➤ High doses of certain supplements may be harmful.

➤ Don't assume "natural" means "safe." The two words are not synonymous. Tobacco is natural, and we know the often lethal long-term risks of using that product.

➤ If you want to ensure that you're getting all you need, eat a variety of foods.

Powder Power

In the previous chapter, we discussed how most people get more than enough protein in their diet. However, occasionally vegetarians or folks on low-calorie diets may be protein-deficient. Even if you fall into that category, there's no reason to run out and buy a tub of that Super Mega Muscle Man Protein Powder you may have seen advertised in a fitness magazine.

In grad school, Jonathan had occasion to examine such a powder. The label of this "miracle" mix of muscle-building power purported to have the ideal combination of amino acids, which are the building blocks of protein. According to the directions, the optimal way to use the powder was to mix it with a glass of skim milk. However, on closer inspection Jonathan and his classmates determined that at least one-third of the amino acids in this miraculous concoction came from the skim milk. Considering that the powder cost a few bucks per serving and the milk retailed for roughly 20¢, all you had to do was down three glasses of skim milk, and you'd have achieved the same effect. If you're totally sold on powders, try evaporated nonfat dry milk. Anti-dairy? Soy milk should fit the bill.

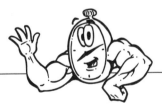

Weight a Minute

Don't believe everything you read. Many of the manufacturers of the supplements advertised in some of the most popular "muscle" and fitness magazines own the magazine they appear in. If that's the case, don't expect an unbiased opinion of a product.

The Creatine Craze

Talk to serious weight lifters, cyclists, swimmers, and a host of athletes from a cross-section of sports and the odds are they've tried creatine.

What is it? And why take it?

Creatine, a nitrogen-containing compound naturally found in our bodies, is made by the liver, kidneys, and pancreas. Creatine helps provide the energy your muscles need to move, particularly when they make movements that require short bursts of explosive energy such as that required in weight lifting.

When your muscles contract, the fuel that initiates this movement is a catchy-sounding compound called adenosine triphosphate (ATP). There is only enough ATP in your body to provide energy for roughly 10 seconds, meaning that for this energy system to continue functioning, the body must produce more ATP. We'll spare you the chemistry lesson, but trust us that creatine acts like an oxygen tank to a high-altitude mountaineer, assisting the body to produce more ATP, which in turn can be used as fuel for more muscle contraction. Since the ability to regenerate ATP depends on one's supply of creatine, it appears that upping creatine levels in your muscles allows for greater ATP resynthesis. If, in fact, all of the above is true, ATP resynthesis prevents your body from relying on your other energy systems, which are not as powerful when relied upon to produce explosive movements.

Does creatine work?

Probably yes, especially for vegetarians, since creatine is found in most meats and fish. However, no matter how much sushi or creatine you ingest, the mere fact that you take creatine won't make you stronger. It's only effective if you work harder in the gym. Since all three of us have tried this supplement, we have a bit of anecdotal information to share.

Deidre, a 122-pound woman who was able to bench press 188, squat 335, and dead-lift 380—all activities that require explosive bursts of energy—says she really couldn't tell if it helped her or not. (How's that for going out on a limb?)

Joe, the marathon kayaker in the group, tried it once and felt nothing. The next time he tried it, however, he said he felt stronger in the gym and was able to recover faster and train harder.

Jonathan, a cyclist who generally isn't in favor of supplements, has been using it during his 1999 cycling season and says he thinks it helps him when competing in short, explosive races, but feels nothing in longer races.

Is it safe? Good question. In the short term, it appears to produce no serious side effects, but it's hard to say over the long haul since there have yet to be any studies to measure its effects over time. Some folks who use it complain about gastrointestinal discomfort or muscle cramps, which is probably due to a lack of fluid intake. Proper hydration should alleviate the problem. In powder form, taking creatine is a bit like eating dishwashing detergent. It comes in pills as well, which are far easier to

84

swallow, but may not be absorbed as effectively. Weight gain often accompanies creatine use because you're likely to retain a little extra water in the muscle as well as experience muscle growth.

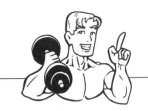

One last tip. Most manufacturers of creatine recommend a "loading" phase of 20 grams a day for the first week or more, followed by a more moderate "maintenance" dose of 2 to 5 grams a day. There has been very little proof that this loading phase actually increases your creatine stores rather than just causing the excess to be excreted by the liver and kidneys. We suggest that you experiment. Go right to the maintenance phase, and see if you feel a difference. If so we've saved you a few bucks (it's nearly $30 a bottle for 120 gel capsules or 500 grams of powder).

Spot Me

Creatine may be a valuable ergogenic aid for some lifters, but there's no need for a "loading phase." While many retailers suggest that you begin your creatine intake with a high dosage, research suggests that there's no need for such a high dose.

DHEA: Yea or Nay?

In 1997, every GNC, health food store, muscle magazine, and gym in the country seemed to be touting *DHEA*—dehydroepiandrosterone—as the muscle-building supplement of the decade. Before you run off to buy a case or two, know this: DHEA, once only available with a prescription, is a hormone produced naturally by the adrenal gland and is a precursor to increased testosterone levels. Since testosterone has legitimate muscle-building and fat-burning properties, advocates of DHEA claim that DHEA can do the same. The only problem is that the majority of the people who made these claims are DHEA salesmen.

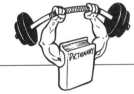

Here's the deal. DHEA levels peak at around 20 to 24 years of age. After age 30, the production of DHEA declines by about 20 percent each decade. Between the ages of 85 and 90, DHEA levels are about 95 percent lower than they were at their peak. So while there is reason to believe that DHEA supplementation may have a positive affect on individuals over the age of 40—and it certainly will aid athletes over the age of 90—there are few (if any) studies performed on humans to suggest that it really works.

Bar Talk

DHEA is a naturally occurring hormone, and a precursor to testosterone. The jury's still out as to whether DHEA has any ergogenic effect in healthy people, or if it's safe.

Given the potential downside of manipulating your hormones, we suggest you leave DHEA on the shelf, especially when you consider that an increase in DHEA in men is likely to increase the risk of an enlarged prostate, abnormal hair growth, and acne.

Burn, Baby, Burn

Another supposed wonder substance is chromium picolinate, a supplement that, according to its advocates, can do anything from help you lose weight to gain muscle mass to speed your metabolism. Scientific evidence, however, suggests otherwise.

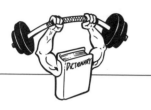

Chromium's role in the body is to help our tissues respond efficiently to insulin, which helps keep blood sugar levels in balance. However, although the natural substance plays an essential physiological role in the body, it's highly questionable whether its supplementation has any *ergogenic* effect on people with normal insulin or blood sugar levels. In other words, you can't live without the stuff, but it's unlikely that taking it in supplement form does much more than improve your ability to swallow pills.

Bar Talk

An **ergogenic** aid is any product that improves athletic or physical performance.

If It's Okay for Mark McGwire

In 1998, St. Louis Cardinals slugger Mark McGwire and Chicago Cubs outfielder Sammy Sosa waged a home run derby the likes of which had not been seen since the Yankees duo of Mickey Mantle and Roger Maris went ballistic in 1961. During the media frenzy surrounding the competition, a reporter supposedly spotted a container of androstenedione in McGwire's gym bag. Before you could say "going, going, gone," the sporting world learned about "andro," which touched off a national debate while at the same time sending sales of the stuff into the stratosphere.

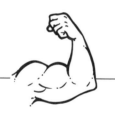

While the supplement isn't prohibited by Major League Baseball, it is on the banned list for Olympic athletes. Some people rushed to state that ingesting it explained why the 6-foot, 5-inch, 250-pound slugger was not only hitting more homers than anyone in baseball history, but also why they vanished into the distance like a golf ball driven by Tiger Woods. (That, of course, didn't explain why Sammy Sosa, a smaller player not on andro, was hitting them almost as often and as hard.)

Flex Facts

When Mark McGwire slugged a record-setting 70 home runs in 1998, many people were quick to point to his use of andro as a possible cause. Well, in 1999 he stopped using the stuff and still hit a mind-boggling 65 homers. McGwire's feats while on andro should not be taken as proof that it works.

Here's what we now know. Androstenedione is a steroid that occurs naturally in the body. Much like DHEA, it is another precursor of the hormone testosterone; taking it creates a small increase in testosterone levels. However, according to the Endocrine Society, an organization that does extensive research on hormones, there isn't any conclusive proof that andro improves athletic performance. On the other hand, there is ample evidence that taking andro leads to increased breast size in men and some studies suggest that taking andro could increase the risk of developing certain cancers and in reducing testicular size in men.

In the end, we just don't know if it works, and there are legitimate reasons to stay away from it, even if you'd like to challenge "Big Mac" for a home run title.

Starbucks Anyone?

In the "old" days, you could get a good cup of coffee in New York City for 50¢. Today, in the era of gourmet coffee shops, half a buck gets you into the men's room. Simply put, coffee has become big business. While you can drop $3.50 for a mocha latte cappuccino at a Starbucks, caffeine—a substance banned by the International Olympic Committee—is one of the cheapest and perhaps most beneficial ergogenic aids out there. (Just for the record: To get booted from the Olympics for abusing caffeine you'd have to top out way above the 100- to 300-milligram dose that is allowable and most beneficial. A cup of brewed coffee contains about 125 milligrams of caffeine.)

Caffeine works to help you in two ways. During aerobic activities it can increase the availability of fat as fuel. And while it won't make you stronger during weight lifting, there is some evidence out there that caffeine helps make the activity *seem* easier.

Before you start swilling shots of espresso, keep the following in mind.

➤ Caffeine can cause gastrointestinal problems.

➤ Drinking too much can make you jittery.

➤ Caffeine is a diuretic. Drink extra water if you're going to work up a sweat.

➤ There are possible links between caffeine consumption and benign fibrocystic breast disease.

➤ If you have an ulcer or irregular heartbeat, your best bet is to stick to decaf.

In the final analysis, each person has a different tolerance for this age-old pick-me-up. Joe, who is a minor coffee fiend, never drinks the stuff before a race, since he feels it dehydrates him and messes with his heart rate. However, he has a friend who is one of the top racers in the country who often has someone hand him a piping hot cup of coffee midway through the race to give him an added jolt. Experiment to see what works for you.

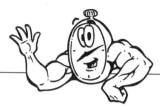

Weight a Minute

HMB (hydroxymethylbutyrate), pyruvate, inosine, branch-chained amino acids, ma huang, bee pollen, ginseng, and guarana are eight rather popular supplements you've probably heard about. None of them impress us for a variety of reasons, mainly because we're concerned about whether they're safe and effective.

The Bar Scene

Flip through any bicycle or runner's apparel catalogue and you're bound to see a host of ads for energy bars, such as PowerBar, Clif Bar, Met-Rx Bar, Balance Bar, PR Ironman Bar, and the list goes on. Each makes bold claims about what it can do for you, from optimizing the body's natural ability to burn stored fat for energy to providing you with a burst of energy. Not only are they supposed to start your engine and keep it running at optimal efficiency, they're designed to taste good. (Unlike their ancestors, which tasted a tad better than the rubber flooring in your gym.) Check out some of these flavors: white chocolate mocha, berry blast, cookie dough, and Kona crunch. Sounds like a get-together at a Ben & Jerry's convention.

These smartly marketed products are good under a variety of conditions, including when you're doing a long training ride, are too hungry to work out but too busy to eat, and as a late-night snack when a piece of fruit just doesn't have enough oomph. Most of these bars are easily digested and pack a fair number of nutrients in a convenient package. When Jonathan wakes up at the obscene hour of 5 A.M. for a bike race, he's usually too comatose to prepare breakfast and simply downs a PowerBar as a prerace meal.

Here are a few energy bar tidbits:

➤ Most bars are fairly high in carbohydrates, which are more readily digested than calories from protein or fat.

➤ Some, however, are extremely high in protein and may not be easy to digest. As we've already said, extra protein often does more harm than good.

➤ Beware of bars that make outrageous claims. These bars are a good source of food to help stabilize blood sugar levels and fight hunger pangs, but they're not going to make you burn fat faster. And they're not going to make you stronger or faster. Six-time Ironman winner Mark Allen didn't run down his competition because he ate PR Bars. (In fact, given his talent and training regimen, he could have eaten a bar of soap and still dominated.)

From A to Zinc

One of the most interesting facts about vitamin and mineral supplementation is that more often than not, if you believe taking them is good for you, it is. In other words, the power of the mind to invest positive qualities in things we believe are good for us is not to be denied. (Studies on the placebo effect are nothing short of remarkable: Patients with inoperative cancer who were given a "miracle" cure [sugar pills] actually saw their cancer temporarily go into recess.)

That said, both competitive and recreational athletes tend to overdose on vitamins and minerals considering that most people who eat a balanced diet get more than enough from the foods they eat. However, the most common vitamins missing in our diets are B_6, B_{12} (typically found in animal products), E (found in vegetable oils), and folic acid (leafy green vegetables and organ meats are good sources). In addition, many women don't get enough calcium and iron in their diet.

While megadosing on vitamins is probably a waste of time and money—and in the case of fat-soluble vitamins and minerals, detrimental—taking a multivitamin can serve as a safe, inexpensive insurance policy against deficiencies caused by poor diet.

The Least You Need to Know

➤ Nutritional supplements are big business. Read the labels and beware of outrageous claims.

➤ Creatine, the most popular supplement on the market today, may give you the boost you're looking for.

➤ DHEA, chromium picolinate, and androstenedione claim to make you stronger and lose weight. We beg to differ.

➤ In moderation, caffeine can make it easier for your body to use fat as fuel.

➤ Energy bars are a good quick snack. They even taste good, but they're not going to make you bigger, stronger, or faster.

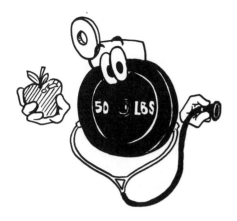

Chapter 9

Getting a Clean Bill of Health

In This Chapter

➤ The importance of a medical checkup

➤ Medical precautions and prescriptions

➤ Handling injuries

➤ The medical benefits of weight training

Here's an amusing paradox: When you're sick or injured, it's nearly impossible to think or talk about anything other than your health or lack of it. When Joe broke his wrist before his kayaking season a while back, he had to put a muzzle on himself not to mention it to perfect strangers. "Excuse me sir, I've broken one of my carpal bones. Care to hear this gripping tale?" Conversely, there's almost nothing more tedious on earth than listening to someone tell you about his health problems. Unless, of course, you have the same condition. In fact, put three guys with broken wrists in a room together, provide refreshments, and they'll entertain themselves till the bones heal.

We note this phenomenon because this chapter, which talks about the importance of consulting with your physician before taking to the gym, focuses on what you need to be aware of, medically speaking, when you embark on a new exercise regimen. Given its clinical nature, this chapter may seem a bit on the dry side. On the other hand, we offer you some important information about how to keep yourself healthy and strong while working out to get even healthier and stronger. If it's been a while since you've had a checkup or exercised on a regular basis, or if you've had (or have) a serious medical condition, you need to take special care. But there's good news: Very few people need to be excluded from working out—although modifications may be necessary. Read on for more info.

The Medical Checkup

The prudent path to follow when you're starting a weight-lifting regimen is to see your doctor for a thorough checkup. Again, this is especially important if you've been inactive for a while, have a bad back, are overweight, or are over 45. To some, getting a checkup is an odious task. Assuming your doctor is a decent sort, it shouldn't be. In health and fitness (as in virtually anything else), knowledge is power. Think of getting a physical not as a burden but as an opportunity to become more powerful. Okay, let's say you haven't been sick in 10 years, you're 29 years old, and the idea of visiting a doctor is as appealing as having a root canal. The generally accepted minimal standard to gauge if you're ready to work out is a seven-question self-evaluation called the Physical Activity Readiness Questionnaire (PAR-Q). Designed for people between the ages of 15 and 69, it was developed by the Canadian Society for Exercise Physiology to see if you've got the mettle to push some metal. The PAR-Q is shown on the following pages.

If you answered "yes" to any of these questions, or if you're older than 69, then head straight to your doctor's office, and tell the doctor you responded in the affirmative to one of the questions on the Physical Activity Readiness Questionnaire. Then let him or her give you a good once-over.

On the other hand, if you honestly answered "no" to these probing questions, then PAR-Q says it's okay to go ahead and have at it—but only if you do so gradually and follow all the safety precautions we'll outline for you throughout the book. (Just to put our prudent approach in perspective: Even if you're in tremendous physical condition, it's unwise to start a new regimen like a lifter possessed. Starting out too fast is a sure way to get injured, even if you're fit.)

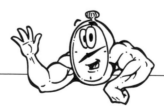

Weight a Minute

If you answered "no" across the board to the PAR-Q on the following pages, it doesn't mean you can't or shouldn't see a doctor. If you have any doubts about that trick knee or the health of your heart, give the doc a call.

PAR-Q & YOU

(A Questionnaire for People Aged 15 to 69)

Regular physical activity is fun and healthy, and more people are starting to become increasingly active every day. Being more active is very safe for most people. However, some people should check with their doctor before they start becoming physically active.

If you are planning to become much more physically active than you are now, start by answering the seven questions in the box below. If you are between the ages of 15 and 69, the PAR-Q will tell you if you should check with your doctor before you start. If you are over 69 years of age, and you are not used to being very active, check with your doctor.

Common sense is your best guide when you answer these questions. Please read the questions carefully and answer each one honestly: check YES or NO.

Yes	No	
❑	❑	1. Has your doctor ever said that you have a heart condition and that you should only do physical activity recommended by a doctor?
❑	❑	2. Do you feel pain in your chest when you do physical activity?
❑	❑	3. In the past month, have you had chest pain when you were not doing physical activity?
❑	❑	4. Do you lose your balance because of dizziness, or do you ever lose consciousness?
❑	❑	5. Do you have a bone or joint problem that could be made worse by a change in your physical activity?
❑	❑	6. Is your doctor currently prescribing drugs (for example, water pills) for your blood pressure or heart condition?
❑	❑	7. Do you know of any other reason why you should not do physical activity?

If you answered

YES to one or more questions

Talk with your doctor by phone or in person BEFORE you start to become much more physically active or before you have a fitness appraisal. Tell your doctor about the PAR-Q and which questions you answered YES.

➤ You may be able to do any activity you want—as long as you start slowly and build up gradually. Or, you may need to restrict your activities to those which are safe for you. Talk with your doctor about the kinds of activities you wish to participate in and follow his/her advice.

➤ Find out which community programs are safe and helpful for you.

continues

continued

NO to all questions

If you answered NO to <u>all</u> PAR-Q questions, you can be reasonably sure that you can: ➤ Start becoming much more physically active—begin slowly and build up gradually. This is the safest and easiest way to go. ➤ Take part in a fitness appraisal—this is an excellent way to determine your basic fitness so that you can plan the best way for you to live actively.	**<u>DELAY</u> BECOMING MUCH MORE ACTIVE:** ➤ If you are not feeling well because of a temporary illness such as a cold or a fever—wait until you feel better; or ➤ If you are or may be pregnant—talk to your doctor before you start becoming more active. **Please note: If your health changes so that you then answer YES to any of the above questions, tell your fitness or health professional. Ask whether you should change your physical activity plan.**

Informed use of the PAR-Q: The Canadian Society for Exercise Physiology, Health Canada, and their agents assume no liability for persons who undertake physical activity, and if in doubt after completing this questionnaire, consult your doctor prior to physical activity.

NOTE: If the PAR-Q is being given to a person before he or she participates in a physical activity program or a fitness appraisal, this section may be used for legal or administrative purposes.

I have read, understood and completed this questionnaire. Any questions I had were answered to my full satisfaction.

Name:_____

Email Address:_____

Date:_____

Most people over the age of 50 or so are concerned about heart disease, and for good reason. Heart attacks and strokes remain the single biggest killer in the United States. Because exercising puts extra strain on your heart and blood vessels, you need to be especially careful to make sure your cardiovascular system is in good working order. Here are the risk factors for coronary artery disease set forth by the American College of Sports Medicine. See where you stack up under any of the following categories:

➤ **Age.** Men over the age of 45; women over 55, or who have premature menopause without estrogen replacement therapy.

➤ **A family history of heart attacks or strokes.** Or sudden death of your father (or another close male relative) before the age of 55. Ditto for your mother (or close female relative) before the age of 65. Genes are powerful, so don't stick your head in the sand if your family's history is sketchy. Go get checked out.

➤ **Cigarette smoking.** Anyone who can read knows smoking contributes to lung cancer, heart disease, and a host of other physical problems. We'll spare you the lecture, but if you smoke and want to work out, see your doctor before you launch a fitness regimen. Of course, it's better to work out and smoke than to just smoke, but our guess is that the more you get into the gym, the less you'll suck the cigarettes.

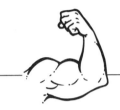

Flex Facts

A "normal" healthy blood pressure is around 120/80. Hypertension, or high blood pressure, is defined as any reading of 140/90 or more. By definition, blood pressure is the pressure exerted on the wall of a blood vessel. The first number, or systolic pressure, occurs as the heart contracts, while the second, diastolic pressure, occurs when the heart relaxes between beats.

➤ **Hypertension.** While exercise is one of the best antidotes for this condition, often curing the condition without the need for medication, you'll need to make sure that you're not stressing an already stressed-out circulatory system. See the doc if you've got any doubts.

➤ **High Cholesterol.** There are volumes written about good and bad cholesterol—what's high, what's low, what's dangerous, and what's not. While your doctor can tell you what's best for you, a good rule of thumb is: If your total cholesterol is over 200 mg/dl or if your HDL or "good cholesterol" is below 35 mg/dl, you are considered at risk. (For the record, mg/dl means milligrams per deciliter.) Again, exercise will have a beneficial effect in increasing your HDL but make sure you're not an egg yolk away from doing yourself serious harm.

➤ **Diabetes mellitus.** The connection between diabetes and heart disease is well known, so if you've been insulin-dependent for more than 15 years, or are over the age of 30 with diabetes, you're considered at risk. The same is true of those noninsulin-dependent diabetics over 35.

➤ **Physical inactivity.** If your job keeps you pasted to your seat most of the day, or if the most arduous thing you've done in a year or more is play badminton at the company picnic, you're considered at risk if you engage in strenuous physical activity.

These risk factors don't mean that you shouldn't or can't work out, but you should exercise a little extra caution before you get started. And the first step you should take should be to the doctor's office.

The Doctor Will See You Now

Weight training can help treat a variety of ailments, especially if combined with a good stretching program and sound nutrition. While we're not going to be so bold as to say that weight training can cure serious maladies like beriberi or foot-and-mouth disease, it often does wonders for an ailing body. Having said that, there are a number of conditions that weight lifting will exacerbate if you lift without medical supervision.

We don't mean to dampen your enthusiasm or frighten you off of the exercise train; in fact, that's the last thing we want to do—well, the second to the last. We're most eager to help you avoid injuries or aggravate a preexisting condition. It may seem obvious, but we'll mention it anyway: When you're having a checkup, make sure to mention any current problems you're experiencing. In other words, don't try to turn the doctor into a mind reader. Once you've had your physical and learned how to safely proceed, find out if the gym you belong to (or are thinking about joining) has trainers who know how to work around your particular condition. (See Chapter 8, "To Supplement or Not?" for more about personal trainers.) Working with a trainer who isn't adept at working with stroke victims or heart patients—if that's your problem—is a big mistake.

Avoiding Risky Business

Okay, so you have high blood pressure or some other medical condition that provides a convenient excuse not to work out. Know this: nine-tenths of the physical restrictions people live with are self-imposed. Recently a man with AIDS ran, cycled, and swam across the United States to prove to himself (and others) that people with this life-threatening disease can do far more than anyone realized. Just to drive home the point further: A man paralyzed from the waist down climbed Yosemite's El Capitan, one of the grandest rock faces in the world. At Joe and Deidre's gym, there's a woman with an artificial right arm who lifts weights.

Let's look at some of the more common afflictions people have to deal with as they pertain to working out.

The Hyper Types

Hypertension, or high blood pressure, is a condition that affects millions Americans by placing chronic, increased stress on the normal function of the cardiovascular system. Often called the silent killer, hypertension is particularly insidious because it often goes undetected until you see the doctor or even have a heart attack or stroke.

Deidre has a photo taken of her deadlifting 365 pounds during a power-lifting competition. What's striking about it, besides the fact that she's lifting the equivalent of a baby elephant, is the terrific strain that shows on her face: Her eyes bulge like Marty Feldman's, and the veins in her neck are engorged like bloated worms. (We call this the Beauty and the Beast syndrome.) While few of us are likely to try to hoist that amount of weight, the fact remains that weight lifting can increase your blood pressure during the actual exercise.

A common mistake is holding your breath during a repetition. We'll talk more about this once we get you into the gym. However, it's worth mentioning now that holding your breath is ill advised—with high blood pressure or without. While competitive lifters like Deidre often hold their breath when they're shooting for a personal record (PR), doing so may cause you bodily harm.

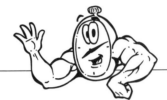

Weight a Minute

Holding your breath while lifting causes an exaggerated and sometimes dangerously high increase in blood pressure. The technical term for holding your breath during a lift is a *Valsalva maneuver.*

Post-Stroke Fitness

For some stroke victims, embarking on a weight-lifting program can be an essential part of their recovery. For others, doing so can be downright dangerous. If you have had a stroke, you need to discuss weight training with your doctor to see which category of patient you fall under.

Typically, if one side of your body is impaired or severely restricted, a knowledgeable physical therapist or trainer will have you work a lot on your unaffected side, since this part of your body will now be working much harder to compensate.

Deidre, who has worked for years as a physical therapist, has done a lot of work with stroke victims, and is continually amazed by the progress people are able to make. One of her most remarkable patients is a woman in her 80s who had a stroke 12 years ago. She was unable to use her right arm and was able to walk with the use of a brace on her right leg and a cane. She walked everyday outside, alone, and was able to cook and clean for herself.

Post–Heart Attack Workout

For some, a heart attack spells the beginning of the end. Victims sense their own mortality and just "try and take it easy," which does little except make them sluggish and more prone to poor health. To others, surviving heart disease is like a second lease on life and a chance to nurture health instead of abuse it or take it for granted.

If you've had a heart attack, or are at high risk for one, your doctor may well suggest that you join a cardiac rehabilitation program—which has strict guidelines for cardiovascular as well as strength-training exercise—or simply encourage you to start exercising slowly. In the latter case, it's wise to work with a trainer or physical therapist who specializes in cardiac rehab. Combining aerobic activity, which can strengthen your heart (which is, after all, a muscle) and a sound diet will no doubt change your life.

Breathing Right

Asthma is a nasty affliction with symptoms that include wheezing, chest congestion, chest tightness, coughing, or shortness of breath. Exercising in cold, dry air is usually the most troublesome for asthmatics, while activities like swimming are often tolerated much better. Usually, a thorough warm-up before exercise can help prevent symptoms, and many athletes with asthma have risen to the top of their game. Just look at former marathon world-record holder Alberto Salazar or Olympic gold medalist Jackie Joyner-Kersee, both diagnosed with asthma. Jonathan also has asthma, but nevertheless may be the best athlete in his apartment building. (Actually, Jonathan, who was severely afflicted with asthma as a child, has benefited greatly from exercise, and though he never rides without his inhaler, his condition no longer prevents him from competing.)

Today, with the advances in medications that can help prevent or alleviate symptoms with few side effects, asthmatics have every reason to exercise if they choose. Your doctor can prescribe an inhaler, which you should keep with you whenever exercising in case symptoms arise.

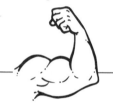

Flex Facts

During the 1992 Summer Olympics, many television viewers were shocked to find out that track and field champion Jackie Joyner-Kersee suffered from asthma. Joyner-Kersee is perhaps the greatest woman athlete ever, and her performance proved that asthma does not prevent exercise, even given the demands of top-level competition.

The Sugar Blues

Diabetes is a disease in which an insufficient amount of insulin (a hormone necessary for the metabolism of blood glucose or blood sugar) is produced by the body. This leads to an abnormally high blood glucose level. When the body functions normally, it releases insulin to counteract the increased sugar as blood glucose levels rise after eating. In diabetics, the body does not release enough insulin (as in the case of Type I, juvenile onset diabetes), or the body is insulin resistant, in which case insulin doesn't do what it's supposed to (as in the more common, type II, adult onset diabetes.)

Like those with asthma, people with diabetes, like New York Knicks center Chris Dudley, are able to work out and function at a high level as long as they are careful to maintain a proper blood sugar level. (The 6-foot, 11-inch Dudley administers four insulin injections to himself each day.) If the blood sugar level dips, extreme hunger pangs and dizziness result. If it's bad enough, blackouts and/or diabetic shock follow.

Since some exercise can have an "insulin-like" effect, there are times when insulin dosages need to be altered after you begin an exercise program. Furthermore, where you inject the insulin may have to be changed since injecting into a working muscle may increase the rate that the insulin is absorbed.

Adult onset diabetes, can be cured or drastically improved by changes in your diet. If you do regulate your diabetes this way, make sure you eat before working out. Talk to your doctor or a nutritionist about the best time to structure your workouts so that they coincide with your normal blood sugar levels.

Building Bones

Years ago it was considered "unladylike" for women to lift weights. Now medical science has come around to tell us that taking to the gym is an effective way for postmenopausal women to combat osteoporosis, a disease that causes the loss of bone density. Proper diet that includes plenty of calcium and magnesium and a gradual weight training program can work wonders to prevent the disease from developing. Once osteoporosis has set in, however, it's important for you to get clearance from your doctor to determine if it's safe to lift weights.

Bum Knees

There seems to be an endless number of things that can cause your knees to ache—from running to poor posture to ballroom dancing. Sometimes postural awareness can cure your knees, sometimes a stretching program will alleviate your pain. If you pursue those remedies and your knees still ache, have your doctor check them out. Once you get

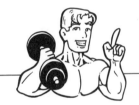

Spot Me

Many people joke that the fragility of the human knee, the largest joint in the body, is ample evidence that God doesn't exist. Aside from being the largest joint in the body, it is surrounded by major muscle groups, (ligaments that promote stability, tendons, and last but certainly not least, cartilage within the knee joint which acts as a cushion and provides the knee with much needed lubrication. A solid strength-training program for your legs, along with regular stretching can help avoid or alleviate knee pain.

the go-ahead, go easy. Very often, strengthening the muscles in your quadriceps and hamstrings will ease your pain.

Oy, My Back

Back pain is one of the most complicated issues in the medical profession. There are literally hundreds of bones, muscles, ligaments, and nerves in the back—any of which can go on the fritz depending on what you're doing and the amount of stress you're under. Consult a doctor if you're experiencing serious trouble. Some people have good results with chiropractors, others respond to massage and/or yoga. A book that has helped thousands of back-pain sufferers is *Healing Back Pain* by Dr. John Sarno.

The basis of Sarno's premise is that anxiety and repressed anger trigger muscle spasm. While the pain is real and often debilitating, the onset is mental. Some people consider Sarno full of helium, others swear by him. Our advice is, if you suffer from chronic back pain that your doctor can't seem to "fix," hobble down to your bookstore and read what he has to say.

Atlas Shrugged

The shoulder is an amazing joint. Maybe the credit belongs to our simian ancestors, who swung through the trees with the greatest of ease, but the range of motion that the shoulder provides the arm is just short of miraculous. Think of a swimmer doing windmills to warm up for a race, or the last time you threw a Hail Mary pass in a touch football game.

But it's because the shoulder is so mobile and flexible that it's also so prone to injury. Shoulder injuries are one of the most common maladies caused by weight lifting—generally from lifting too much weight with too little form. Weight lifting can also aggravate an existing minor injury.

The two "itises"—*tendonitis* and *bursitis*—as well as *rotator cuff* tears, are all common injuries that are brought on by repetitive activity, such as racket sports and swimming. They all result in the same symptom: shoulder pain. It's normal for your shoulders to feel sore after serious exertion, like helping your cousin

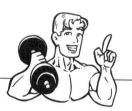

Spot Me

Along with improving the flexibility of your back muscles, strengthening your abdominal muscles can often help alleviate back pain. Stay tuned for Chapter 19, "Armed but Not Dangerous," where we'll cover abdominal exercises.

Ruth move to a fourth-floor walk-up or playing a game of ultimate Frisbee. But if it's been business as usual and you experience shoulder pain at rest or on movement, see your doctor.

One last bit of advice on a question that comes up far too often about the merits of working out when you're feeling under the weather. Ready for this political answer? Sometimes it can help, and sometimes it can hurt. Generally speaking, if all you have is a cold, and all your symptoms are above your neck (sniffles, tickly throat, etc.) a moderate workout can help clear your head. If your symptoms have spread to your chest or include fever or body aches, working out is likely to worsen the condition, so we suggest you rest, recover, and have at it when you're feeling better.

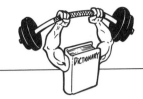

Bar Talk

Anything that ends in "itis" means inflammation. Therefore, **tendinitis** is an inflammation of the tendons (the connective tissue that connects bone to muscle), and **bursitis** is an inflammation of the bursa (which are padlike sacs found between tendons and bones that act to reduce friction).

The Least You Need to Know

➤ If you've been sick or injured, or haven't exercised in years, get a physical before embarking on a new exercise regimen.

➤ Haven't been sick in years? Take the PAR-Q before you hit the gym.

➤ Once you've received medical clearance, ailments like diabetes and asthma shouldn't hold you back.

➤ Fortify your brittle bones, tricky knee, and bad back with a well-designed strength-training regimen.

Part 3

Ready to Roll

Now the fun starts. In Chapter 10, we'll take you on a guided tour of the gym—from soup to nuts, or rather machines to shower stalls. To the uninitiated, gyms can be confusing institutions of higher fitness; we'll familiarize you with the basics you'll need to know before you get started.

In Chapter 11, we'll discuss safety issues to make sure you leave the gym in one piece. This is the chapter that you should not miss and one that beginners often take a long time to learn. We'll also fill you in on gym etiquette to make sure you don't make any enemies early in your workout career.

Finally, in Chapter 12 we stress the importance of getting and staying flexible— perhaps the most neglected aspect of most people's fitness regimens. We hope we'll convince you that stretching isn't a waste of time but an invaluable part of becoming fit. And then we'll give you a thorough routine to help keep you limber and injury-free.

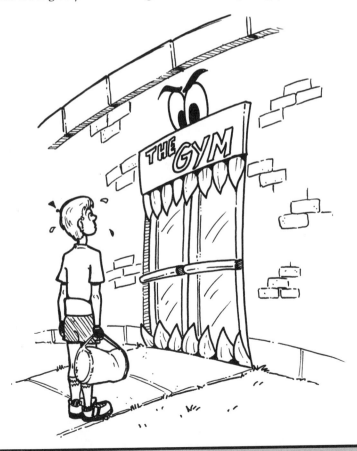

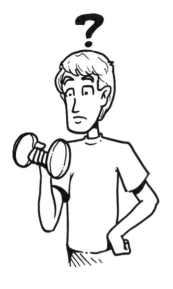

Chapter 10

Virgin Territory

In This Chapter

➤ Finding your way around the gym

➤ Do you need a trainer?

➤ Don't be dazzled by those high-tech machines

➤ Freeweights: What goes up

With few exceptions, the first time you do anything—go to school, kiss that special someone, jump out of an airplane—you're liable to feel anything from uncertainty to downright terror. (Kissing a blind date while skydiving really can cause sweaty palms!) For many people, stepping into a gym for the first time can be an intimidating experience. There's music blaring, sweating bodies basking in their own reflected glory, and the drone of machines working in the background. In fact, one of the reasons people say they delay starting an exercise program isn't because they lack the motivation, but because they're nervous about being in such a foreign setting.

Relax! Gyms represent an athletic cross-section of the world you've just stepped in from. It is populated by people like you and me, so once you spend a little time inside the mirrored walls, our bet is you'll look back and laugh at those first anxious moments. And we'll help you along the way in this chapter.

Heading into the Gym

When Deidre first stepped into a gym, she remembers feeling a whole lot of apprehension. As a kid she was so timid, so painfully shy, that she avoided most challenges she longed to try: gymnastics, track, singing, and piano lessons. ("Had I nurtured the interests I had as a kid," she says, "I probably would've been as addicted to playing the piano as I am to lifting.")

In 1985, she impulsively walked in off the street to check out a gym. At the time, she didn't know the difference between a leg press and a printing press. However, one day after a long-term relationship ended and she was feeling low, she saw some women working out through the window of a second-floor Manhattan gym, and thought, "What the heck!" It was the first time she'd ever been inside such a sweaty place. Luckily for a tenderfoot like Deidre, she stumbled into a small gym specifically geared for women, staffed with competitive bodybuilders who were supportive, knowledgeable, and amusing. Less than 10 years after that uneasy start, she won the New York State Powerlifting Championship, setting a state record (314 pounds) in the squat.

What Deidre didn't know then (but knows now) is that gyms are no longer the province of muscleheads or die-hard jocks. The best way to approach whatever gym you decide to join is to sign up as if you belong—because you do.

Those First Anxious Steps

Just about any gym worth its soap dispenser will offer a complimentary orientation to new members. Members like it because it's a good way to familiarize themselves with this labyrinth of machines and freeweights. Gym management likes it because it allows them an opportunity to encourage you to hire a personal trainer for training sessions.

While it's a no-brainer to take advantage of the free tour, the question as to whether you should sign on for training sessions requires a more complex answer. If you read this book, you'll be knowledgeable enough to work out well. However, if you're the type of person who likes the personal touch of another human urging you on, or if you have some doubts about whether you'll stick to it, then by all means hire away. (Doling out cold, hard cash is usually incentive enough not to miss your scheduled appointment.)

On the other hand, another effective strategy is to work out for a few weeks after you join, put into practice what you've learned from these pages, and then hire a trainer to check on your progress as well as answer any questions you may have.

As we mentioned in Chapter 1, "Let's Get Physical," before you hire a trainer, make sure you're comfortable with the trainer you choose. Check out his or her credentials. Explicitly tell her your goals and feel reasonably confident that she's on the same page as you are. We know a trainer—he's a former bodybuilder and powerlifter with a winsome smile and smooth rap—who trains everyone (and we mean everyone) as though he or she were an aspiring powerlifter and/or bodybuilder. This is like a mechanic taking your station wagon and putting mag wheels on it. Client: "I'd like to tone up and lose a few pounds." Trainer: "Good, we should be able to double the size of your quads in two months." Allow a trainer to guide you, but don't let him impose his goals on you.

In addition, if you have any specific medical concerns, find out if the trainer has experience working with someone with a similar condition. Most of all, try to find out if you like the person you trust your body to. Credentials alone don't make a good trainer; this is, after all, a human science. Interpersonal skills are of the utmost importance.

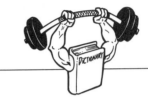

It might sound odd, but if you notice that the trainer can't keep his eyes off of his reflection in the mirror when he talks to you, you might want to consider someone else. We know one qualified trainer, an amateur bodybuilder with the body of a gladiator, who is so enamored with his own image that he often practices his bodybuilding *poses* even while his clients are lifting. While he's doing his job, it has to be disconcerting to feel as if you're in the way of his viewing pleasure—sort of like listening to someone who always refers to himself in the third person.

Bar Talk

Posing is a facet of bodybuilding where the competitor demonstrates his or her physical assets by assuming various positions that show off his or her muscularity and proportion.

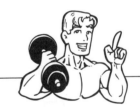

There's another way to take advantage of a trainer that gym personnel don't often tell you about. When Jonathan worked as a personal trainer, he had several clients with whom he met just once or twice a month. Generally speaking, those who chose this intermittent schedule were self-motivated types who didn't need a trainer to keep them on track day-to-day. In addition, economic necessity sometimes ruled the day—paying a trainer anywhere from $25 to $100 an hour two or three times a week can get expensive. Others didn't have the time to show up at a prearranged time week after week. Nevertheless, Jonathan was able to offer constructive advice once or twice a month that improved their progress and ensured that they hadn't developed any poor habits.

Spot Me

If you feel intimidated (psychologically or physically) by your trainer, report it to management and find another trainer. You're paying them for a service, and you should never feel ill at ease.

In This Room

We know a gym in Brooklyn that's adequately equipped, but extremely nontrendy. New members are given a cursory tour by either an overweight woman who smokes, a Spanish-speaking guy who maintains the equipment, or a hulking powerlifter who can bench press a barnyard animal but is unintelligible in any language. In other words, they show you the lay of the land, and you have to hire a trainer to figure out the nuances of how to use what and when. The point is, not all gyms will make your orientation as seamless as a guided tour of the Louvre. Don't worry too much about this bare-bones approach. After reading this book, you'll know your way around just about any gym even if you're blindfolded.

If your orientation tour is tip-top, a qualified trainer will show you the place from soup to nuts—machines, stretching room, locker room, steam room, sauna, whirlpool, juice bar, you name it. In addition, he or she should show you (or at least schedule an appointment to do so) how the equipment works, what muscles each works, and how to adjust it to fit your body. While this whirlwind of information can seem over-whelming, don't worry. It's that way for just about everyone without a degree in Exercise Physiology. Besides, no one expects you to remember everything you're shown at first glance. Just try to absorb the basics. We'll help you with the rest.

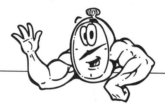

Weight a Minute

If you use the steam room, sauna, or whirlpool after a workout, remember to "cool down" to bring your heart rate and blood pressure back toward resting levels before entering. If you don't, you run the risk of passing out. In addition, it's not recommended that pregnant women or people with heart conditions use them.

Right now, we're going to introduce you to some of the equipment available to you, namely the "machines" and the "freeweights." Each of these techniques has its bene-fits and drawbacks and, as you'll see, most weight lifters use a combination of the two. Let's get started.

Machine Power

High-tech machines are the meat and potatoes of any modern gym. Freeweights are as timeless as the pyramids, but in the last decade strength training machines have evolved significantly. Depending on the gym you join, you're liable to be confronted by a variety of contraptions: BodyMaster, Cybex, Icarian, Hammer Strength, Nautilus, and a variety of others with equally important names. Which is best, and what should you use when? Here's a sound question you may be pondering: "If three different machines all work the chest, why does the gym offer three different machines?" Actually, we have no idea. (Just kidding.) While most of the machines use stacks of weights to provide resistance, brands like Keiser use hydraulic resistance. LifeFitness has machines that use magnetic braking for resistance and are harder in one direction than in the other. Others like Nautilus vary the resistance throughout the range of motion while still other machines have constant resistance.

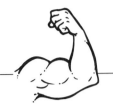

Flex Facts

Arthur Jones built the first Nautilus prototype more than 50 years ago, and the first unit was sold in 1970. Jones is a very opinionated and controversial figure within the fitness industry, but there is no argument that before Nautilus, it was freeweights or nothing. Without the advent of Nautilus machines, gyms today would be very different places.

Sound question number two: "Which is best?" Deidre and Joe have had the "privilege" of listening to Jonathan's unabridged lecture on the theoretical pros and cons of different types of equipment. If at the end of three scintillating hours you're still conscious, he'll excitedly conclude that there's really not much difference at all. Huh?

The bottom line is that your muscles don't really have a discerning intelligence. In other words, a biceps doesn't know whether air pressure, a weight stack, a metal plate, or a side of beef is strapped to your wrist. It knows that there's a task to accomplish and recruits as many muscle fibers as necessary to get the job done. As long as the machine you sidled up to offers enough resistance and can be adjusted to fit your body, you'll be adequately challenged. (By appropriate resistance we mean that the heaviest weight isn't too light and the lightest weight isn't too heavy.)

With most machines, a weight stack provides the resistance. The amount of weight is adjusted by inserting a pin in the stack. In some cases, smaller "fractional" plates can be piled on top of the stack to allow you to make more gradual increases.

Here are some of the pluses of using machines:

➤ Safety. If you're on your sixth *rep* (or repetition) in your second *set* and unable to complete a seventh, you simply lower the weight to its starting position. There's no need for a spotter and no risk of dropping the weight on your head.

➤ Ability to work harder. Unlike freeweights which require you to stabilize as you move, a machine allows you to concentrate solely on pushing or pulling the weight without fear of hurting yourself. This should allow you to squeeze out a few extra reps.

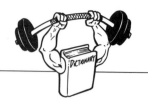

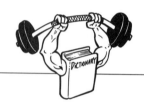

➤ Ability to increase the weights in smaller increments. Typically, the lightest plate you can use in freeweights is a $2\frac{1}{2}$ pounder, which means a five-pound increase on the bar whenever you want to add any weight. Some of the newer machines, on the other hand, can be adjusted in one-pound increments.

➤ Variable resistance. Certain machines decrease the resistance during the phase of the exercise when your muscles are the weakest. This helps eliminate the *sticking point* and allows you to become stronger through the entire movement.

➤ Fewer opportunities to cheat. With their padded features and adjustable parts, machines are built to isolate the muscle you're working. This reduces your tendency to move other body parts to "cheat" or assist you as you increase the weight, which translates plainly and simply into bad form.

Here are a few of the disadvantages of machines:

➤ While machines are easily adjusted to accommodate just about everyone, really small and/or large people may find it a poor fit.

➤ Unlike freeweights, which reinforce bilateral symmetry, some machines allow you to favor your dominant (or stronger) side. This perpetuates any disparity between your dominant and weaker sides.

➤ Machines restrict you to a specific movement and therefore don't allow you to vary the exercise.

Ultimately, you can get stronger using machines, freeweights, or a combination of the two. There's no reason to restrict yourself to one or the other, but we suggest leaning toward machines as you begin.

Lift Free or Die

As we mentioned earlier, freeweights consist of anything with a barbell and/or dumb-bells. That includes the Olympic bar, a seven-foot long bar weighing 45 pounds; dumbbells that come in various shapes and range in weight from 3 to 150 pounds; and plates, circular metal weights that range from 2.5 to 45 pounds, which fit on the end of a barbell. You're also likely to come upon a variety of other funky-looking spe-cialty bars and attachments that are used for a variety of exercises. We'll explain what these do later; for now let's stick to the basics.

There's a subtle difference that serious lifters typically make between machines and freeweights. Their thinking goes something like this: "Freeweights are for serious lifters; guys who train hard and often." According to the lore of the earnest lifter, machines are "too easy" or "easier" and therefore not as efficient at building strength as freeweights. While there is a small grain of truth to that logic, the funny thing is that when you watch these guys, or better yet, query them on their routines, you find out that they also partake of the machines. For example, just about every macho dude uses a lat pull-down machine, a leg-extension and curl machine as well as a leg-press machine, and so on. So while they feel emotionally wed to the cold hard steel, in fact, just about everyone who works out regularly uses a combination of the two.

As we'll discuss later, we'll have you using a combination of machines and freeweights in your workout routine. (Remember, your muscles really can't tell the difference.) It is, however, important to note that freeweights require more vigilance on your part. Apropos of the "what goes up must come down" theory, hoisting even a five-pound dumbbell over your head means you can do bodily harm to yourself or your lifting brethren. When you watch someone bench press 315 pounds or squat twice his body weight as Deidre did, the concentration needed to control this weight is intense. (This might account for why serious lifters consider freeweights more "real." They're also counting the adrenaline rush they get.) In short, anytime you lift a free weight, or in fact stand next to someone doing the same, you must be mindful of the risks at hand.

Here are the major advantages of freeweights:

➤ Bilateral strength gains—no compensation for your weaker side by your stronger.

➤ A near-infinite variety of exercises and the ability to train nearly any muscle in the body.

➤ Can be used by anyone regardless of size, shape or strength.

➤ Easily duplicated from one gym to another. While machines vary, as long as there is gravity, weight will be weight.

➤ Less expensive for home use.

Here are a few of the negatives:

➤ Requires more concentration and focus, if you think of that as a negative

➤ Increased risk of injury. If you're lifting without a spotter or using shoddy form, the risk of injury increases dramatically.

➤ Harder and sometimes more intimidating to learn

Despite the differences between machines and freeweights, both are highly effective training tools. People who disdain one over the other are either arrogant, not accurately assessing their workout, or unaware of how similar they actually are. When used together, you double your fitness options and add welcome variety to your workout.

The Least You Need to Know

➤ Entering a gym for the first time can be intimidating, but that's part of the challenge.

➤ Hiring a personal trainer should be an option when you join, not something you feel obligated to do.

➤ There is an endless variety of fitness machines, but in many ways they are remarkably alike.

➤ Freeweights require that you lift with a keener focus, but they're not just for hard-core types.

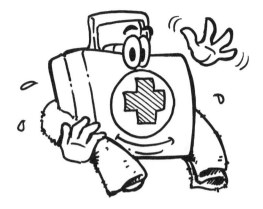

Safety First

After finishing several sets on the bench press years ago, Joe and a friend were removing 45-pound plates from either side of the barbell. Protocol dictates that each person removes the plates more or less at the same time. Joe, however, wasn't paying attention and removed all the weight from his end before his friend grabbed his side. The weighted side made like a seesaw and the plate fell smack on his friend's big toe. Later on they had a good laugh about "Crack-a-toe-a," but at the time Joe's momentary lapse left his friend hobbled for weeks.

Understanding safety issues in the gym is extremely important. People do get injured in health clubs, and more often than not it could have been avoided. Jonathan has lost count of the number of times he's had to sprint from one end of the gym to the other to pull a bar off the chest of a beefy dude who thought a spotter was reserved for the scrawny types. There aren't a lot of rules, and they're not terribly complicated, but they are specific to this unique environment where motivated individuals (many of whom are wearing headphones) are hoisting large metal objects overhead.

This chapter will teach you proper gym etiquette, describe correct form, and explain common safety concerns like making sure that the barbell collars are in place, being mindful where you drop your weights, and the right way to "spot" for someone. The key is consideration and awareness. If you were only in danger of hurting yourself, that's one thing, but you become a threat to others if you start turning toes into pancakes on a regular basis. This is one of the most important chapters. For your own sake, please read it.

Form, Form (and Form)

Hang out in a gym long enough and you hear a litany of complaints—injured shoulders, stiff backs, tweaked biceps, and strained hamstrings. The causes are many and varied, but the biggest culprit is bad technique. Proper technique is the key not only to making solid strength gains, but also to maintaining health over the long term.

Generally speaking, using good form means lifting *less* weight than you might think you're able. Proper form requires you to isolate the muscle or muscles you're trying to build, which makes the exercise harder to perform.

We'll give you a complete description of the proper way to execute each exercise we recommend in the appropriate chapters, but you should keep in mind that the actual amount of weight you lift is in many ways insignificant. Instead, what's important is how you lift that weight. Remember that you're lifting to improve your body and mind, not to pump up your ego. Lifting slowly through a full range of motion is your ultimate goal. If you practice proper technique from the beginning, you'll build a solid base—strength from the inside out. Slow, controlled movements and proper breathing are a few of the key components we'll be stressing.

What Goes Where?

The first time you walk into a gym you might feel like a city slicker dropped off in the middle of a forest. The texture of the landscape is so foreign you might feel dizzy with anxiety and confusion. But don't feel bad: To the uninitiated the gym is a jungle, and you don't know where anything goes or what any of these shiny metal contraptions do.

Fret not! Once you learn the lay of the land, you'll waltz through the establishment like a deer bounding through the woods. In the section that follows, we'll discuss the typical layout of most gyms, where you'll find what, and what you should do with it once you're done using it. Here's a theoretical tour of a typical gym.

The Machines

Most gyms are set up just like a supermarket—all the equipment that's used for a particular body part is together just the way all the dairy products are in one aisle. Generally, machines will be grouped so the machines that work larger muscles like chest and back come first, followed by those that work the smaller muscles like biceps and triceps. (As we'll explain later, that's the logical progression for you to follow in your routine.)

Sometimes, larger gyms will have full lines of more than one brand of machines. If that's the case, you may find all the machines of one line grouped together and the other company's machines in another area. The point is that most gyms have a logical plan that's easy to discern once you know what to look for.

The Freeweights

The dumbbell racks are usually set up in front of a mirror according to weight, with the lighter weights on the top tier—say 5 to 50 lb. barbells—and the heavier weights on the bottom tier. (The heaviest dumbbells we've seen in a gym are 150 pounders, which work well as anchors for ocean liners but which you shouldn't even consider trying to lift for some time.)

Dumbbell racks in tiers.

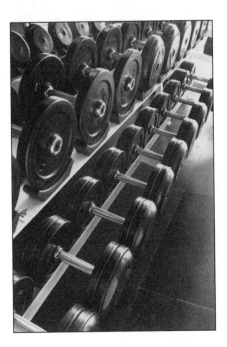

115

There are also odd-looking treelike objects (vertical racks) that are usually set up adjacent to the location of a barbell. These racks hold metal *plates* and are (we hope) arranged so the *plates* that weigh the same amount are grouped together. These plates can be as light as 2½ pounds and as heavy as 45 pounds. Unfortunately, when you're short on time the five-pound plate that you really want invariably is buried under six 45-pounders, a task nearly as arduous as digging out from under a train wreck!

Plates and bar on a tree.

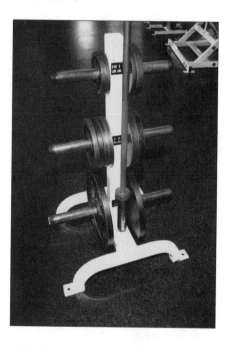

The Bars

The long 45-pound bar used in almost all commercial gyms is called an Olympic bar. These hefty rods of steel are usually found either on the various benches and racks or propped up in a corner. By adding plates to the bar and securing them with collars, you can control the amount of weight you lift for any given exercise. Some folks may use the bar alone when they bench press, while others load as much as 500 pounds onto it. Assuming you're not working out with someone significantly stronger or weaker than you are (requiring you to remove and replace hundreds of pounds of weight), changing the weight is relatively easy. You just remove the collars, add or subtract weight, and continue on.

For those who aren't ready for a 45-pound bar on a particular exercise, lighter, shorter versions of the Olympic bar are usually available. They are the same diameter and just as compatible with the same set of plates.

Some of the larger and better-equipped gyms will have "fixed" barbells in addition to Olympic bars. These bars are already loaded with plates in 5-pound increments and save you the time and trouble of loading and unloading the bar. These usually come in increments from 20 pounds up through 100 pounds. Beyond that, you're back to the bare Olympic bars.

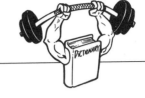

The Pins

Unlike freeweights, which are as basic as a hammer and anvil, there are more variables to concern yourself with when it comes to weight machines. In fact, you're bound to encounter machines from lots of companies (Cybex, Nautilus, Bodymaster, Paramount, Universal, and more). Luckily they are more alike than they are different.

Almost all of them are adjusted with pins. Pins are metal rods used to adjust a stack of weights on a particular machine. By placing the pin into a notch on the stack, you set how much weight you'll attempt to lift. Some pins fit straight into the weight stack while others need to be inserted at a certain angle. Other machines require that you push a button before removing or inserting the pin.

> **Bar Talk**
>
> **Plates** are what you add to each side of a bar to increase its weight. Plates that you'll see in most gyms come in denominations of $2\frac{1}{2}$, 5, 10, 25, 35, and 45 pounds.

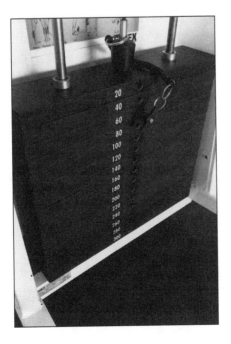

Weight stack using a pin.

Much like socks in a dryer, pins often disappear mysteriously. (Where they go, no one seems to know; since they have virtually no other use, theft is not a viable explanation.) If you're unable to find a pin for the machine you're using contact a staff member.

One important note: Never take a pin from one machine to use with another unless it's of the same model. Since the size and configuration of machines and their weight stacks vary, using the pin from a Universal machine on a Nautilus machine is ill advised. Often the pin will pop out and you'll be in for a rude surprise.

Ask First, Lift Later

Some people are comfortable asking questions when they're lost or confused, while others (usually men!) remain silent, even if it means they must wander aimlessly for hours. Much to our surprise, we consistently see people working out who clearly are clueless when it comes to the nuances of a particular machine. "Nuances my ear," you say. "This is a gym, not an art gallery!" Well, okay, let's just say that just about every piece of equipment can be adjusted in a variety of ways. For example, many benches can be set to a different angle; certain machines can be adjusted to your specifications; and some bars are better suited for certain exercises than others. It can be confusing until you learn which end is up.

Just as you wouldn't wander aimlessly around your workplace during the first week on the job, you shouldn't work out at the gym trying to figure out each piece of equipment for yourself. It seems rather obvious, but when in doubt, ask someone who clearly knows what's what—preferably a staff member.

One way to avoid confusion when you first start out is to take advantage of new member orientations. During these orientations, a staff member will take you through each workout apparatus and show you how to adjust it to your level of skill and your specific physique. In addition, many gyms offer a workout log with each setting and adjustment recorded on a card to help guide you during future visits. You can consider this a road map to terrain that will soon become as familiar to you as your own backyard.

Similarly, you shouldn't be shy when it comes time to ask someone to be your spotter. (A spotter is someone who stands by to help you control the weight should you reach failure in the middle of a repetition.) This ensures that you don't get stuck under a weight that's too heavy for you to remove. While a good spotter can help you squeeze out an extra repetition or two and help you get the most out of each exercise, the most important role a spotter plays is to ensure safety. One of the advantages of machines over freeweights is that machines are generally safer and, unless you want someone to help you squeeze out a few extra repetitions, don't require a spotter for the sake of safety.

When do you use a spotter?

➤ If you're doing an exercise that you can't walk away from if you "fail" in the middle of a rep.

➤ If you want to get a little extra out of your workout, your spotter can help you do a few *assisted reps* instead of quitting as soon as you're out of gas.

➤ If you want to see how many repetitions you can get at a certain weight. Say, for example, you want to bench press 135 pounds 12 times but aren't confident you can do more than 10.

Finally, if a spotter isn't available, wait until a staff member or trusted fellow exerciser near you is available. In the meantime, don't just sit around; consider whether another exercise can do the trick by working the same muscle in a safer fashion. (As you'll see later, just about every freeweight exercise has a machine equivalent.)

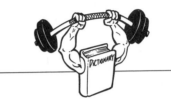

Bar Talk

When a spotter helps you do a few repetitions that you couldn't finish by yourself, they are known as **assisted reps.** The key to getting the benefit from assisted reps is to work as hard as you can, and make sure that the spotter only helps you enough to keep the weight moving.

The Collars

They're called collars, but they're really more like cufflinks. Collars are metal clips that you put on the barbell to keep the plates from falling off the bar and onto a part of the human anatomy. They also ensure that you don't break the plates, the floor, or anything else should they come flying off the bar due to recklessness and gravity.

There are several types of collars. The following are the most common:

➤ **Squeeze**   This is a flexible metal circle with two handles. When you squeeze the ends, the circle becomes larger, enabling you to slide it on the barbell. Once released, it compresses to keep the plates in place.

➤ **Metal**   Often found in serious "muscle" gyms, the collars slip over the bar and are secured by twisting a threaded L-shaped nut that presses against the bar.

➤ **Olympic**   These are the sturdiest types of collars and involve two wing nuts that open and close to clamp down on the bar and hold the plates. These monsters weigh five pounds each, so remember to include their weight when adding up the weight of your bar.

Although Olympic collars are preferable when using a hefty amount of weight, it doesn't really matter what type of collar you use—as long as you use something. At some point in your gym career, you're likely to see some thick-chested guy lifting serious weight on the bench press without collars to secure the weight. With each bounce of the bar on his chest (a big no-no), the plates drift farther and farther toward the end of the barbell. This is a disaster in the making—especially if one of these behemoths is squatting 500 pounds. If one of the plates comes sliding off, it would be next to impossible to maintain balance. With that much weight on the shoulders, a serious injury to the lifter is inevitable, and anyone in the way of the plates is in trouble, too. (For whatever it's worth, we've rarely seen a woman shun collars on an exercise where it was necessary. If we have to shame the guys into proper collar use, so be it.)

Use collars on a barbell no matter how light the plates.

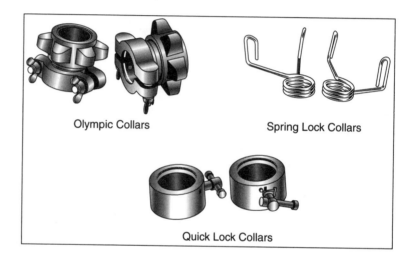

Olympic Collars

Spring Lock Collars

Quick Lock Collars

Miss Manners Says

As a whole, human beings are a sensitive lot. The lack of civility in any locale—rush-hour traffic, waiting in line at the post office, or at your desk at work—is often quite upsetting. The gym is no exception. The importance of functioning politely and courteously in a setting in which you're likely to see many of the same faces day after day can't be stressed enough. Of course, the basic manners of normal society apply in the gym: no belching, releasing gas, or other discourteous behavior is acceptable. However, there are a few particular items of gym protocol that you should know in order to make everyone's life under the fitness roof more enjoyable—including your own.

Deidre and Joe know a hulking chap who was offended by a woman who refused to let him "work in" with her. (We'll discuss "working in" in a moment.) Here's a man who's worked out faithfully for more than 20 years, a man who has a shaved head and more muscles than most Rodin sculptures—in short, an intimidating figure—and yet her rude dismissal left him as wounded as a little boy excluded from a game of pickup basketball. "I can't believe that," he muttered over and over as he got madder and madder. The point is that civility is important—on the road, in the workplace, and in the gym.

We also know a man who often bellows so loud in the gym on his last few repetitions that one fears for anyone with a weak heart. Lest you think we're exaggerating, the roar is an obnoxious combination of a martial arts expert breaking bricks and an elephant orgy. Simply put, it's noise pollution. Joe once politely informed him that this was considered "unorthodox" and he essentially countered by saying, "Hey, I pay my money, I can hoot as loud as I want." True enough, but most people consider him a self-involved goofball.

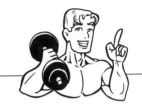

Spot Me

Relative silence is golden. Rather than yell or groan like a sumo wrestler in action, try to limit your vocalizing to heavy breathing or a mild grunting. Hooting like a madman is a great way to attract attention, but useless in helping you lift the weight. Be civil: Keep the weight up and the volume down.

Lightening the Load

Without question, one of the most common mistakes that people make in the gym is leaving "their" weights on the bar when they're finished using them. Even if you're only using a pair of 10-pound weights, it's still rude to leave them.

Actually, the people irked most by this lack of gym courtesy are the staff members who work there. (Jonathan, who has worked in gyms for the last 12 years, often does more lifting while cleaning up after gym members than he does in his own workouts.) People who regularly abuse their bit of gym protocol say they're "too busy" or "they plan to use the bar later in their workout." Sorry. Imagine a slender woman (who is probably just as busy) spending time hoisting 45-pound plates off a bar that you just used. Be fair, put back what you put on.

May I?

"Working in" with another person who is using the same piece of equipment you desire is one of the subtle practices in the gym that you'll need to learn in order to feel at home. Let's say you want to do three sets of biceps curls on the biceps machine. If there's no one waiting to use it, it's just fine to sit down and wait until you're ready to lift for your next set. If, however, there's someone waiting to use the machine, it's common courtesy to ask him if he'd like to "work in" with you. (That's if he doesn't ask you first.) Unless you were just about to start your next set, proper gym etiquette dictates that you get off the equipment and allow the polite interloper to do a set. Once he's finished a set, it's your turn. While it often can seem like an inconvenience, working in with someone ensures that you don't dawdle between sets, which means you're likely to get a better workout. In the spirit of cooperation, it's a good idea to replace the pin at the weight the other person was using. Ditto on the seat height if you moved it.

Wiping It Clean

Here's another bit of obvious advice that's often ignored. Wipe your sweat off the piece of equipment you've just used. Surprisingly, it's a practice that's frequently ignored. It's standard practice to work out with a small towel, bandana, or piece of paper towel. Some people place the towel between them and the seat or bench they're up against. Some just wipe it down after they're done. As long as the sweat is gone, either way is just fine.

The "sweating-on-the-equipment" phenomenon can be a touchy one, and some people clearly go overboard, audibly sighing as they wipe the very machine you've just thoroughly toweled off. Our experience is to let them do the extra housework and hope they get to a therapist who can help them deal with their intense reaction to the thought of someone else's perspiration.

Keep It Clean

Gyms have their own unique aroma. People sweat when they lift weights, run on treadmills, ride stationary bikes, and toil away on stair climbers, VersaClimbers, and rowing and cross-country ski machines. Just writing about it is enough to make one break into a cold sweat. All this sweat can turn a poorly maintained gym into a very, how shall we say, *pungent* environment. Most gyms, however, wash their machines with aromatic cleaning fluid as well as vacuum and scour the locker rooms.

While sweating is basic to a gym, don't push your luck by wearing workout gear that you've worn three days in a row. This is a good way to earn nicknames like "The Stinky Guy." And it's not advisable if you're planning to run for political office. In fact, wearing foul clothes will:

➤ Make it difficult to build friendships—at least friends with a sense of smell.

➤ Make finding a spotter tougher than finding Godot.

➤ Make you the topic of gym gossip.

➤ Make it highly unlikely someone will work in with you.

Of course, as we just said, this is a gym, not an opera house. The idea is to go there and sweat. And while no one expects you to leave smelling like a daisy, it's important that you and your clothing at least start out nose-friendly. If you haven't showered in 45 hours, avoid sleeveless shirts and please don't use the gym as the place to find out if your new deodorant's 48-hour guarantee really works.

The Least You Need to Know

➤ Proper technique and attention to detail will ensure your safety in the gym.

➤ Learning what goes where is easier than you might think.

➤ How do you learn all the nuances of all of those machines? Ask.

➤ Working in. Wiping off. Smelling clean. It's downright civilized.

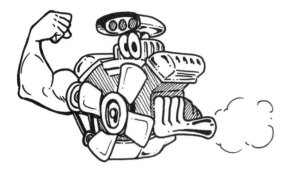

Chapter 12

Revving the Engine

In This Chapter

➤ Begin a stretching program

➤ Stretching easily and breathing hard

➤ Learning how to stretch different muscles

Steve Ilg, a highly sought-after professional trainer and author of *The Winter Athlete* (Johnson Books, 1999), has been a nationally sponsored multisport athlete who has excelled in technical rock and ice climbing as well as in Nordic skiing, cycling, and snowshoeing. He is also a yoga teacher and Joe Glickman's coach. Often when he's asked what's the best way to stay flexible, he replies, "Renounce your furniture. Learn the Asian squat and make use of it." While it might sound absurd or amusing, it makes sense. If you toss your chairs and tables, reduce the amount of desktop work you do, and eat your meals seated cross-legged on the floor, your lower back and hips will be far better off than the compressed lifestyle to which most of us are accustomed.

While getting rid of your furniture might be good for your overall flexibility, it's likely to make your family and friends think that you've either had a momentous religious experience or you're absconding with company funds and heading to Mexico. Assuming that you keep your dining room set and Lazy Boy lounger, you'll be well served to do the next best thing—embark on a regular stretching program.

"But I hate to stretch," you say. Sure, stretching hurts. At least when you start. And wine tastes like cough medicine the first dozen times you try it. However, the more you do it, the more limber your body becomes. Eventually, you'll get so accustomed and even fond of that self-lubricated sensation that you'll crave it like a Frenchmen does a fine Bordeaux.

If you're like the three of us—highly motivated fitness addicts leading busy lives—here's the way you probably think: Time is precious, gotta get in and out of the gym as soon as possible. However, let us assure you (and we're speaking from experience here), if you don't stretch and continue to work out, your body will rebel. Again, to quote Mr. Ilg, "More than a fitness quality that allows you to gain something, kinesthetic training enables you to release something that is already within." To borrow terminology from the martial arts: Lifting weights is *hard* training; stretching is *soft*. Do both, and you're armed and dangerous.

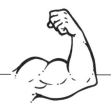

Flex Facts

In Chapter 1, "Let's Get Physical," we told you that Dr. Wayne Westcott found that a strength-training program increased golfers' club speed. In a further study, he found that adding a flexibility program to the strength training doubled the increase in club speed.

It might sound dramatic, but almost more than anything else we tell you in this book, warming up and stretching are crucial if you're to stay healthy and achieve your fitness goals. Joe, who spends a lot of time crunching his 6-foot, 4-inch frame into a narrow, tippy kayak, suffered from a number of chronic, nagging injuries—the most pernicious being sciatica (a painful condition caused by compressing the sciatic nerve, which is located right behind the back pocket of your pants) in his left leg. Two weeks into his daily stretching routine, the pain virtually disappeared even though he continued paddling. Ditto for the achy feeling he experienced each morning in his lower back.

This chapter will guide you through the basics of warming up and stretching—the two most neglected aspects of the fitness game.

How Long Do I Stay on This Thing?

Years ago, runners and cyclists were taught to head out the door and hit the pavement at full stride—or at least to reach peak efficiency as fast as possible. (Hence the "no pain, no gain" theory.) While this might work if you're a marine in boot camp, it's a great way to tweak cold muscles and ensure that you're on the disabled list faster than you can say illiotibial band syndrome. (IBS is a common running injury that affects the tissue that runs from the hip to the knee, often alleviated by stretching). In time, virtually all aerobic athletes learned the virtue of a proper warm-up. And you should too.

Warming-up is the perfect catchall phrase for what you should do right after you enter the gym and change into your workout gear. Pick your favorite piece of aerobic equipment and ease into an easy-to-maintain rhythm for approximately 10 minutes (although five minutes is better than nothing).

Here are our favorite machines to warm up on:

➤ **The Schwinn AirDyne.** This bicycle uses your arms as well as your legs.

➤ **The Concept II rowing machine.** This machine works your whole body.

➤ **The Nordic Track.** This machine simulates cross-country skiing. It's gentle on the joints but works your entire body.

➤ **A treadmill.** Put it on an easy setting and tread lightly.

How fast should you go? That depends on how fit you are. In other words, if you're breathing heavily you're going too fast. If your pulse is the same as it is while you're reading this book (unless you're reading it as you ride the exercise bike), you're going too slow. Your aim is to raise your body temperature as well as increase the blood flow to your muscles and joints. Just as you begin to sweat, it's time to move on to the next crucial stage of working out: stretching.

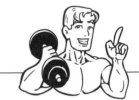

Spot Me

Do your warm-up at a pace that will allow you to break a light sweat. Again, it should be nice and easy, no racing heartbeat or gasping for air.

Hey Stretch!

When you've finished warming up, head to the stretching area. Typically, this is a small, quiet room littered with mats. You'll know you're in the right place when you hear the loud "whoosh" of people exhaling.

Again, we can't overstress the importance of stretching to the quality of your workout as well as the quality of your life. Here's where you'll stretch each major muscle group. If the mere thought fills you with dread, it's all the more reason to suck it up and face your tight hamstrings.

While kids are naturally as loose as Gumby, age and our sedentary lifestyles shorten our muscles. Think about it: You sit for hours each day, and lie virtually motionless in bed for eight or so hours at a time. Riding a bike, running, and clicking the keyboard of a computer shortens your muscles over the course of a lifetime. Without stretching, the natural length of a muscle is changed, which can lead to weakness and muscle imbalances, which can in turn lead to structural changes as you get older. Just thinking about it conjures up images of the Hunchback of Notre Dame.

As we said earlier, the way to counteract this process is to stretch. Simply put, stretching maintains the flexibility that's compromised as we age. Flexibility is important in both everyday activities like turning your head before you make a left-hand turn onto

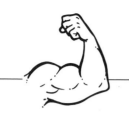

Flex Facts

One of the best indicators of back pain and/or potential injury is the *sit-and-reach* test, where a subject sits on the floor with straight legs and bends forward at the waist toward his or her toes. If your fingertips can't reach your toes, it's a sure sign that you need to work on your hamstring and lower back flexibility. If they can't reach your knees, get yourself to a yoga class.

the highway or bending over and picking up your two-year-old child, as well as in athletic endeavors like fielding a ground ball or shushing down the ski slopes without pulling a muscle.

In her work as a physical therapist, Deidre saw countless injuries that were directly related to decreased flexibility. Not surprisingly, virtually every one of these people complained about lower back pain. Care to guess how well they did on the sit-and-reach test? If you said "badly," you win a tube of Ben Gay. Once they were given a comprehensive stretching routine, their symptoms usually disappeared.

Now while Deidre told her patients to stretch like there was no tomorrow, she lifted weights each day and diligently skipped stretching herself. The result? During her powerlifting career she suffered from chronic lower back pain. When she was evaluated, she was told that the flexibility of her lower back musculature was that of a 75-year-old driving instructor. When she began to stretch on a regular basis, this nagging injury receded into the background.

Easy Does It

One of the reasons why motivated types like Jonathan and Joe postponed stretching for so long is that they viewed it as a cardio- or strength-training session. In other words, they saw it as a contest they waged with themselves (a particularly male condition known as *machismo*). This ability to try less hard is particularly irksome for these achievement types since they are so conditioned to believe that harder is better.

Here's where the *train hard, train soft* mindset must come in. The key words when it comes to flexibility training are *gradual* and *easy!* And, as we'll discuss in a moment, the operative phrase is "belly breath." Stretching consists of several fluid, graceful movements that you do in concert with focused breathing. Done correctly, you should experience mild discomfort in one or more muscle groups, but not pain. Again, if there is pain, there will not be gain.

Why? There are defense mechanisms inside your muscles called muscle spindles. The muscle spindles are quite sensitive to stretch. If your muscle stretches too far too fast, the muscle spindles pull back to shorten the muscle and prevent muscle or tendon damage. It's precisely because of this self-protective mechanism of the muscle spindles that it's so important to stretch correctly. Try too hard and you may actually end up with less flexibility rather than more.

To Do and Not to Do

While most of us did it in high school gym class and army boot camp, bouncing while you stretch has gone the way of the beehive hairdo. It might have seemed like a good idea at the time, but we know much better these days.

If you bounce while stretching you're likely to engage those defensive mechanisms again, or, worse yet, override them and pull a muscle. To state the obvious, don't bounce. It won't help your flexibility.

The three most important things to remember about basic stretching are:

1. Stretch to the point where you feel a gentle tension in the muscle. While that sounds like a contradiction in terms, it's really another way of saying that you should ease into a mild state of discomfort that is well short of pain.

2. Hold the stretch for 20–30 seconds.

3. As you hold the stretch, breathe deeply, stretching just a little farther with each exhalation.

It seems redundant to mention, but it's crucial to remember to breathe while you stretch. Breathing helps to deliver fresh blood to your muscles. Get into the habit of practicing this deep-belly breathing. It will help you immensely when you lift weights. However, it's common practice to hold your breath as you move deeper into a stretch. Be mindful of this—it's a sign that you're pushing too hard or are resistant to the task at hand—and return to your breath. Not only will this help you to relax, it will allow you to stretch a little farther with each exhalation.

Deep breathing is not something that we do naturally at rest. In fact, most of us breathe shallowly from the chest and don't use our *diaphragm*. Try this now: Place one hand on your abdomen and one hand on your chest. Take a deep breath through your nose and fill your abdomen with air (you should feel your hand rise with your abdomen. Complete the breath by filling your chest with air (you should feel your hand rise with your chest). Now exhale through your mouth, expelling air from your abdomen first, then your chest. Repeat this slowly five times. You may feel a little dizzy or light-headed, but that's normal since you're not used to such oxygenated air.

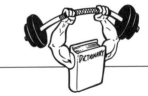

Bar Talk

The **diaphragm** is a muscle used in respiration; with each inhalation, it contracts and flattens; with each exhalation it relaxes and elevates.

Of course, you're not going to place your hand on your abdomen or your chest while you stretch or lift weights. (It's challenging enough to lift with two hands, let alone one.) Instead, practice inhaling deeply through your nose and forcefully out through your mouth. Once you realize the positive effect this has on your stretching (not to mention your sense of well-being), it will be a standard part of your workout.

Now that we've convinced you of the importance of getting (and staying) limber, let's take a look at some of our favorite stretches. Starting a routine is a little like working your way into a great book. The first 50 pages may seem laborious, but once you get into it, you'll be hard pressed to put it down. Do the following for two weeks. You'll be surprised how grateful your stiff body feels.

Torso Stretch

Improving and maintaining a flexible trunk (torso) is extremely important for obvious reasons. If you've ever seen an elderly person (or someone with a back injury) bend down to pick up a piece of paper you'll know what we mean. If your torso becomes stiff, simple tasks like turning and reaching are compromised. In fact, you often hear of people who say that they *threw out* their backs lifting a pot of water. In fact, that was merely the straw that broke the camel's back.

Here is what you need to do to stretch your torso:

1. Stand with your feet shoulder-width apart and toes pointed straight ahead.
2. Keep your knees bent slightly.
3. Place one hand on your hip for support while you extend your other arm up and over your head toward the ceiling.
4. Now slowly bend at your waist to the side where your hand rests on your hip.
5. Move slowly, gracefully, and continue to breathe.
6. Hold the stretch for 20-30 seconds.
7. Repeat on the other side.

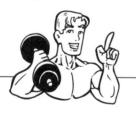

Spot Me

For people who have scoliosis (sideways curvature of the spine) the torso stretch is a good stretch for the opposite side of the curvature. For example, for a left-sided scoliosis, stretch the right side.

Pec Stretch

Here is what you need to do to stretch your pectoral muscles, the muscles of your chest that pull your arms forward:

1. Stand up or sit on a bench and interlace your fingers behind your back.
2. Lift your arms up behind you until you feel a stretch in the arms, shoulders, and chest.
3. Keep your chest out and chin in.

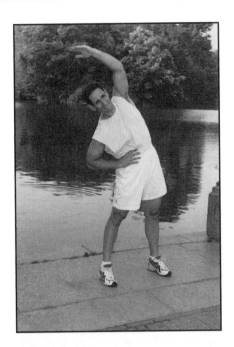

Torso stretch.

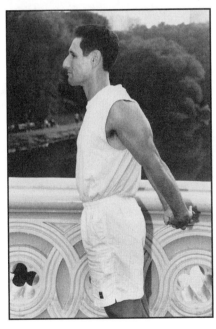

Pec stretch.

This is a good stretch to do at any time, especially if you are at a desk and find yourself slumping.

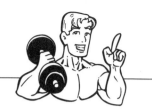

Spot Me

The pec stretch is a great stretch for people who suffer from asthma. Asthmatics tend to take on a forward chest posture, probably from difficulty breathing. This stretch opens up the chest muscles, freeing the muscles used for breathing.

Spinal Twist

The spinal twist is great for limbering the muscles that align your spinal column. It also stretches the buttocks and hips. Here's how to do it:

1. Sit with your left leg straight on the floor.
2. Place your right foot flat on the floor over your outstretched left leg, and rest it to the outside of your left knee.
3. Place your left elbow on the outside of your upper right thigh just above the knee.
4. With your right hand resting behind you, slowly turn your head and look over your right shoulder. At the same time, rotate your upper body toward your right hand and arm.
5. During the stretch, use the left elbow to keep your right leg stationary with controlled pressure to the inside. As you turn your upper body, think of turning your hips in the same direction without lifting your hips off the floor. You should feel a stretch in your lower back and side of hip.
6. Hold for 20–30 seconds.
7. Breathe deeply. Repeat on the opposite side.

Spinal twist.

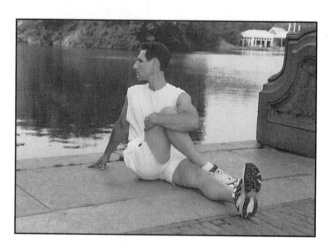

Groin Stretch

Tight groin muscles are a common source of strains in sports with sudden stops, starts, and turns. The groin is defined as the depression between the thigh and the trunk and consists primarily of tendons from your *adductor* muscles.

Here is what you need to do to stretch your groin muscles:

1. Sit with your spine straight.

2. Put the soles of your feet together and grab your toes.

3. Bending from the hips, gently pull yourself forward until you feel a good stretch in your groin. Do not make the initial movement for the stretch from the head and shoulders; move from the hips. You may also feel a stretch in your lower back.

4. Hold for 20–30 seconds.

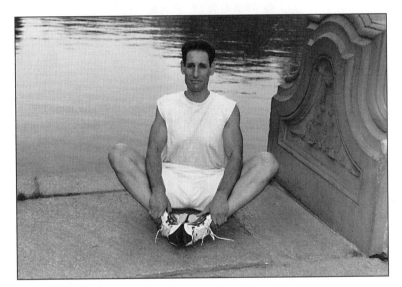

Groin stretch.

Quadricep Stretch

The quadriceps (or "quads") are a group of four individual muscles—rectus femoris, vastus medialis, vastus lateralis, and vastus intermedius, if you must know—that attract so much attention when you walk around in shorts. They work together to straighten the knee. The rectus femoris is the only muscle of the four that also flexes the hip. Your quads are the workhorses in activities like running, stair climbing, squatting, and lunging.

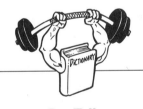

Bar Talk

The **adductor** muscles are the muscles that draw your leg in toward your body from an outward position.

To stretch these large muscles, do the following:

1. Stand near a wall for support.

2. Bend your right knee and hold the top of your right foot with your left hand,

133

gently pulling your heel toward your buttocks. Make sure that your knee is pointing down toward the floor.

3. Keep your hips and shoulders level.

4. Hold for 20–30 seconds.

5. Breathe deeply throughout the stretch and then switch to the other leg.

Quadricep stretch.

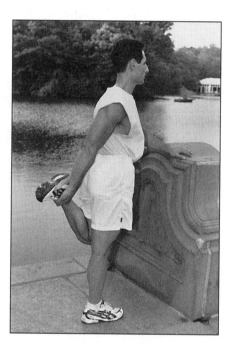

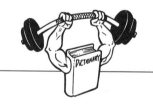

Spot Me

The reason that you hold your foot with your opposite hand is that the natural angle of the patellofemoral joint is not straight as you bend it; it turns inward with end-range flexion.

Hamstring Stretch

The hamstrings are three individual muscles that oppose the quads—the biceps femoris, semitendinosus, and semimembranosus. They work as a group to bend the knee and to straighten the hip. Tight hamstrings, a condition so common that it sounds like the official name, can often contribute to low back pain. Keep them loose, and you'll feel like a new person.

Here is what you need to do to stretch your hamstrings:

1. Sit and straighten the right leg.

2. Place the sole of your left foot against the inside of the right thigh.

3. Slowly bend forward from the hips toward the foot of the outstretched leg until you feel a gentle stretch.

4. Hold for 20–30 seconds.

5. Once the initial discomfort has diminished, bend forward a bit more.

6. Visualize your chest against your knee.

7. Hold for another 20–30 seconds.

Hamstring stretch.

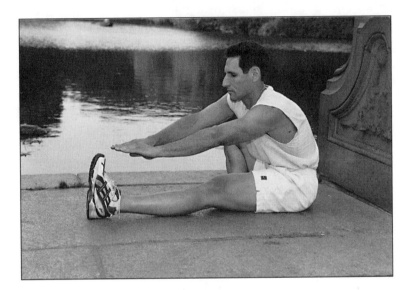

Again, when the stretch becomes more comfortable, lean forward for the last time for another 20-30 seconds. Repeat this three-part move on the other leg. Remember to relax and focus on your breath.

Hip Flexors

Next we have the hip flexor, as it is called in lay terms; to medical types it refers to the iliopsoas muscle, which flexes the hip. The hip flexors are instrumental in running, especially sprinting, as well as cycling and stair climbing.

Here is how you work your hip flexors:

1. Kneel on both knees.

2. Extend one leg forward so that the knee of the forward leg forms a right angle directly over the ankle.

3. Gently lower the front of your hip downward so that the front leg lies on the ground like an L.

4. Hold for 20–30 seconds.

5. Switch legs and work the other hip.

Hip flexor stretch.

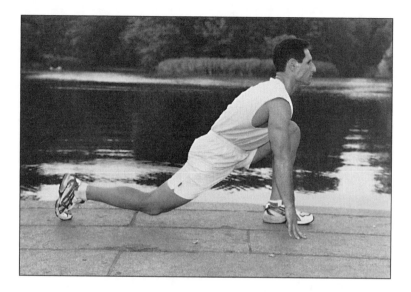

Be careful of this stretch if you have knee problems. Here's a fine alternative to that stretch:

1. Stand facing a support high enough that your hip and knee form a 90° angle.

2. Bend your left knee and place your left foot on the support.

3. Your grounded foot should be pointed straight ahead.

4. Keeping your back straight, lean your hips forward until the heel of your standing foot lifts slightly from the floor.

5. You should feel a slight stretch in the front of your right hip. Hold for 20–30 seconds.

6. Repeat on your other leg.

Calf Stretch

To stretch your gastrocnemius (the calf to you and me), do the following:

1. Stand on a solid support and lean forward against a wall with your head resting on your hands.

2. Place one bent leg forward and extend the other leg with a straight knee behind.

3. Slowly move your hips forward, keeping your lower back flat.

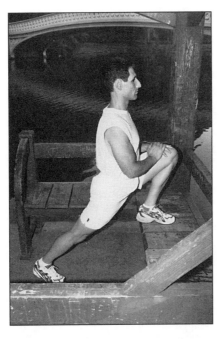

Alternative hip flexor stretch.

4. Be sure to keep the heel of the straight leg on the ground with your toes pointed straight ahead.

5. Hold for 20–30 seconds.

6. Don't bounce, make sure you breathe, and repeat on the other side.

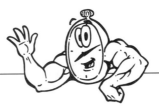

Weight a Minute

For any stretch where you have to bend your knee, make absolutely certain that your knee doesn't "overshoot" your toe. The knee should never be farther forward than your toes, otherwise there's too much stress on the knee.

Here's a wrinkle to the gastrocnemius stretch to work the deeper calf muscle as well as the Achilles tendon:

1. Assume the position we just described for the gastrocnemius stretch, but lower your hips downward as you slightly bend your back knee and bring it forward just a touch.

137

2. Be sure to keep your back flat.

3. Try to keep the heel of your back foot down.

4. Hold for 20–30 seconds.

5. Switch legs and stretch the other side.

Gastrocnemius.

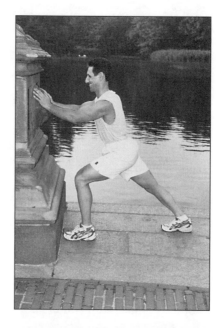

Soleus.

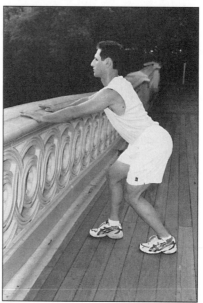

Back and Hip Stretch

Here is what you need to do to stretch your lower back and the side of your hip:

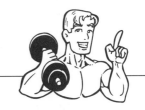

1. Bend one knee at 90 degrees and, with your opposite hand, pull that bent leg up and over your other leg, as shown.

2. Turn your head to look toward the hand of the arm that is straight out with palm down (head should be resting on the floor, not held up).

3. Placing the other hand on your thigh (just above the knee), pull your bent leg down toward the floor until you feel the right stretch feeling in your lower back and side of hip.

4. Keep feet and ankles relaxed and make sure the back of your shoulders are flat on the floor.

5. Hold for 20–30 seconds and repeat on the other side.

Spot Me

Tight hamstrings and tight calves (also called the gastrocnemius) can be the source of a knee condition called patellofemoral syndrome. Symptoms can include pain during prolonged sitting and walking down stairs. Getting these muscles flexible can help alleviate this problem.

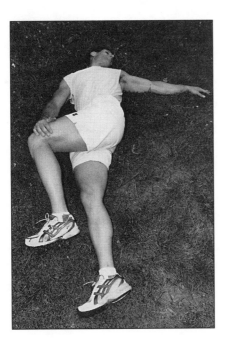

Lower back and side of hip.

139

Here is what you need to do to stretch your middle back:

1. Stand and interlace your fingers out in front of you at shoulder height.

2. Turn your palms outward as you extend your arms forward as if pushing something away from you.

3. You should feel a stretch in your shoulders, middle of upper back, arms, hands, fingers, and wrists.

4. Hold for 20–30 seconds and repeat twice.

Middle back.

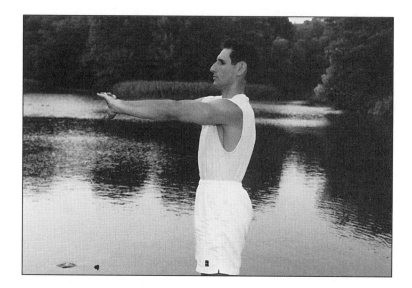

The Least You Need to Know

➤ Age and a sedentary lifestyle make stretching a necessity.

➤ Stretch to the point where you feel a gentle tension in the muscle.

➤ Hold your stretches for at least 20 seconds.

➤ As you hold the stretch, breathe deeply, stretching just a little farther with each exhalation.

➤ Whether you're hustling after a bus or trying out for the Bolshoi Ballet, you'll feel and perform far better if you're limber from the waist down.

Part 4

The Workout

It's funny how many people who start lifting have little or no idea what muscles they're working. "I want to work these things," they'll say, pointing to their deltoids. In Chapter 13, we'll give you an anatomy lesson so that you know what you're doing when the lifting begins.

Chapter 14 gives you a rundown of how you can expect your muscles to develop and respond when the fun starts. We also underscore the importance of proper form and technique—the foundation of any lifting program.

Chapters 15 through 20 are the guts of the how-to section. You'll find a complete list of weight-lifting exercises for your entire body. Each exercise is accompanied by photos and a thorough explanation of what to do. Why is it important to hold your elbows here or your knees there? This section, which tells you how and why, is your own personal trainer in print.

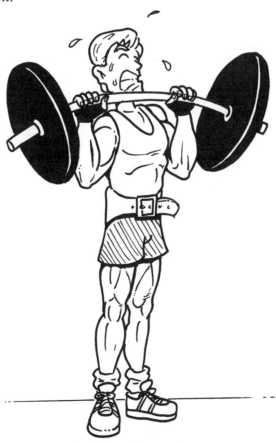

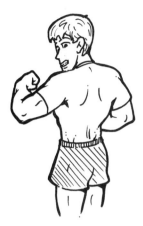

Gluteus What?

It seems each sport, club, fraternity, family (or any other subset of society at large) has its own lingo; its own code words that the initiated use as shorthand. Cyclists "hammer," "jam," or "bonk"; street hoop junkies "slam," "dish," and do battle in "the paint." The gym, of course, has its own jargon. Words like *pecs, quads,* and *lats* are tossed around like five-pound barbells. While these code words may sound like snippets of conversation between two narcotic cops, they're actually abbreviated versions of the technical names for various body parts.

When Joe was a child, his uncle gave him an anatomy book that he had used during medical school. Each page revealed another complete system: circulatory, nervous, muscular, and so on. As a child, pondering how these separate systems functioned as one filled him with wonder. Even as a busy adult, when you pause to consider the human body, only the most jaded mortician wouldn't be awed by the complexity of this amazing machine. Since you're going to be spending a fair bit of time working your muscles, we think it's important to be able to visualize what's going on beneath your epidermis. In fact, the better you understand how your muscles work, the easier it is to appreciate what we're talking about when it comes to particular exercises. In addition, gaining an appreciation for human anatomy might help ensure that you maintain solid technique and not injure yourself.

In this chapter, we've provided you with charts so that you can familiarize yourself with these roughly 600 muscles that compromise your body, the very muscles you'll become intimately involved with in the near future.

Know What and Where It Is

Here's a partial list of common code words you'll hear at the gym:

➤ **Pecs** (pectoralis major). This is the body part Fabio made famous. In ancient Greece, soldiers were chided: "What do you want, a medal or pecs to pin it on?" The muscles of your chest, the pecs move the upper arm down and across the body.

➤ **Lats** (latissimus dorsi). Check out a world-class swimmer or kayaker from behind, and you'll see the sweeping expanse of muscle from the armpit to just above the waist that resembles a highly agitated cobra. The lats pull the upper arm back and down.

➤ **Quads** (quadriceps). From the waist up, Jonathan looks like a fairly normal athletic citizen. (Of course, looks can be deceiving.) However, from the waist down, he looks a bit like two loaves of bread with too much yeast. Why? As a cyclist who averages 50 races and 7,500 miles a year, his quads are his biggest allies. The quads' main function is straightening the knee.

➤ **Hams** or **hammys** (hamstrings). Look at baseball's all-time stolen base leader Rickey Henderson stride to the plate and you'd swear that his striped pants are stuffed with pads. While his quads are large, his hamstrings, which are made up of three separate muscles that run from just beneath the backside to the back of the knee and are responsible for bending the knee, are as inflated as a side of beef. In fact, all superior sprinters and NFL running backs have these sweeping, sculpted strands of muscle.

➤ **Bi's** (biceps). Large biceps ("guns"), the muscle that bunches up into a ball between your elbow and shoulder, are the classic symbol of masculine strength. What do Arnold, Popeye, and Mr. Clean have in common? Big biceps! Without them, the tattoo business would be in dire straits. The biceps are to the arms what the hamstrings are to the legs—they bend your elbow.

➤ **Tri's** (triceps). The opposing muscle to the more famous biceps, triceps push while biceps pull. This lopsided triangle of muscle on the posterior side of your upper arm is most visible when you do a pushup. The job of the triceps is to straighten your elbow.

➤ **Traps** (trapezius). If you've ever seen the heavyweight boxing champion Evander Holyfield sans shirt, you're likely to have noticed these two Brahma bull-like lumps that sprout from under his ears and connect to the tops of his shoulders. These pronounced loaves of muscle help shrug your shoulders and pull your shoulder blades together.

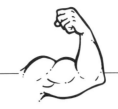

Flex Facts

The word **deltoid** is derived from the Greek word *delta*, which means triangle. Take a look at a well-developed pair of delts and you'll see why.

➤ **Delts** (*deltoids*). Atlas shrugged them and David Robinson, the seven-foot center for the 1999 NBA Champion San Antonio Spurs, has a huge pair as well. It's the shoulder muscle, a large triangle-shaped muscle that covers the joint and serves to raise the arm laterally.

➤ **Abs** (rectus abdominis). Also known as the tummy, gut, and stomach, which actually is a misnomer. Your abdominals run from the lower rim of the rib cage to the pelvis. Your stomach is the organ that digests your food. Well-developed abdominals ("a washboard stomach") à la Bruce Lee not only look great but they will increase your athletic potency tenfold.

➤ **Glutes** (gluteus maximus). Buttocks, tush, backside, derriere, and many more are synonyms for this old trusted friend. Once developed, these oft-neglected muscles provide lots of oomph for forward propulsion.

Here's a nuance of gym vernacular that you should know about. Typically, when someone is asked what body parts he's working on a particular day, the answer is something like "Chest and back; shoulders and arms," and so on. Rarely will you hear someone say, "I'm working my pecs and delts." However, when lifters refer to a particular body part, they more often than not use the abbreviated Latin names we've just mentioned. For example, "Wow, your lats are huge." Or, "Your abs are ripped." Or, "Your quads look like a chicken that needs a tan." (Just for the record: The first two are highly complimentary; the latter is a solid insult.)

The following is a chart of the muscles of the front (anterior aspect) and back (posterior aspect) of the body.

Anterior and posterior muscle chart.

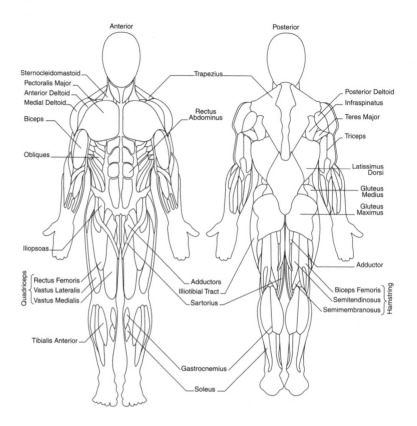

Walking Tall

At first glance, lifting weights is less risky than, say, waterskiing or rock climbing. All you need to do—once you join a gym—is walk in and start lifting. Herein lies the rub. In sports like waterskiing with obvious objective hazards, the risky elements are obvious: fast boat, hard water, big ouch. Assuming you don't drop a barbell on your forehead, the risk in weight lifting tends to be cumulative—the proverbial drop in a bucket that one day overflows and stains the carpet.

Take a chap we know at the gym—a short, bearded muscular guy who trains hard. No matter the exercise, he piles on a lot of weight and gives it the old heave-ho. The problem, however, is that he's often twisting and straining and using other body parts to assist him as he reaches failure. Not long ago he was complaining to Joe about his sore left shoulder. While he reduced the amount of weight he used on the bench (a notorious shoulder wanker), he continued lifting like a man paid by the pound. The moral of the story? Arthroscopic surgery that will keep him out of the gym for six weeks.

As we've now said many times, it's very important, before we have you hoisting weights, that we make sure that you will be able to execute all of these exercises with sound form and technique. That means proper posture and attention to your breathing. If you start using shoddy technique, you're likely to build a house of cards. One day a strong wind rushes through and you're reduced to rubble. And remember, it's harder to unlearn bad habits than it is to learn good ones. So learn it here, the right way.

Be Erect

Woody Allen once said that his brain was his "second favorite organ." While most men would probably agree, when it comes to your overall health, your back is the most important body part you have, principally because it's the core to which everything (muscles, nerves, etc.) is attached. As a private-practice physical therapist, Deidre saw many ailing patients who complained about back pain after a particularly strenuous gym workout. The biggest culprit? Lousy technique.

Try this exercise:

1. Stand against a wall so the back of your head and your buttocks are flush against it.
2. Now take one step forward, tighten your stomach muscles, and keep your buttocks in the same position—almost as though you have a tail tucked between you legs.

Correct standing posture.

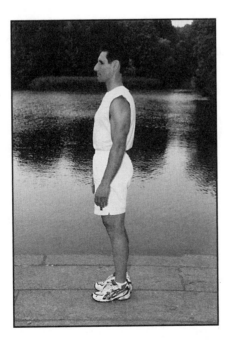

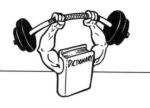

Bar Talk

Lordosis refers to the natural inward curve of the lumbar or lower spine. In some people, especially those with potbellies, the curve is greater than normal and can be the source of back pain.

This is the position you should maintain while performing any standing weight-lifting exercises. At first you might feel like a Buckingham Palace guard or an English schoolmarm, but once you get used to feeling comfortable like this, you'll be righting a lot of postural wrongs. The bottom line here is that when you're properly aligned, your abdominal muscles help to protect the back and decrease excessive *lordosis*, a condition that can be a source of back pain. While bad posture is enough to injure your back, start stressing your skeleton with weights and the plot only thickens.

Sitting Bull

As we have mentioned, an excessive amount of sitting can wreak havoc on our skeletal structure. Let's set the record straight: We aren't antisitting—in fact, we sat throughout the writing of this book; however, too many of us sit too much of the time—for hours at work, in front of the television, in the car to Grandmother's house, and more. Most often we are sitting in chairs that are improperly fitted for us and, if you're a desk jockey who talks on the phone a lot, this unnatural position adds another wrinkle in the bad posture formula. Toss in a good dose of stress—"What, the order won't be here till Tuesday?"—and you understand why massage is such a striving business.

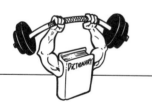

Bar Talk

The **erector spinae** muscles run along either side of the spine and are instrumental in good sitting posture.

Twenty-five percent of the patients in Deidre's physical therapy practice had back (upper and lower), shoulder, or neck pain from sitting either too much or improperly. How can such a passive activity as sitting cause so many problems? Here are some reasons:

➤ There is more pressure on the lumbar spine when we sit than when we stand.

➤ When we slouch in a chair or couch, the *erector spinae* muscles are overstretched for an extended period of time, which weakens them. Weak muscles tend to spasm because they have to work harder to perform simple tasks like sitting straight.

➤ Serious slouchers crane their necks forward in order to see what's in front of them. This puts significant pressure on your *cervical spine* and can cause weakness, spasms, and headaches.

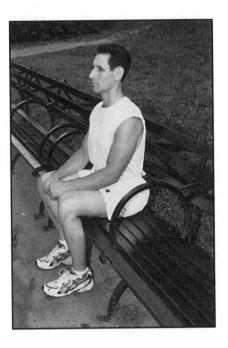

Proper sitting posture.

Here's more good news: poor posture can also cause shoulder problems. How? Try this: Slouch in a chair and raise your arms overhead. Now sit up straight. Notice a difference in your range of motion? Slouching does not allow proper engagement of your rotator cuff muscles, which can weaken them over time and lead to problems such as *impingement syndrome*. Impingement syndrome is a painful shoulder condition that can be caused by several factors, including a weak rotator cuff. As you raise your arm, an arc of pain radiates in the shoulder. Often strengthening the weak muscles in the area resolves the problem.

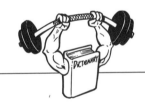

Bar Talk

The **cervical spine** is the part of your spine that attaches your head to your body. When someone says, "He's lost his head," he's indirectly talking about the cervical spine. It is comprised of the first seven vertebrae from the base of your skull (C1) to the largest protrusion that you can feel (C7).

Bend Right

Let's assume for a moment that after reading the various skeletal maladies you haven't quit your job, sold your furniture, and moved to a yoga ashram to find postural enlightenment. Instead, let's hope you at least recognize the importance of sitting up correctly and the subsequent importance of stretching. Unfortunately for the poor unsuspecting weight lifter, there's another danger lurking in the shadowy recesses of your neighborhood gym: improper bending—probably the number-one cause of lower back pain. Luckily it's also the most preventable.

Our backs are built to withstand a tremendous amount of pressure. Our spines, flexible pieces of architectural genius, act as shock absorbers to counteract forces that occur from walking, running, skipping, hopping, driving, sky diving, weight lifting—well, you get the point. However, our backs are not built to withstand the rigors of bending all day long, especially when picking up heavy objects.

If you continually bend the spine of a book in the opposite direction it was meant to go, it eventually weakens and breaks. This is more or less what happens with your spine when you continually use your back incorrectly, day after day, year after year. In her private practice, Deidre heard countless times, "I just bent over to pick up my shoe, and my back gave out." Well that may be the way it seemed, but that's not the way it happened.

"How," you may ask, "should I bend if not from my back?" Ironically, most of us know how to bend correctly because we have ample practice doing so when we have a stiff and sore back. When your back is ailing, you make sure you use your hips and your knees to lower your body to the ground and to raise yourself back up again. Your legs have the largest muscle groups in the body for a reason.

All of this has considerable practical application to the time you spend in the gym, because you have to bend to pick up weights and you have to bend to put them back. To state the obvious: It is very important that you do this correctly.

Try this exercise:

1. Stand against a wall with your feet shoulder width apart, roughly six inches from the wall.

2. Begin to slowly slide down the wall while bending your knees.

3. Now step away from the wall and lower yourself into a deep knee bend while keeping your back straight.

This is how you should use your back at all times, whether picking up a gum wrapper or a 45-pound barbell.

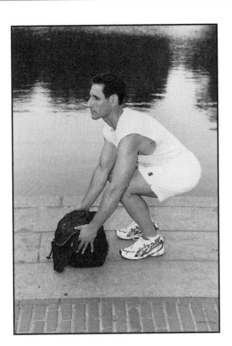

Proper bending and lifting technique.

In and Out

Joe's coach, Steve Ilg, is a big proponent of training an athlete's mind, body, and spirit. Peppered throughout his training schedules are small reminders that pay huge dividends. Here's one to keep in mind whenever you train: "Spine erect, breath full and deep, yet soft."

Breathing properly allows you to merge with the activity at hand. This might sound like a line from *Kung Fu,* but it's one of the most important techniques you can use. Why? The link that connects the body and the mind—a hard-to-describe but easily felt connection—is the breath. Not only will this help you lift more and better, it is also a key way to alleviate boredom in the gym.

Conversely, breathing shallowly or even holding your breath is like working out while wearing a corset. Done under extreme stress, holding your breath can cause you to black out by cutting off oxygen to the brain. And you increase the chance of having a stroke by aneurysm.

Try this exercise:

1. Inhale deeply through your nose, and then exhale through your mouth. Repeat this five times. (If you're not used to breathing from your diaphragm, you may feel a little dizzy.)
2. Now, sit in a chair with your arms by your side.

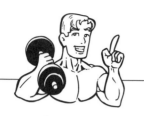

Spot Me

When you're lifting weights, remember to forcefully exhale in the concentric or power phase. This will ensure that you breathe through the most difficult part of the exercise when the tendency is to hold your breath. To help you to remember, keep this in mind: Exhale on effort.

3. Inhale through your nose.

4. Now raise your arms until they are shoulder-level and exhale through your mouth.

5. Next lower your arms while inhaling through your nose.

This little exercise is a way to introduce you to how you would be breathing in the gym while performing shoulder raises.

Up Three, Down Three

Earlier, we referred to the use of momentum as a way to "cheat" when lifting (read: men eager to lift more than they should). This use of body English (cheating) makes the exercise easier and puts a ton of stress on various joints in your body. While it may help you lift more weight, this jerkiness ensures that you're not giving the specific muscle group proper attention. By using the technique of "up two and down four," you will effectively remove momentum from the gym and put it back in Physics 101 where it belongs.

Here's how this simple but effective technique works: Stand with your arms by your side. While bending your elbows, count "one-and-a," "two-and-a." By the end of "three-and-a," your elbows should be fully bent. Pause for one count at the fully contracted position. Now reverse the process and straighten your elbows. As you do so, count "one-and-a," "two-and-a," "three-and-a." By the end of "three-and-a," your elbows should be straight. (We recommend you do this silently unless you're a bandleader or kindergarten teacher.) This count helps you to move slowly, establish a good rhythm, and ensure that you're depending entirely on the muscles you should be working.

Here's a quick checklist of reminders you should take with you on each trip to the gym:

❏ Perform all standing exercises with proper standing posture.

❏ Perform all sitting exercises with proper sitting posture.

❏ Bend from your hips and knees, not your back.

❏ Breathe properly, in through your nose and out through your mouth.

❏ Remember the count—three seconds on the positive phase of the lift, a one second pause, and three for the negative.

Improper Technique

Here's a solid bit of irony. After reading the preceding information you may decide that it's easier to perform exercises improperly, and you're probably right. When you enlist other muscles to assist you, hold your breath, or use momentum to your advantage, the exercise becomes easier but at a cost—safety and effectiveness.

We want to make this very clear so that when you see incorrect technique you know it. Furthermore, we don't care who's doing it—the huge guy with the bulging biceps or the trainer, yes the trainer, who is showing an exercise to a novice who doesn't know a dumbbell from a doorbell.

We know a trainer who advises all of his clients improperly. In fact, when Deidre hears him tell clients to "throw your back" into a biceps exercise or recommend they perform leg extensions at breakneck speed, she's tempted to walk over and hand the client her physical therapy business card. While the majority of trainers know their stuff, this is a good reminder that you shouldn't take everything a trainer teaches you as gospel. Don't be afraid to challenge them and have them explain their thought process if it's something that you don't understand. If we question our doctors, we can certainly question health club trainers.

Cheers

Water, water everywhere, but alas, few of us drink enough of the stuff. This is even more applicable for people who work out. The key fact to remember is that by the time you're thirsty, your body is already dehydrated. The trick is to head that thirsty fiend off at the pass and stay topped off in the first place.

If you notice that you're lethargic, sore, experience muscle cramps or irritability after a particularly hard workout, the odds are you're dehydrated. Again, as we said earlier, it is recommended that you drink at least 80 ounces of water per day even if you don't exercise that day. Remember, now that you are increasing your activity level, you must drink more water to maintain proper hydration.

While we don't expect you to keep track of how many ounces of water you consume, an easy way to tell if you are hydrated is to note the color of your urine. If you're well hydrated it will be virtually colorless (unless, of course, you take vitamins). If it's a concentrated yellow and you don't take vitamins—drink up, mate!

You can do as we say, or learn the hard way. Take Deidre, the powerlifter who preached the virtues of stretching but who hardly stretched, until she was so compromised she had to in order to get out of bed in the morning. Before training for the New York City Marathon in 1999, she still wasn't convinced she needed to drink more than a few glasses of water a day—until she completed a nine-mile run that left her wiped out with fatigue and muscle soreness for two days. After several demonstrative vows of "liquid repentance," she heeded this traditional hydro warning and drank the appropriate amount of water for a week before her next long run. Much to her surprise, she felt much better during and after the run. As you no doubt know, there's nothing worse than the zeal of a recent convert!

The Least You Need to Know

➤ Proper attention to posture—sitting, standing, and bending—is essential.

➤ Understanding the importance of proper breathing further ensures the mind/body connection.

➤ Remember that by the time you're thirsty, your body is already dehydrated; the trick is to stay topped off in the first place.

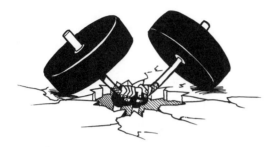

Now What?

In This Chapter

➤ Understanding physiology fact and fiction

➤ Determining how long, how much, and how often

➤ Learning what's in a rep

Strength training is part art, part science, and part luck. The science is how to lift and when. On the physiological front, we know a lot about what happens when you follow specific training guidelines. The art is applying this knowledge to your body. For example: How hard do you lift? Are you able to back off when you're tired and push harder when you're stuck at a plateau? Does your diet complement your fitness goals or sabotage them? And there are a host of other factors that govern the way one progresses in the game of fitness. The luck part revolves around one word: *genetics*.

In other words, there are a lot of variables that surround a lifting program—some you can obviously control, some you can't. In this chapter, we'll discuss the various x-factors involved so that you have a better understanding of how you can best progress in the gym. For example, here's a question that continually stumps people: Why will two people who work out together, doing virtually the same routines, progress at different rates? Read on.

That Was Intense!

Having said that, of all the variables in your lifting program, how hard you work—let's call it the intensity factor—is the single most important one that you can control.

In this chapter and the chapters that follow, we'll give you plenty of tips on how to safely increase this intensity factor so that you get better results faster.

Of course, there are the variables that aren't under your control: age, gender, muscle fiber types, and a few other genetically determined variables that play a major role in your strength development. We'll talk about what they are and how you can work with them instead of getting frustrated and giving up.

Here's the how and the why.

It's Quality, Not Quantity

There are no real differences between the muscle fibers of men and those of women. On a pound-for-pound basis, women are capable of becoming as strong as men. (When Deidre competed as a powerlifter, on a pound-for-pound scale she routinely outlifted most of the men at the meets.) However, because men tend to be larger and have a greater percentage of lean tissue (lower percentage of body fat), men generally have greater strength potential. Dr. Wayne Westcott put it best: Men are stronger than women due to muscle quantity, not muscle quality. While there are differences between the sexes, the methods used to train women need not be any different than those used for men. And in fact, the glut of *women's exercise* programs arises more from a marketing angle than from genuine need.

How Long?

Consider this scenario: Tim and Tom, identical twins, are seated on opposite sides of a seesaw. If Tim sits all the way at the end while Tom sits three feet from the end, Tom will be airborne despite the fact that they are exactly the same size. It's an issue of simple physics.

Now picture two workout partners who have been training together for one year. Let's say they're doing biceps curls. If both lifters are using the same weight and lifting with the same intensity, one may outlift the other by a substantial margin. Why? Again, it's physics, since the lifter with the shorter arms will have much less work to do. Clearly, there's no reason for the longer-armed lifter to alter his training program—and reducing your arm length is far too drastic a course to follow—but it would explain why the shorter-armed chap is progressing at a faster rate.

Now here's one you've probably not spent a lot of time pondering: tendon length. Remember that tendons attach muscle to bone. Let's consider the biceps curl again to show how tendon length can affect strength. The biceps muscle runs from the shoulder to a point just below the elbow. Sparing you the physiological details, you might be interested to know that if your tendon attaches farther from the elbow, it's analogous to being at the far end of the seesaw. Similarly, an attachment closer to the joint is analogous to being in the middle.

Of course, there's nothing you can do about where your tendons attach to the bones; however, this will help you understand why you and your training partners don't always progress at the same rate. Since many people get discouraged when their partners progress faster, it's good to know why not all arms were created equal. Other than the fact that everyone is different, here's the good news: Lift diligently and intelligently and you'll get stronger. In short, you'll be building the body that you've always dreamed about.

Fiber Types

Back in Chapter 3, "What Goes Where and Why," we told you about the different muscle fiber types—fast-twitch and slow-twitch—and their different characteristics. Remember that it's the fast-twitch fibers that have the greatest potential for size and strength gains, so if you were to build a perfect weight lifter, he or she would be chock-full of fast-twitch fibers. The problem—if in fact this is a problem—is that you can't choose the fiber type that you're born with (ditto on the length of your limbs and tendons). While weight training can modify a muscle fiber's characteristics, the fact is that you can't make a fast-twitch into a slow-twitch or vice versa.

If you went to the lab to construct the perfect weight lifter, you'd use lots of fast-twitch muscle fibers, short arms and legs, and long tendons. When six-footer Jonathan accompanied Deidre to her powerlifting meets, he felt like Kareem Abdul-Jabbar at a jockey convention. At a bicycle race he looks like one of the herd. (This may explain why he went into bicycle racing rather than competitive lifting.) Nevertheless, he lifts diligently in order to improve his cycling performance. On the other hand, Deidre, who carries 122 pounds of sculpted muscle on her 5-foot, 3-inch frame, has the ideal muscle type and body for hoisting prodigious amounts of weight. Did she have to train like a Trojan to become a world champion? Definitively yes. Could she have been a comparatively good cyclist or basketball player? House money says no.

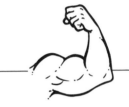

Flex Facts

Some Eastern Bloc countries do muscle biopsies on young children to determine whether they have predominantly fast-twitch or slow-twitch muscle fibers. This information allows them to direct the kids to sports that favor their particular physiological makeup.

Your next question might be: If you can't change these things, why even bother discussing them? For the simple fact that knowing about these variables can help prevent unnecessary frustration in the weight room. As we mentioned earlier, everyone can get stronger from weight lifting, but each person responds differently even if the stimulus is the same.

Now that you know about some of the things we can't alter, let's talk about some of the things we can. Luckily, no matter what your genetics, height, or body type are, the body is an amazing machine that adapts beautifully when called upon. If you run a lot, your legs will respond; if you swim or kayak a lot, the upper body snaps to attention. The same is true of lifting weights: lift right, lift often, and the gains are there to be had.

Get With the Program

While there are unyielding universal truths when it comes to developing a strength-training program, it's just common sense to tailor your routine to you—and not some prototypical lifter who may have different goals, time constraints, and so forth.

In the next chapter, we give you a variety of exercises to work all of your major muscle groups. Don't know how to awaken your dormant latissimus dorsi? No problem—we offer step-by-step instructions. And later on we give you suggestions about which exercises are most appropriate for you given your specific goals. After all, if you want to improve your 10K running time, buffing up your biceps isn't time well spent. Strong hamstrings—well, that's a muscle of a different color.

For now, let's go over some of the fundamental aspects of a sound training routine.

What to Do?

For virtually every body part we'll discuss, we'll show you a few exercises. For every exercise that we show you, there are usually at least two or three more—some good, some not so good—that you could do instead. In most cases these exercises are interchangeable. They're not really all that different. The most important thing to do is to make sure that you train all your major muscle groups and that you train them in the right order. Right order? Yes. As we mentioned earlier, if, for example, you train your biceps first, your arms are likely to be too tired to offer proper assistance when you work your back or shoulders. As a rule, it's best to work the larger muscles first and work in descending size order. This means that if you were going to hit all your major muscle groups on a particular day, you'd start with, say, your hips and legs and move down the list as we suggest below:

➤ Hips and legs

➤ Back

➤ Chest

➤ Shoulders

➤ Biceps

➤ Triceps

➤ Abdominals

No, that's not written in stone—for instance, there's no real problem with switching chest and back or biceps and triceps—but it's a good guideline.

Schedule

When it comes to weight lifting, more is not always better. For instance, while your initial temptation may be to take your ambitious mind and eager muscles to the gym as often as possible, that strategy can actually work against you. Again, one essential key is to know when to work out and when to rest. Too much of one or the other and you've upset the apple cart.

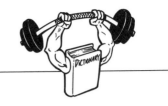

Bar Talk

A **split routine** is a strength-training program in which you divide your body's muscles into two or more groups. On the first day of a split routine you train muscle groups A and B; the following day it's on to groups C and D.

If you recall what we said in Chapter 3, as you lift, you're actually fatiguing and wearing down the muscle tissue. It's during the recovery process that your muscles actually grow bigger and stronger. So as you can see, you should never train the same muscles on consecutive days since it's actually counterproductive.

That's where a *split routine* comes in. This is a program in which you train different muscles on different days. So while you might lift on consecutive days—chest, shoulders, and triceps on Monday; legs, back, and biceps on Tuesday—you'll be using different muscles each day. Not only does this allow ample time for your muscles to recover, it means you'll be doing fewer exercises on any given day. This prevents burnout, allows you to spend less time lifting on each visit, and means you'll be able to work more intensely on the exercises that you will do. Right now, don't sweat the particulars since we'll talk lots more about split routines in Chapter 23, "High Tech."

At the other end of the "too many" spectrum, if you train too infrequently, the strength gains you made in one session will be lost by the next. That means even if you do the best routine in the world on January 1 and little or no training until February 1, the result would be minimal at best in the strength gains department. That should come as no surprise, but we hear people who lift twice a month lament the fact that they're not making much progress.

So what is the ideal frequency? That varies from individual to individual and has a lot to do with how hard each training session is. Here's another immutable rule to note: A hard workout will require more recovery time than an easy one.

Individual strengths and weaknesses aside, two workouts per week is good; three may be better. Whenever possible, we advise beginners to aim for three workouts. If you manage to do two, fine; however, if you're shooting for two, the tendency is that you miss one and compromise your gains. There's another reason why three sessions may be better than two. Early in your workout life, one of our primary goals is to get your brain and body used to the exercises. At this stage we're less concerned with intensity than frequency. So don't worry about your body's ability to tolerate three workouts a week. Once you make going to the gym a regular part of your life—when your weight-lifting workout becomes part of your regular routine—we'll up the intensity and really start to see significant gains.

Reps

The repetition, or *rep,* is the basic unit of any weight-lifting program. Think of each rep as the nails that a carpenter uses to hammer the studs of a house. While you need to know the big picture, the walls will fall down if you don't pay proper attention to which nail goes where. The point is that unless we first focus on each and every rep, other variables like how many reps per set, how many sets per exercise, and the choice of exercise don't really matter.

How Fast?

Since it's quite important that each and every rep be performed with proper technique, let's do a quick rep check review.

A good guideline to follow while you're performing that perfect rep is to count to three during the positive or concentric phase, hold for a count of one, and count to three for the negative or eccentric phase. By controlling the speed, you accomplish a couple of productive things:

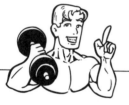

Spot Me

A good way to gauge if you're doing an exercise too fast is to try to stop at various points along the range of motion. Done correctly, you should be able to stop on a dime without momentum carrying you further than you want.

➤ First (and foremost), you maximize your safety and minimize the stress on your joints.

➤ You also ensure that momentum is a nonfactor, which means that you stress the muscles as much as possible and get the best bang for your buck.

➤ Finally, by keeping constant form for every rep of every workout, you're able to measure your progress.

For those of us who are goal-oriented (which tends to be just about everyone who works out regularly) or for those who just like to know that something is working, doing each rep as we just described is vital.

Consider the following scenario. On January 1, you do a biceps curl with 15-pound dumbbells and are able to do 11 repetitions in a 3-1-3 cadence with textbook-perfect form. If by March 1 you're up to 13 reps, with the same weight and form, clearly you have made progress. On the other hand, if you never pay any attention to anything other than how much weight you hoist and how many reps you've done, an increase in how many reps you do could be due to changes in form rather than strength gains. This type of approach highlights our "lift to gain strength, not demonstrate strength" philosophy. While it's not the best way to impress your musclehead friends in the gym, it's a great way to get strong and healthy while staying injury-free.

How Many Reps?

Now that we've established how you should perform each rep, let's examine how many reps you should do in each set. Walking around your local gym, you're likely to hear all sorts of different theories. Odds are that few, if any, are based on fact. Many will be based on refined analytical thinking that goes something like this: Big Bob does sets of 25 for each exercise and he's bigger than anybody else in the joint. That must be the way to go. Or: I read a bodybuilding magazine that said Ms. Olympia never does more than five reps per set, so that's what I do. Again, how big and strong you get is largely a factor of genetics. Just because Bob the Bruiser is as broad as a barn door doesn't mean that you will be, too. In fact, there are guys out there who get big just by looking at a dumbbell rack.

Wander around the gym a little longer and you're also likely to hear another bit of misinformation that goes something like this: Using high weight with low reps builds bulk, but low weight and high reps helps build definition. Sometimes people will even tell you that lifting like that will actually elongate the muscle. Not so!

Here's the scoop. First of all, your muscle isn't going to get any longer by lifting weights—it attaches to a tendon, which attaches to a bone, and that's that. As for the notion that high reps will define or tone your muscles any more than low reps, wrong again. There are just no medical facts to substantiate such a statement. Too many other factors like genetics and nutrition come into play; and besides, it's intensity, not the number of reps, that makes most of the difference.

Where this supposedly correct fact came from we don't know. Perhaps it derives from the fact that a long set often produces a burning sensation in your muscles—flashback to Jane Fonda in a leotard encouraging you to "feel the burn"—but that's just due to an increase in the *lactic acid* in

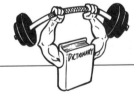

Bar Talk

Muscular fatigue and a burning sensation during strenuous exercise is often due to a high concentration of **lactic acid,** which accumulates in the blood when the energy demands of an exercise exceed the supply or utilization rate of oxygen.

your blood stream, and doesn't indicate that fat is being burned. Muscles look defined when there's a minimal layer of fat covering them. It's as simple as that. So the question remains: How many reps should you do? For most exercises, a range of 10 to 12 repetitions at a three-second, pause, three-second cadence is appropriate. When you can perform more than 12 well-executed reps at a given weight, it's time to up the weight by about 5 percent. The last rep of the set should always be a challenge—a noble effort we refer to as *elegant failure*.

How Many Sets?

Once again, ask five different so-called experts about the optimal number of reps to do and you're likely to get five different answers. In fact, this question produces quite a bit of controversy; controversy we must add that is based on fiction rather than on fact.

Traditionally, lifters have performed two or three sets per exercise, though often you hear about people doing as many as five or six. However, if you read the copious number of studies on the subject, most of them seem to indicate that one set (yes, one set!) can be just as effective and far more efficient than doing multiple sets. By effective, we mean that you can get every bit as strong. By efficient, we mean that you can gain that strength in a fraction of the time. If you use that extra time to do your cardiovascular training, to stretch, or to practice your sport, you're upping your fitness quotient twofold.

When Jonathan played junior varsity basketball at Hunter College, he observed many of the varsity players spending several hours a day in the weight room. While they got plenty strong, they also shot a measly 65 percent from the foul line. Those players probably would have been much better served by cutting their lifting time in half and practicing their shooting.

Now, we're not saying that you can't or won't get strong from two, three, or more sets per exercise—of course you will—just that you can get as strong from one set, too. Again, whether you do one set or 10, the most important thing to keep in mind is that the last repetition of any set should be difficult. That's why it's important to avoid what we call the *magic number syndrome*. This occurs when people stop at a given number of reps (usually 10, 12, or 15) even though they've got a lot of gas left in the tank. If you reach your tenth rep and you can do another rep or two without sacrificing form or safety, do it. Remember that you're not a Swiss watch but an evolving work-in-progress.

How Much Weight?

The question of how much weight to lift is probably asked more than any other question in weight lifting.

Now that we've established that a range of 10 to 12 reps is ideal for most exercises, we need to find the weight that will allow you to do that many without compromising your form. As we said before, early on your goal is to learn to do the exercises with the proper technique. In this initial phase of your lifting life, you should err on the side of caution when picking a weight to start with. A rule of thumb to keep in mind is that generally, the larger the muscle, the more weight you can handle. And as you'll quickly learn, you can move more weight with your legs than with your arms.

In the next chapter, we begin to give you step-by-step instructions on how to actually perform these exercises. When you get started with each of them, begin with the lightest weight possible. If it's a machine, set it to one plate to get the feel for it and then add a little more. Right now we want you to focus on technique without worrying about completing the lift. For exercises that require dumbbells, use relatively light ones to accomplish the same aim. And for exercises with a barbell, try using the Olympic bar without weight, or even a lighter one if necessary.

In any event, be sure not to strain or push too hard during your first few workouts. Once you get the feel of things, you can gradually start to increase the weight during the next few workouts. Be patient. Increase the weight a little each time until you find a weight that will be challenging by the tenth or eleventh rep. Once you've found that weight, stay with it until you can do 12 good reps. When you can do 12 solid reps without straining a vital organ, it's time to increase the weight. When you bump up the weight, try for about a 5 percent increase. Adding that extra weight should make reaching 10 a challenge again.

Here's another issue to keep in mind. If you've been lifting for six months and find you're unable to perform 12 reps even though you did so last week, don't worry. The key is form, concentration, and intensity. As long as you reach elegant failure on your ninth, tenth, or eleventh rep, you've making progress. Lack of sleep, stress, and a myriad of other factors will impact on how you feel on any given day, so cut yourself some slack as long as you're working hard.

How Much Rest?

The amount of rest to take between exercises is as fundamental a concern as any other, but for some reason it is the one issue that is often overlooked. For example, most gym veterans can tell you how much weight they use and how many reps they do for any exercise, but few pay much attention to how much rest they take between sets.

From a physiological point of view, there's no real reason to take more than three minutes between sets. By that time, your ATP (remember, ATP is your body's source of immediate energy) is about 99 percent replenished and your body is as ready as it's going to be. From a practical point of view, there's no reason for a beginning lifter to wait that long between sets. Two minutes allows your muscles ample time to recover and gives a workout partner time to change the weight and do a set, without wasting undue time.

While we don't want to make working out into a stressful bit of time management, you should be aware that when you're not thinking about time, two minutes flies by. In fact, very often people have *brief* chats between sets that last anywhere from 4 to 15 minutes. Ask them how long they take between sets and they assume it's only a few minutes. Before you know it, the workout that should take you 45 minutes to an hour has stretched to $1\frac{1}{2}$ hours. As a result, it's good to time yourself between sets early on. Once you find a rhythm, your body will know the appropriate amount of rest to take.

For certain advanced programs like circuit training (Chapter 23, "High Tech"), super-sets (Chapter 22, "Getting Fancy"), bodybuilding, or powerlifting (Chapter 24, "And the Winner Is ..."), we will vary the rest interval that we recommend. But for now let's stick with two minutes.

Spotter, Please

Remember, a spotter is someone who is ready to help the lifter in case he or she can't complete a lift. As someone who has chosen to lift a heavy object—often over your precious head or neck—it's your responsibility to make sure you have a spotter whenever you're doing an exercise that may jeopardize your health and welfare. Probably the two most important exercises to have a spotter for when you're using freeweights are the squat (Chapter 15, "Below the Waist") or bench press (Chapter 17, "Chest or Bust"), but they're not the only ones. Again, if you can't lift the weight, you're in serious trouble.

Even when you're using a machine or doing freeweight exercises where your safety isn't jeopardized by the absence of a spotter, a helping hand can help you get more out of an exercise in two ways.

How? Everyone has exercises that he or she finds particularly difficult. Let's say for you it's shoulder presses. (For an illustration, see Chapter 18, "The World on Your Shoulders.") Oftentimes, just having someone stand next to you provides the extra motivation to focus and finish the set with good form and maximum effort. Second, a spotter can help you get a few extra reps out of any exercise by offering the barest assistance. We've had spotters who nudged the weight with two fingers who provided invaluable help.

As the lifter, it's your responsibility to tell the spotter what you're going to do. Let him or her know how many reps you're hoping to do, if you want a spot on the *lift off* (when you first pick the weight off the stand), and so on. It's also your job to never give up on a lift. Jonathan has helped spot powerlifters bench pressing over 400 pounds. While he couldn't lift close to that much by himself, as long as the lifter doesn't *bail out* on him, he'll never have to. In fact, even if the bruising powerlifter can't moose out that last rep, as long as he gives it his best effort, Jonathan only has to help out with the last few pounds.

Sooner or later, you'll be asked to switch places and act as a spotter. In that case, it's your job to ensure the lifter's safety. Here's the key: Never agree to do something you can't. And if you're not sure what's expected of you, ask. A good spotter is like a good baseball umpire—as unobtrusive as possible. Aside from an inattentive one, an over-anxious spotter is the next biggest sinner. Once you've ensured that the lifter doesn't drop 200 pounds on his esophagus, the spotter's job is to make sure that the weight keeps moving with as little assistance as possible. Remember, you're doing the lifter a disservice if you provide too much assistance.

If you see the weight stop moving, give it a little nudge. (On most exercises that use a barbell, you're usually best off by lifting the bar itself. In the case of exercises that use dumbbells, it's usually preferable to nudge the lifter's elbows.) Once you've done it a few times, you'll get the hang of it. The most important things to keep in mind are to always pay attention, don't jump in too soon, and stay close enough to the lifter to help out whenever needed.

Now that you understand the various x-factors of weight training, let's move on and teach some specific exercises to you.

The Least You Need to Know

➤ Understanding why no two different lifters are alike should clear up a lot of questions as well as potential frustration you may feel.

➤ The anatomy of a repetition is of the utmost importance.

➤ The nitty-gritty of a strength-training program: how many reps, how many sets, and how much weight?

➤ Offering assistance to your fellow lifters is a standard part of gym etiquette.

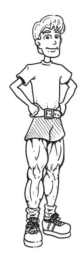

Chapter 15

Below the Waist

In This Chapter

➤ Determining nice Calvins

➤ Two great free weight exercises to build your legs

➤ Seven leg machine exercises for buffer gams

Okay, anatomy fans. What's the largest group of muscles in your body? Back? Wrong. Chest? Nope. Abdominals? Sorry. In fact, the largest muscles you have are located below the waist. Most people when they think of their legs, think of the muscles in two major groups: upper and lower or thighs and calves. There is, of course, a lot more going on in those sturdy legs of yours. So that you know what we're talking about when we recommend the exercises that follow, here's a quick tour of Leg World.

One of these muscle groups is the *gluteus maximus,* or glutes, a wide band of muscle that covers your entire butt area. If you've ridden a horse too long or cycled for hours at a time, these are the muscles that doth protest too much. They are also the muscles that are featured in all of those salacious Calvin Klein jean ads. ("Nice Calvin's" is another way of saying, "Nice gluteus maximus!") The glutes, of course, can do more than sell pants. Their primary function is to extend your legs from your hips when your leg is bent. In other words, when you're running for the bus.

Located opposite your glutes are your *hip flexors.* Although there are several muscles that contribute to the act of hip flexion, the largest is called the *iliopsoas.* These muscles don't receive much attention. In fact, in all of our years of going to the gym we've never heard someone say, "Hey, nice iliopsoas." (We think this is a shame, but there's not much we can do about it.)

The iliopsoas is a strong muscle that doesn't need much concentrated work because it receives quite a bit of work on a daily basis with walking, running, and climbing stairs. In fact, since we tend to sit so much it is the muscle that is often too tight. As a result, this muscle is usually better served by being stretched than by being strengthened. If it becomes too tight, this tricky muscle that runs from the lumbar spine to the inside of the uppermost part of the long bone in the thigh (femur), can pull your pelvis forward and put stress on your lumbar spine. The result? Serious lower back pain.

On the sides of your hips are the hip abductors, the main one being the *gluteus medius.* This muscle works to move your leg away from your body—while pushing off during inline skating, for example. Their companions, located on the inner part of the thigh, are the *adductors,* which draw your leg toward your body.

The big boys in the band are the *quadriceps,* or quads. These are the muscles that span the entire front part of your leg. If you're an NFL running back or a professional cyclist, odds are that your quads are like large loaves of bread. The quads are comprised of four muscles (hence the name quadriceps) that work to straighten your lower leg from a bent position. One of them, the *rectus femoris,* crosses the hip joint and works to bend as well as flex the hip.

Opposite the quadriceps are your *hamstrings,* or hams, which cover the entire posterior aspect of your upper leg. The hamstrings are actually three muscles that work in concert to perform two actions: to extend your leg from the hip when your leg is straight, and to bend your lower leg from the straight position.

Finally, there are your *calves,* the muscles located near the bottom of the legs. One of them is the *gastrocnemius* (or gastroc). This diamond-shaped muscle works to push you up on your toes. The other muscle, the *soleus,* is deeper and comes into play when your knees are bent and you need to lift your heel. The third muscle, located on your shin in the front of your leg, is called the *tibialis anterior.* This is the muscle that rears its ugly head when you come down with a case of shin splints. It functions to lift your toes from the floor. Think back when you've been speeding down the highway and seen flashing lights in your rearview mirror. The muscle that pulls that lead foot off the gas pedal is the tibialis anterior. In fact, the next time you're stopped by a cop for speeding, tell the officer that you have chronically tight tibialis anteriors. If that doesn't work, hope that you have a pregnant woman in the car.

What's the Point?

These are comments we hear all the time: "I'm a swimmer—why do I need strong leg muscles?" Or, "I cycle a lot so I don't need to work my legs." Or, "I'm a runner and don't want to do leg exercises because my legs will get too big"—or any number of other faulty lines of reasoning.

Here are good reasons why lifting weights with your legs will serve you well:

➤ Strong leg muscles are the key to injury prevention in sports from cycling to running. In fact, weak leg muscles are the number-one reason that runners are unable to complete proper training for a marathon or finish the actual race itself.

➤ Strong legs will help your performance on the field. For example, some people think that a pitcher like Roger Clemens can throw a baseball nearly 100 miles per hour because he has an exceptional right arm. Of course he does, but much of his velocity comes from his powerful thighs.

➤ Strong muscles protect your hip, knee, and ankle joints from a lifetime of stress—from running, jumping, and going up and down stairs.

➤ They look good when you wear shorts. Similarly, just think about how weird it looks to have a great upper body and itty-bitty legs.

➤ For the elderly, keeping the legs strong is important for balance, walking moderate- to long distances and moving from a sitting to a standing position.

Now that we've convinced you that you need strong legs, let's show you how to get them.

Freeweights

In general, most of the lower-body exercises we recommend for you will use machines; however, with only two freeweight exercises you could develop an extremely effective lower-body routine. These exercises—the squat and the lunge—involve not only your legs but your entire body to stabilize you during the performance of the lift. Oh yeah, one sobering note: Both of these exercises are difficult.

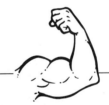

Flex Facts

The squat is one of the three lifts done by competitive powerlifters. (More on the sport of powerlifting in Chapter 24, "And the Winner Is ....") Using support gear like wraps, suits, and belts (the stuff we discuss in Chapter 6, "Strain in Style"), competitive lifters squat farther down than parallel to the ground—the depth we recommend for you.

Squat

Ah, the beloved and dreaded squat. The squat, a lower-body exercise that requires you to shoulder a barbell and literally squat, is a great way to strengthen your legs. When the 122-pound Deidre was powerlifting at the world-class level, she was able to do eight repetitions with 185 pounds. In competition, her personal record is 330 pounds. Each time she did these, however, she thought, "Dear Lord, don't let me crumble under this stack of iron." While no sane person (at least no sane 122-pound person) will attempt to do that much weight, the point is that squatting is a demanding exercise. Despite its incredible payback, it is extremely important that you pay strict attention to your form—and that you never lift more than you can safely handle. We'll omit squats from beginning programs, but we'll keep them in the arsenal for when you get the hang of things.

A few other words of warning: Work with a spotter whenever possible, and make sure that you're good and warmed up. Squatting when your legs are stiff is a great way to court injury. If a spotter isn't around, be sure to use an apparatus that's designed for squatting. A cage, such as the one pictured in the following figures, is designed to catch you if you can't get up from the squatting position.

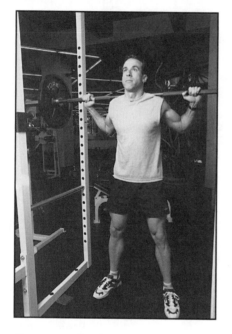

Squat start/finish position.

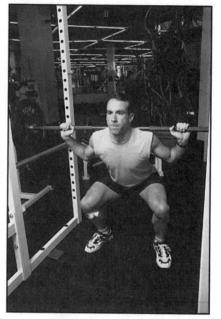

Squat middle position.

Here is how you properly perform a squat:

1. Stand underneath the barbell with your feet slightly wider than shoulder width apart.

2. With your arms holding the barbell with a grip about six to eight inches from your shoulders, lift the barbell off the rack.

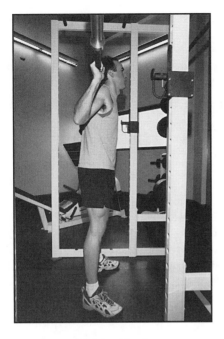

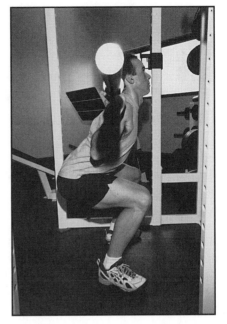

Squat start/finish side view.   *Squat middle position side view.*

3. Take one step backward so you don't hit the racks as you squat, and keep your toes pointed slightly outward.

4. Keeping your back straight, begin to bend your knees until your thighs are parallel to the floor. Don't squat deeper. However, if you squat too little you're not maximizing the benefits of the exercise—remember that a greater range of motion ensures full strength gains.

5. Return to your starting position.

The following is a list of don'ts:

➤ Lean forward as you squat.

➤ Squat without a spotter or safety rack.

➤ Place the bar across your neck.

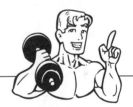

Spot Me

While some trainers consider it safer to do a **quarter squat** where you only bend to about 45°, we question whether that's the case. When you cut the range of motion that far, there's a tendency to greatly increase the weight that's used, which puts much more stress on your back.

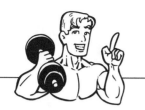

Spot Me

To work on keeping your back straight and your chest up, you may want to practice squatting with a broomstick.

The following is a list of do's:

➤ Keep your abdominals tight.

➤ Keep your weight on your heels, not on your toes.

➤ Maintain an upright posture.

➤ Place the bar across your upper back.

Lunge

Lunges use the same muscles as squats do. However, you don't need nearly as much weight since you're exercising one leg at a time. Lunges also require more concentration. Space out and you're likely to lose your balance. Whether you do lunges or squats is a personal preference since you don't need to do both. Deidre eschews lunges because she'd rather get both legs done at the same time. Because Jonathan has a strength deficit between his right and left legs, he does them a lot more for the left leg.

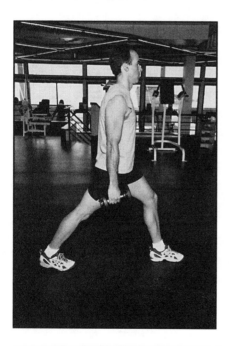

Lunge start/finish position.

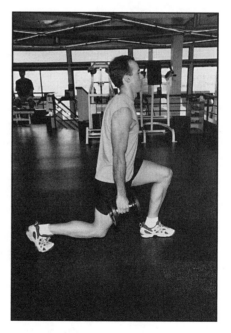

Lunge middle position.

Here is how you properly perform a lunge:

1. While holding a dumbbell in each hand (palms facing the outer thighs), stand with your feet slightly less than shoulder width apart.

2. Now move your right leg approximately one stride length in front of the left. The exercise is called *lunge*, but it is more aptly named *controlled lunge*.

3. Bend your right and left knees until your right thigh is parallel to the ground.

4. Return to the starting position. Repeat with the left leg.

The following is a list of don'ts:

➤ Lean forward.

➤ Let your knee pass forward of your big toe in the middle position.

The following is a list of do's:

➤ Keep your abdominals tight and back straight.

➤ Keep your torso upright.

Keep in mind that this exercise can also be done with a barbell.

Machines

The muscles in your legs are strong. Consequently, after a while the amount of weight you'll be lifting is likely to be rather high. That's where machines come in handy. Working with substantial amounts of weight requires greater levels of caution and vigilance. Using machines virtually eliminates the fear of getting squashed by the weight. It also ensures that you can work to failure and not worry about having a spotter.

Leg Press

The leg press machine is one of our favorites because you can safely work both legs at the same time even while using a lot of weight. However, don't be fooled just because it's a machine; we know of people who have injured both their back and their ribs. How? For some reason, people have a tendency to load on a lot of weight. By stacking on too many big plates, the overloaded sled comes crashing down as soon as they release the break. The obvious point? Don't add more weight than you can safely control for 10 to 12 repetitions.

The keys to a safe workout on the leg press machine are as follows:

➤ Select an appropriate amount of weight that you can safely do on your own.

➤ Bring the sled down slowly. Maintain control.

➤ Don't allow your lower back to rise up off the seat pad. If this happens, then you are bringing your knees too close to your chest.

Leg press start/finish position.

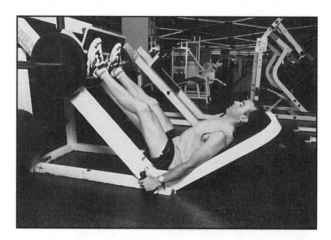

Leg press middle position.

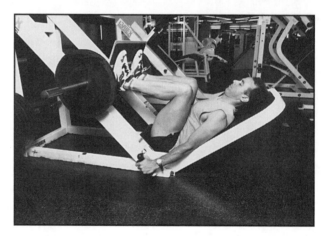

Here is how you properly perform a leg press:

1. Position yourself on the machine, and place your feet on the sled approximately shoulder width apart.

2. Point your toes outward slightly.

3. Grasp the handles that are on either side of the seat.

4. Disengage the brake, and slowly lower the sled as far as you can without your lower back coming up off the sled.

5. Pause for a count of two and slowly return to the starting position.

The following is a list of don'ts:

➤ Lock out or snap your knees at the top of the movement.

➤ Arch your back.

➤ Allow your buttocks to lift off the seat.

The following is a list of do's:

➤ Keep your abdominals tight.

➤ Bear weight on the midfoot to heel portion of your feet, not the toes.

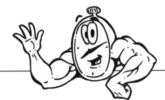

Weight a Minute

This exercise may be contraindicated for people with hyperextended (excessive backward bend) knees.

Leg Extensions

Want quads like Lance Armstrong's? Do leg extensions. (Of course, it would help if you rode a bicycle 500 miles a week.) Okay, perhaps you won't build the legs of a Tour de France champion, but done diligently, leg extensions are among the best ways to build powerful upper thighs. Be very careful not to do more weight than you can handle for 10 solid repetitions. If you overextend yourself on this machine, you could end up with patellar tendinitis (an inflammation of the tendon just below the knee caused by overuse).

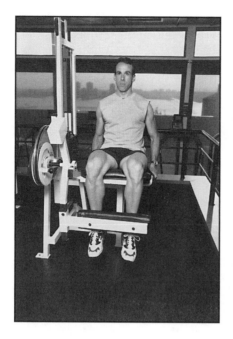 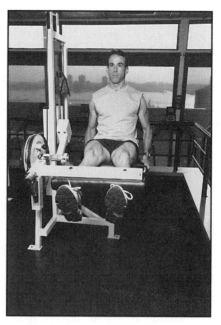

Leg extension start/finish position.   *Leg extension middle position.*

Here is how you properly perform a leg extension:

1. Sit down with your back against the back pad, and position your shins behind the lower leg pad.
2. Grasp the handles on either side of the seat.
3. Straighten the lower legs as high as possible.
4. Return under control to the initial starting position.

The following is a list of don'ts:

➤ Jerk your legs up rapidly.
➤ Allow the weights being lifted to slam down against the weight stack between repetitions.
➤ Lock out or snap your legs straight.
➤ Swing your trunk back and forth.

The following is a list of do's:

➤ Keep your back against the back pad.
➤ Focus on your quads.

Leg Curls

Leg curls are to your hamstrings what leg extensions are to your quads. Since muscular balance is so essential, it's important to build both your quads and your hams so that one doesn't overwhelm the other. Again, remember to stretch your hamstrings before doing this exercise.

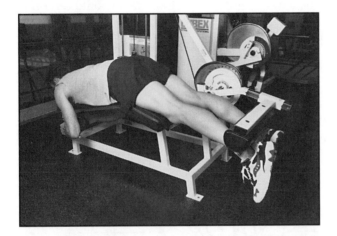

Leg curl start/finish position.

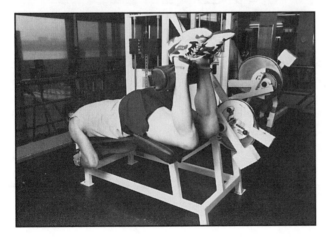

Leg curl middle position.

Here is how you properly perform a leg curl:

1. Lie face down on the bench and place your lower legs underneath the roller pads.

2. The tops of the kneecaps should be positioned just over the edge of the bench pad and not on the pad itself.

3. Grasp the handles on either side of the bench.

177

4. Pull the heels up as close to the buttocks as possible.

5. Slowly return to the initial starting position.

The following is a list of don'ts:

➤ Arch your back or lift your pelvis.

➤ Lie with your head in the left- or right-side position. You should rest on your forehead.

➤ Allow the weight stack being lifted to slam down on the remaining weight stack between repetitions.

The following is a list of do's:

➤ Make sure that you attain an angle of 90° or less at the midposition.

➤ Keep your hips on the bench.

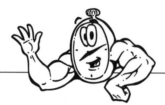

Weight a Minute

Leg curls are not recommended for people with low back pain or hyperextended knees. Some gyms have a leg curl machine on which you sit rather than lie that would be more appropriate for people suffering from back pain. For people who have hyperextended knees, a standing leg curl machine would be better. If you don't have these options, do the following: For lower back pain, place towels beneath your abdomen to give your back support. For hyperextended knees, adjust the rotary arm so that there is a slight bend to your knees.

Calf Raises (Standing)

Much of your ability to continue to do even the most basic activities is due to muscular endurance. Muscular endurance is related to muscular strength. So if you want to continue to walk up stairs with a spring in your step, you'd better begin to strengthen those gastroc muscles.

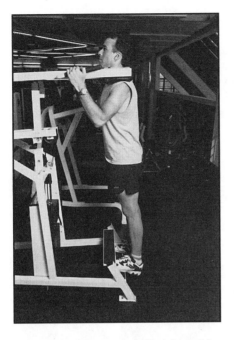 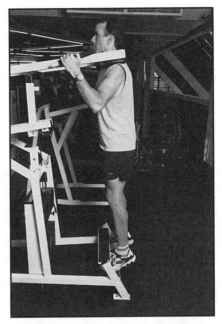

Standing calf raise start/finish position.   *Standing calf raise middle position.*

Here is how you properly perform a standing calf raise:

1. Stand on the bottom step so that the balls of your feet are on the edge of the step and the heels extend over the edge.

2. Position your shoulders beneath the pads, and place your hands on either side of the pads.

3. Keeping your legs straight, rise up onto the toes as high as possible.

4. Return slowly to a position where your heels are hanging down as far as possible. This will ensure a good stretch.

The following is a list of don'ts:

➤ Arch the back.

➤ Rock back and forth.

➤ Perform the exercise rapidly.

The following is a list of do's:

➤ Keep your abdominals tight and back erect.

➤ Keep your legs straight.

➤ If it burns, you're doing it right.

179

Calf Raises (Seated)

As we explained earlier, the soleus muscle is engaged while the knee is bent. It follows that the way to strengthen this muscle is to do so while the knees are bent. This muscle is extremely important, especially if you're a runner. It is a deep muscle (located close to your lower leg bone), and deep muscles are called into play with endurance activities. If they are weak, they fatigue and can become extremely painful.

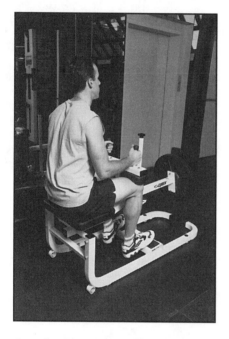

Seated calf raise start/finish position.

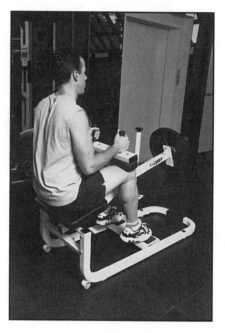

Seated calf raise middle position.

Here is how you properly perform a seated calf raise:

1. Sit on the seat with your knees under the kneepads.
2. Position the balls of your feet on the edge of the foot plate.
3. Disengage the brake, allowing your heels to hang over the edge.
4. Rise up on your toes as high as possible.
5. Return slowly to a position where your heels are hanging down as far as possible to ensure a good stretch.

The following is a list of don'ts:

➤ Rock back and forth.
➤ Perform the exercise rapidly.

The following is a list of do's:

➤ Keep your abdominals tight and back erect.

➤ Remember, burn baby burn.

Hip Abduction

Since our muscles don't work in a vacuum, you don't really need to isolate your hip abductor muscles, because they are busy stabilizing and working while you're performing exercises like squats and lunges. However, there is no harm done if you choose to isolate these muscles.

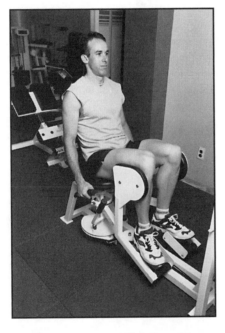

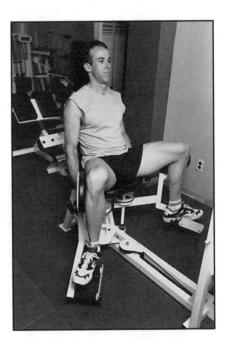

Hip abduction start/finish position.   *Hip abduction middle position.*

Here is how you properly perform a hip abduction:

1. Sit on the machine with your back against the back pad and your outer legs against the thigh pads.
2. Secure the belt if there is one.
3. Push the legs apart as far as possible by pushing against the thigh pads.
4. Return slowly to the initial starting position.

The following is a list of don'ts:

➤ Bend forward as the exercise is performed.

➤ Allow the weight stack to slam down on the remaining weight stack between repetitions.

The following is a list of do's:

➤ Keep your abdominals tight and back erect.

➤ Keep your head and trunk against the back pad.

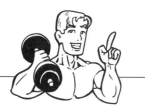

Spot Me

People with relatively short legs may require an additional back pad for this exercise.

Hip Adduction

Again, our muscles are not islands unto themselves; these muscles are working in conjunction with others while doing squats, leg presses, or lunges. However, if you are involved in a sport that overstretches and/or overuses the adductors, you will definitely need to isolate them with these exercises. When Deidre powerlifted, she developed adductor tendinitis in both legs because she constantly overstretched her adductors with her wide-stance deadlifts.

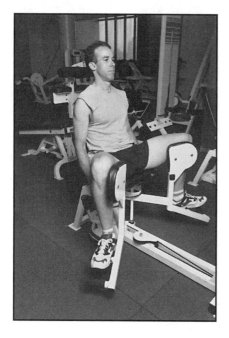

Hip adduction start/finish position.

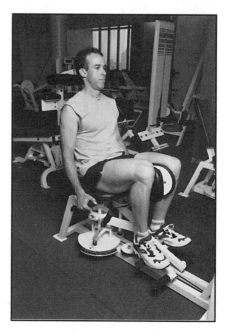

Hip adduction middle position.

Here is how you properly perform a hip adduction:

1. Sit on the machine with your back against the back pad and your inner legs against the thigh pads.
2. Secure the belt if there is one.
3. Bring the legs together as close as possible by pushing against the thigh pads.
4. Return slowly to the initial starting position.

The following is a list of don'ts:

➤ Allow the weight stack being lifted to slam down on the remaining weight stack between repetitions.

The following is a list of do's:

➤ Keep your abdominals tight and your back erect.
➤ Keep your head and trunk against the back pad.

Don't be surprised to see people (usually women) doing hundreds of reps of abduction and adduction exercises in the hope of burning fat and *slimming* their thighs. The problem is that when a muscle works hard enough it gets *bigger*, not smaller. (Those guys doing biceps curls all day aren't trying to get their arms to shrink!) Furthermore, the muscle that's exercising has nothing to do with where fat is burned. So, while there are reasons to work these muscles, shrinking your thighs isn't one of them.

The Least You Need to Know

➤ Everyone—old folks and swimmers—will benefit from strengthening his or her legs.

➤ Squats and lunges are great all-around freeweight exercises for the legs.

➤ There are several machines designed to strengthen all the muscles in your legs.

Flip Side

If you've ever spent any time thinking about your back, as we have, it's rather funny what an overactive (and underused) mind comes up with. While there's nothing inherently funny about a back, it's a rather odd body part. Here's a large group of muscles that are integral to our strength and well-being, but we rarely get to see it and consequently think about it far less than we do our chest, shoulders, and abdominals. *Latissimus dorsi* (or lats) are what gives us that "V-shape"—that rear-view bystanders get to admire while we stare straight ahead. The lats are broad muscles that span the area from just behind each armpit to the center of your lower back. These muscles are key for hoisting yourself up while rock climbing, rowing, and performing pull-ups—to name just a few.

For men, large lats provide that wide expanse of muscle that resembles the top of a manta ray. Many women who weight train notice that well-developed lats offer the illusion that their waist is narrower. In fact, it's not; it only appears that way, but few women we know complain about this complimentary illusion.

Just above the lats are the traps or *trapezius* muscles (traps). These powerful muscles run from just below the back of your skull, to the edge of your shoulders, and down through the center of your back. When you shrug your shoulders you're using your traps. (As we mentioned earlier, former heavyweight Evander Holyfield has traps like a Brahma bull; in fact, his entire back looks like an anatomical chart.)

What else is going on in that back of yours? The rhomboids—major and minor—span the area between your spine and your shoulder blades. Along with your traps, the rhomboids retract or squeeze your shoulder blades together. The rhomboids are shaped like a Christmas tree and are attached to the innermost part of the shoulder blades (scapula). Any exercise that brings the shoulder blades together will work these muscles.

Why Bother?

Aside from looking good, strong back muscles are important for maintaining good posture and vice versa. Meaning: Good posture equals a strong healthy back, and a strong back contributes to good posture. Slouching over stretches the muscles, making them work harder during the day. Since overworked muscles fatigue and often spasm, keeping your muscles at their proper working length and strength will prevent this. (Again, assuming you pay attention to your posture.)

Here are three other reasons to train your back:

➤ Strong upper back muscles allow you to maintain an erect sitting posture without fatigue. Slouching, a bad habit that accounts for untold amounts of chronic back pain, puts these muscles in an overstretched position. This weakens them and leads to muscle spasms, headaches, and backaches.

➤ Strong lats can help you scale that rock wall or give you more power while on the rowing machine, in a swimming pool, or while you paddle a canoe or kayak.

➤ Strong upper back muscles prevent muscle strength imbalances and protect the shoulder, especially in sports where emphasis is placed on the anterior shoulders and pectoralis muscles like swimming, tennis, and pitching.

Freeweights

The lats, being so large and expansive, respond well to both freeweights and machines. As a matter of fact, you can probably work them much harder with machines than with free weights, because you're able to use a little more weight and not have to concentrate on form quite as much as you would with free weights. However, it is still important to use both, especially when you concentrate on the smaller back muscles like the rhomboids.

Following are a number of exercises that help to develop overall strength as well as specific back strength.

Deadlifts

One of the three powerlifting exercises, the *deadlift* is one of those good news/bad news deals. First the good news: The deadlift is one of the best overall body exercises that you can do. Every muscle is involved during the dead lift—upper back, hips, quads, hamstrings, abdominals, you name it. Now the bad news: It's an advanced lift and must be performed with perfect form or you'll risk injury. While we'll omit it from beginning programs, it can become a valuable weapon in your back-training arsenal as your strength training progresses.

The most important thing to keep in mind during this lift is that the back must be held as erect as possible. Never allow your chest to go over the bar—this will bring your body forward as you lift the weight, causing you to use your low back for most of the lift instead of your hips and legs. As you pull the weight, think of pushing your feet through the floor so that you really get your legs into it.

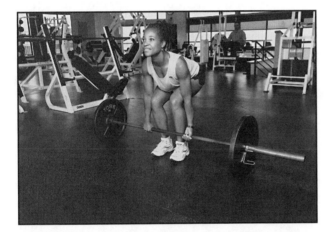

Deadlift start/end position.

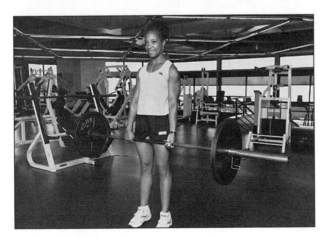

Deadlift midrange position.

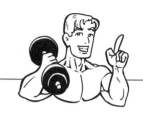

Spot Me

When deadlifting with 45-pound plates, the bar begins just below your knees. The problem is that most people must learn the exercise with significantly less weight than that, which lowers the bar and increases how far you need to bend to get the bar. Try starting off using dumbbells instead of a barbell to avoid back strain associated with bending too far.

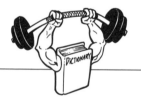

Bar Talk

In the alternating grip or **reverse grip,** you hold the bar with the fingers of one hand facing your body, and the fingers of the other hand facing away from your body. This improves your ability to hold the bar without it slipping out of your hands.

Here is how you properly perform a deadlift:

1. Place your feet slightly wider apart than shoulder width.

2. Reach down and grasp the bar on the outside of the legs with a *reverse grip.*

3. Lower the hips until the thighs are close to parallel to the floor.

4. Flatten your lower back and look up slightly.

5. Make sure that your weight is on your heels, not your toes. Form is of the utmost importance here, so make sure the first time you do this awesome lift you do it with just the bar.

6. Stand upright by straightening the legs and upper body; pause and then slowly return to the initial starting position. Think of yourself as a piston or as an arrow being shot out of the bow.

7. Look up toward the ceiling because that is where you want to go. (Typically, your body goes where your head and eyes go.) If you look straight ahead, you may come out of the lift going forward. Look up and you'll usually come out going up.

8. As you lower the bar to the starting position, be sure to keep the bar close to your shins. In fact, the bar should actually graze your shins throughout the lift.

The following is a list of don'ts:

➤ Lift your hips too quickly. This will transfer most of the effort to your lower back. The legs, hips, and lower back should be working together with most of the work done by your legs and hips.

➤ Snap or lock out your knees as you straighten your legs.

➤ Lean back excessively.

➤ Bounce the weight off the floor between repetitions.

The following is a list of do's:

➤ Keep your abdominals tight and your back as erect as possible.

➤ Keep your shoulder blades pulled together—this will help keep your back erect.

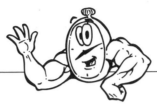

Weight a Minute

Don't attempt this exercise if you have lower back problems. People with long torsos often have difficulty performing this lift because the lower back often becomes the pivot point.

Pull-Ups and Chin-Ups (Gravitron)

If we were in jail and could have just one apparatus, we'd pine for a pull-up/chin-up bar. These simple exercises, which happen to be uncommonly difficult, are (along with the push-up and sit-up) very effective exercises when your access to equipment is limited. (By the way, what's *up* with exercises that end in *up*? They seem uncommonly arduous.) Here's the skinny on pull-ups: Don't try once or twice and give up. Pull-ups and chin-ups are hard for nearly everyone, so don't get discouraged. If you stick with it, you'll improve rapidly. The keys are effort and focus. Since pull-ups and chin-ups are among the most difficult exercises you'll do in the gym, this often discourages people, and that's a shame since it's such a thorough strength-building exercise. If weak arms and gravity have got you down, try doing an assisted chin-up or pull-up on a machine that allows you to lift only a percentage of your body weight. The *Gravitron* was the first of this type and is still the most popular, but many others can be found in gyms nowadays. To use them, you stand on a platform that pushes up to help you hoist your body weight. The directions are fairly simple; the rough equivalent of getting candy out of a vending machine—only much better for you.

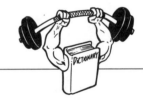

Bar Talk

The **Gravitron** machine allows users to select either a percentage of their body weight or an amount of plated weight to assist them with the pull-up/chin-up. For example, if you weigh 150 pounds, you can set the machine to give you 50 percent assistance with the exercise so you'd be pulling or chinning 75 pounds. Or you can select plated weights to give you 70 pounds of assistance.

189

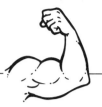

Flex Facts

At age 63, South Korea's Lee Chin-Yong holds the world record with 370 consecutive pull-ups. Not impressed? Robert Chisnail performed a record 22 consecutive one-armed pull-ups on a gymnastics ring!

Here's how effective this exercise can be. Because a strong back is essential for a kayak paddler, Joe regularly does pull-ups as part of his strength-training regimen. (In fact, most paddlers do.) For years, he and a mate were running neck and neck in virtually every marathon race they did. However, one season Joe's paddling mate began whipping him regularly on the water. The difference? His friend had gone on a mad pull-up crusade, doing 20 sets of 10 repetitions regularly while Joe watched late-night TV.

Sound like a lot? It is; however, Joe has another friend who can do 100 consecutive pull-ups. This amazing specimen has a back as wide as a barn door and happens to be one of the best paddlers in Australia.

The point is that adhering to a regular pull-up regimen will have a major impact on your lats.

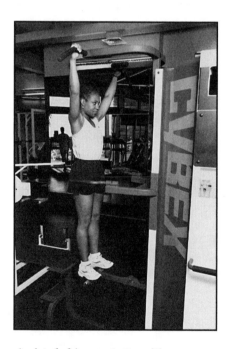

Assisted chin-up start position.

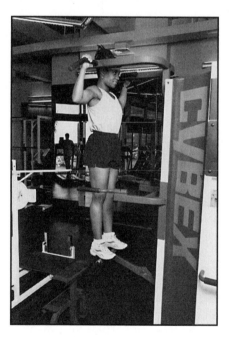

Assisted chin-up finish position.

Here is how you properly perform an assisted chin-up:

1. Grab hold of the chin bar with your hands several inches wider apart than shoulder width.

2. Keep your palms facing away from the body. Lift your feet off the floor and cross your legs at the ankles.

3. Pull your body to the heavens and touch the upper chest to the bar. (Most people try to inch their chin over the top. By focusing on your chest you ensure you really work your back.)

4. Pause briefly and return gradually (don't drop down) to the initial starting position with your arms fully extended to get a good stretch.

Concentrating on your breathing is extremely helpful. Remember on the positive or upward phase to exhale smoothly; reverse on the way down.

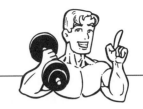

Spot Me

The difference between the pull-up and the chin-up is the hand position. For pull-ups, palms face away from the body. For chin-ups, palms face toward the body. The underhand grip tends to stress the biceps muscles more, while the overhand emphasizes the muscles of the back more.

The following is a list of don'ts:

➤ Arch your back as you lift your body.

➤ Swing your legs or pull your knees up to help you reach the bar.

➤ Drop from the top position.

The following is a list of do's:

➤ Keep your abdominals tight.

➤ Perform all repetitions in a slow, controlled manner.

➤ Breathe, breathe, breathe.

Row, Row, Row

Dumbbell rows emphasize the lats, middle traps, and rhomboids. The key to performing dumbbell rows is choosing a weight that allows you to squeeze the shoulder blade back on the positive phase of the movement, with control. If you have to jerk the dumbbell up with your body, you're not performing an effective set, meaning your muscles are not getting any stronger no matter how much weight you're hoisting.

Another key to performing this exercise effectively without causing harm is to keep the leg on the side you are working on on the floor. This lends support to your back as you are leaning forward. (Unsupported forward flexion is a major cause of lower back pain.)

With so many back exercises available, must you do this one? It depends on what you feel comfortable with. You certainly don't need to perform every single back exercise there is. The variety is to give you a mental break from doing the same things all the time. Deidre never does dumbbell rows. Why? Because even though she trains as regularly as a Swiss watch, she's pretty lazy and would rather work both arms together than one arm at a time (hence she favors cable rows or pull-ups). Once you learn the ropes you'll see that whether you do this or any of the other exercises is really a matter of personal preference.

Dumbbell row start/finish position.

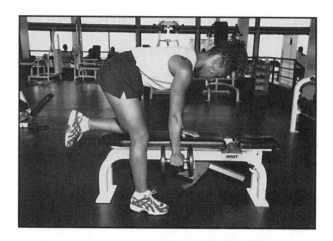

Dumbbell row midrange position.

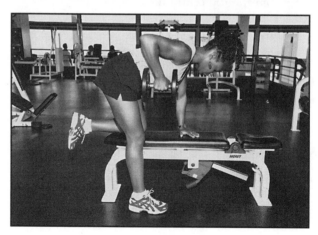

Here is how you properly perform a dumbbell row:

1. Place the left hand and the left knee on a bench and position the right foot on the floor at a comfortable distance from the bench.

2. Reach down with the right hand and grab the dumbbell.

3. Lift the dumbbell off the floor, keeping the right arm straight. The right palm should be facing the bench.

4. Keeping the upper arm near the torso, slowly pull the dumbbell up to the right shoulder as if you were sawing a piece of wood.

5. Pause briefly and gradually return the dumbbell to the starting position.

6. Repeat with the left arm (with the right hand and right knee on the bench).

The following is a list of don'ts:

➤ Arch your back.

➤ Move the shoulder excessively.

➤ Swing your body in an effort to hoist the weight.

➤ Twist your torso.

The following is a list of do's:

➤ Keep your abdominals tight and your back erect.

➤ Keep your shoulder and torso down and parallel to the floor.

Upright Rows

Many people think of the upright row as a shoulder exercise. In fact, it is a good way to work your deltoids and biceps, but it's a great way to hit the top section of your trapezius, which is why we've included it in the back section.

Here is how you properly perform an upright row:

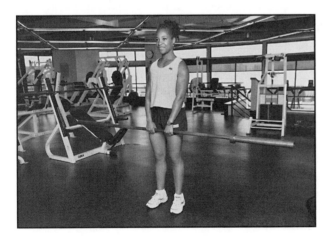

Upright row start/finish position.

1. Stand with feet shoulder width apart.

2. Hold the dumbbell slightly less than shoulder width apart with your palms facing your thighs.

193

Upright row midrange position.

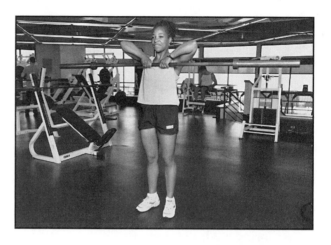

3. Pull the bar up until the hands are about level with the shoulders. The elbows should be slightly higher than the hands.

4. Pause briefly and slowly return to the initial starting position.

The following is a list of don'ts:

➤ Allow the bar to move away from the body while performing the repetition.

➤ Rock the body back and forth in an effort to lift the weight.

The following is a list of do's:

➤ Keep the abdominals tight and back erect without leaning backward.

➤ Keep your elbows higher than your hands throughout the range of motion.

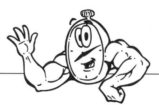

Weight a Minute

People with shoulder impingement syndrome (a painful condition in which various structures are compressed in the shoulder joint when the arm is raised) should not perform this exercise.

Shrugs

While the upright row works your biceps and deltoids in addition to your trapezius, shrugs work the traps without involving those other muscles. Shrugs may look like a silly, insignificant exercise, but they're a great way to strengthen the traps. (To the uninitiated, someone doing shrugs looks terrifically undecided.) For anyone involved in contact sports or ones where neck and head injuries are a possibility, the added neck stability that shrugs can develop can be crucial.

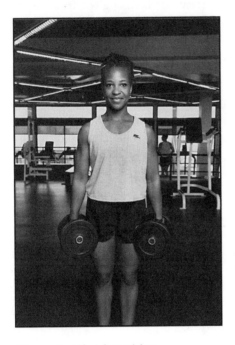

Shrug start/finish position.

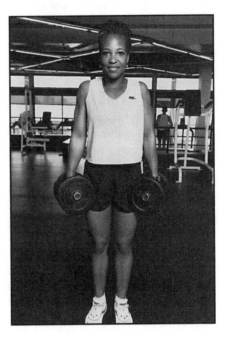

Shrug midrange position.

Here is how you properly perform a shrug:

1. Stand with feet shoulder width apart.

2. Hold the barbell wider apart than shoulder width with palms facing your thighs.

3. Keeping the arms and legs straight, move the bar as high as possible by trying to touch your shoulders to your ears.

4. Pause briefly and slowly return to the initial starting position.

The following is a list of don'ts:

➤ Let your range of motion decrease as you get tired.

➤ Rock your body back and forth in an effort to lift the weight.

The following is a list of do's:

➤ Keep your abdominal muscles tight and back erect without leaning backward.

➤ Perform this exercise with a barbell for a change.

Machines

To keep you amused and active, should someone else be using the freeweights you're after, we'll include a list of our favorite back exercises that you can perform on machines.

Lat Time

Lat pull downs are a standard part of virtually every lifter's routine. Done correctly, a lat pull down will turn a blocky or narrow back into that much-sought-after V-shape. Furthermore, if you're a swimmer, rock climber, rower, or any type of athlete who would benefit from a powerful upper body, this exercise is for you.

There are two types of lat pull-downs:

➤ Behind the neck

➤ To the chest

With the behind-the-neck exercise, there is a tendency to jut the neck forward, putting it in an awkward position, especially if the lifter is using too much weight. For this reason, we prefer the chest variation because the neck is kept in a more stable position.

Here is how you properly perform a lat pull-down:

1. Grab the bar with palms facing away from the body, slightly wider apart than shoulder width.

2. Sit on the seat with your knees under the pads. (Remember to adjust the pads if your knees don't fit snuggly yet comfortably.)

3. Pull the bar behind your head to the base of the neck.

4. Pause briefly and slowly return to the initial starting position.

The following is a list of don'ts:

➤ Jut your chin forward; keep it tucked to avoid neck problems.

➤ Come out of your seat on the way up.

➤ Swing your body back and forth in an effort to lift the weight.

➤ Slouch as you bring the weight down behind your neck.

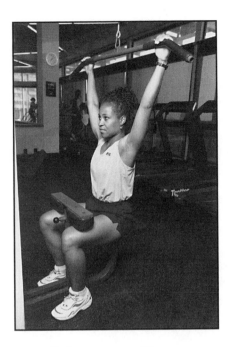

Lat pull-down start position.

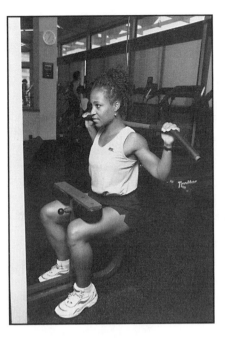

Lat pull-down finish position.

The following is a list of do's:

➤ Keep your abs tight and your back erect.

➤ Squeeze your shoulder blades together as you bring the weight down behind your neck.

➤ Control the weight throughout the range of motion.

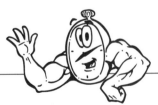

Weight a Minute

Lat pull-downs are contraindicated for those with shoulder impingement syndrome because it can aggravate the condition.

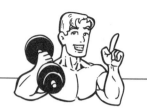

Spot Me

There are several different handles available for this exercise. Experiment with them until you decide which one feels the most comfortable.

Cable Rows

The cable row machine works the lats, the middle traps, and the rhomboids. You should remember to keep your back erect even as you lean forward to return to the start position. As you pull the handle toward you—the initial pull is where your lats are worked—remember to keep your chest up and squeeze your shoulder blades together. (This is where the traps and the rhomboids are worked.) Like virtually every exercise we recommend, cable rows should be performed slowly, with the exhalation coming on the positive phase of the movement. (In this case, the pull toward the chest.)

Cable row start/finish position.

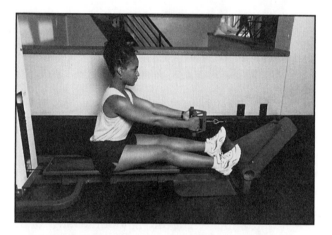

Cable row midrange position.

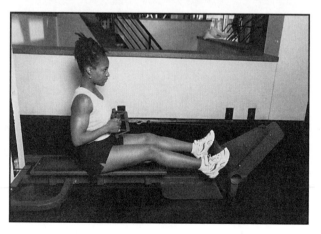

Here is how you properly perform a cable row:

1. Sit down and place your feet against the foot platform.
2. Grab the bar and lean back slightly.
3. Pull the bar to your midsection.
4. Pause briefly and slowly return to the starting position with arms fully extended.

The following is a list of don'ts:

➤ Swing your upper body back and forth in an effort to lift the weight.
➤ Allow the weight stack that is being lifted to slam or bounce against the remainder of the weight stack between repetitions.
➤ Perform the exercise rapidly.
➤ Arch your back.

The following is a list of do's:

➤ Keep your abdominals tight and back erect.
➤ Keep your knees slightly bent.
➤ Squeeze your shoulder blades together at the finish position.

Extension

Most of the exercises in this chapter have focused on the muscles of your upper and middle back, but we've yet to get to the *erector spinae* muscles of your lower back. Strengthening those muscles is crucial in ensuring proper posture and in the prevention of lower back pain. Considering that the majority of people experience lower back pain at some time in their lives, it's not a bad idea to do whatever's possible to decrease your chances of being a statistic.

The back extension machine is an effective way to work those muscles. While they vary from manufacturer to manufacturer, most will have a seat belt-like mechanism to help hold you in place. Use it!

Here is how you properly perform a back extension:

1. Begin in the forward-most position allowed by the machine.
2. Using the muscles of your lower back, press against the roller pad.
3. Pause at the fully extended position and slowly return to the starting position.

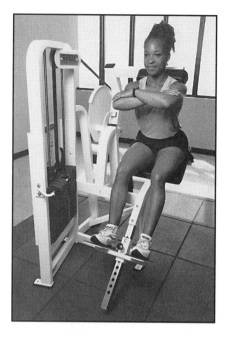
Back extension start/finish position.

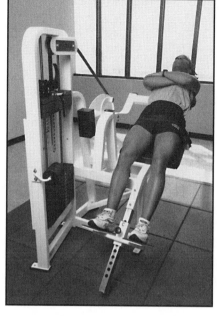
Back extension midrange position.

The following is a list of don'ts:

➤ Push with your legs.

➤ Throw your head back.

The following is a list of do's:

➤ Keep your head in a neutral position.

➤ Control the weight in both directions.

The Least You Need to Know

➤ Our back is our physical foundation.

➤ Lats give athletes that seductive swooping V-shape.

➤ Out of sight shouldn't mean out of mind. Many people neglect their back muscles in favor of the muscles on the front of their body.

➤ Strengthening your lower back may help prevent chronic pain.

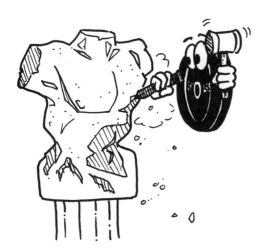

Chest or Bust

Bulging arms and a chiseled chest may be the ideal for American men, but the bench press—one of the three powerlifting disciplines—is generally the signature lift that men use to demonstrate how strong they are. Often you'll hear weight lifters ask each other, "What's your bench?" the way runners ask each other how fast they can run a 10K.

Oddly enough, the bench press, the exercise that builds the muscles in your chest, may be the most abused and overpopularized lift of them all. Why? A thick sculpted chest is the body part men often assume will impress women. (Says Deidre, "A nice chest is attractive but the ability to speak in complete sentences is much more of a turn-on.") Since this lift has become such a *benchmark* of strength, too many men put too much weight on the bar too much of the time. The result often leads to shoulder injuries as well as bruised egos.

Pecs to Flex

The *pectorals* (pecs) are the muscles that span the upper chest wall. They are largely responsible for pushing and throwing movements. There are actually two pectoral muscles—the *pectoralis major* (the muscle we're concentrating on for weight-lifting purposes) and the *pectoralis minor,* which depresses the scapula (or shoulder blade); the pectoralis minor often gets extremely tight in people who have poor posture and needs to be massaged to get released.

Why strong pecs? Because of the following reasons:

➤ If you play baseball or any other sport involving throwing, strong pecs can give you that added oomph.

➤ If you're a swimmer, building your pecs will get you from one side of the pool to the other a bit quicker.

➤ If you are taking boxing classes or practicing the martial arts, strong pecs can make your punch a little harder.

Freeweights

The following are some basic exercises to get you started in the gym. Remember:

➤ Do them all slowly and elegantly—your muscles and joints will thank you.

➤ Breathe out as you push, breathe in as you return to the starting position.

The Bench

The bench press, also known as the chest press, is a standard part of virtually every strength program. Its primary focus is on the pectoralis major muscles, though it also works the front of the deltoid and the triceps. As we mentioned earlier, don't get caught up in the "How much can you lift?" game. Focus on form and the strength gains will take care of themselves.

Here is how you properly perform a bench press:

1. Lie on your back with your feet either flat on the floor or, if your feet don't touch the floor, without your back arching.

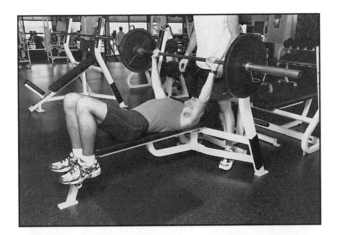

Bench press start/finish position.

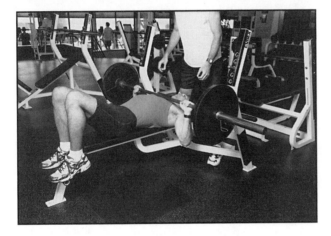

Bench press midposition.

2. Bend your knees and put your feet on the bench itself. (When you put your feet on the bench you reduce the potential stress on your back and isolate the muscles a bit more. It also means you'll use less weight.) In either case, keep your back flat.

3. Grab the bar with a grip slightly wider apart than shoulder width.

4. Lift the bar from the uprights or have a spotter assist you.

5. Slowly lower the bar to your chest, stopping at the highest part of your chest (at the nipple line); then return to the initial starting position.

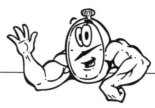

Weight a Minute

As we mentioned, people will often ask you, "What can you bench?" The temptation to try a maximal lift on a bench press (or any other lift) is one we urge you to ignore. One-rep maximal lifts place an enormous orthopedic stress on your body and tend to shoot your blood pressure through the roof. Leave maximal lifts to competitive lifters.

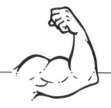

Flex Facts

Performing the bench press is significantly different for powerlifters than it is for non-competitive athletes. In competition, powerlifters arch their backs, dig their feet into the floor, and grind their shoulder blades into the bench. This anchoring gives them enough leverage to drive the bar up off their chest in order to successfully make their one repetitiion max.

The following is a list of don'ts:

➤ Arch your back.

➤ Lift your buttocks off the bench.

➤ Move your legs or feet—keep them stationary for better support.

➤ Snap or lock out your elbows at the end range position.

➤ Bounce the barbell off your chest.

➤ Hold your breath.

The following is a list of do's:

➤ Keep your abdomen tight and your back flat.

➤ Use a firm but relaxed grip.

Goin' Uphill

The incline bench press works on the upper part of your pecs. Bodybuilders tend to focus on defining every single muscle possible so they will perform flat, incline, and decline bench presses to bring out the pecs as much as they can.

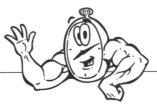

Weight a Minute

The suicide grip (or thumbless grip) refers to gripping the barbell with your thumb on the same side of the barbell as your four other fingers. Some lifters find this more comfortable, but it is extremely dangerous because there is the possibility that the bar will slip from your hands. We don't recommend it.

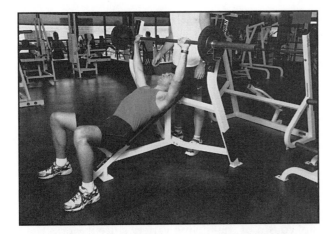

Incline press start/finish position.

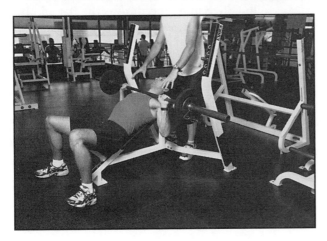

Incline press midposition.

Here is how you properly perform an incline press:

1. Lie on the bench and place your feet either flat on the floor or on the footrest (if one is present).
2. Grab the bar with a grip slightly wider apart than shoulder width.
3. Lift the bar from the uprights or have a spotter assist you.
4. Slowly lower until it touches the upper part of your chest, just below your collar bone; then slowly return to the initial starting position.

The following is a list of don'ts:

➤ Lift your buttocks off the bench.
➤ Arch your back.
➤ Move your legs or your feet.
➤ Bounce the barbell off your chest.
➤ Snap or lock out your elbows at the end range.
➤ Hold your breath.

The following is a list of do's:

➤ Keep your abdomen tight and your back flat.
➤ Make sure to lower the bar to just below your collarbone.

Down We Go

The decline bench is the kissin' cousin of the incline variety since it works the lower part of your chest. Essentially, you follow the same procedure as the flat and incline bench. The tricky part is sliding under the bar without smacking your head.

Here is how you properly perform a decline press:

1. Lie down on the bench, putting your feet under the support provided.
2. Grab the bar with a grip slightly wider apart than shoulder width.
3. Lift from the uprights or have a spotter assist you.
4. Slowly lower the bar to your chest just below the nipple line; then return to the initial starting position.

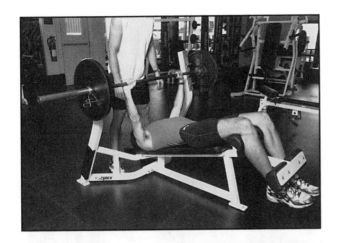

Decline press start/finish position.

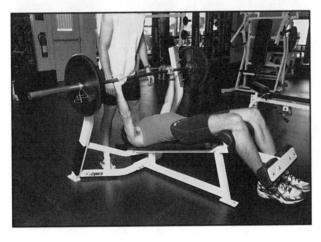

Decline press midposition.

The following is a list of don'ts:

➤ Lock your elbows out as you straighten your arms.

➤ Bounce the bar off your chest.

➤ Arch your back.

➤ Hold the bar with a Suicide Grip!

The following is a list of do's:

➤ Keep your abdominals tight.

➤ Keep your head on the bench.

➤ Lower the bar to your nipple line.

Dips

Most people find dips extremely difficult, with good reason—they are. They also happen to be one of the best exercises for your chest and upper body that money can buy. If you can't do even one, don't despair. Nowadays, most well-equipped gyms have an *assisted dip machine* that helps you by pushing up as you stand on a platform. Better to use the help than to use bad form with your full body weight.

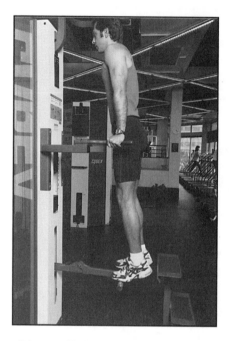

Dip start/finish position.

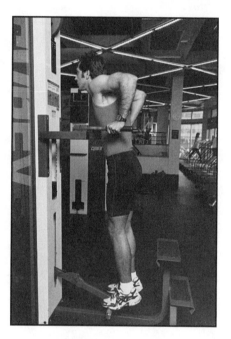

Dip midposition.

Here is how you properly perform a dip:

1. Stand between the two handles, bend your knees, and hold yourself up by keeping your elbows straight. If you're using an assisted dip machine, keep your feet flat on the platform.

2. Slowly bend your elbows, lowering your body as far as you can comfortably— ideally, until your upper arms are parallel to the floor; then return to the initial starting position with a smooth outward breath.

The following is a list of don'ts:

➤ Snap or lock out your elbows as you push yourself up.

➤ Arch your back.

➤ Allow your elbows to jut out toward the side; keep them pointed directly backward.

The following is a list of do's:

➤ Keep your chest up.

➤ Keep your chin tucked and your eyes focused on an object directly in front of you.

➤ Keep your knees bent.

Push, Please

The push-up is perhaps the most classic of all strength-training exercises. Think back to grade school when you did that first facsimile of what Marines and Navy SEALs do more of than any other exercise. While the push-up is as common as a pigeon in New York City, it is a deeply personal and important exercise to incorporate into your regimen, especially considering the fact that you can do it anywhere, at any time. Deeply personal? Yes, since it requires you to call on that part of yourself that refuses to quit called *willpower.*

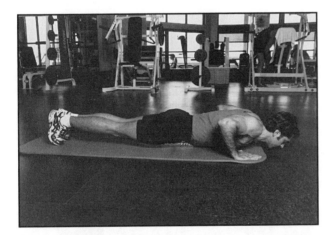

Push-up start/finish position.

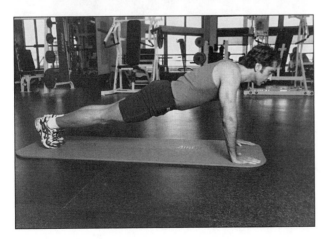

Push-up midposition.

Here is how you properly perform a push-up:

1. Lie on the floor with legs together and hands on the floor pointing forward and just outside the shoulders.

2. Keep the back and legs straight.

3. Slowly pull your body from the floor until your elbows are straight, then slowly return to the initial starting position. Concentrate on keeping your back straight and your rhythm even.

The following is a list of don'ts:

➤ Allow the back to sag while assuming the up position.

➤ Snap or lock out the elbows while at the end range.

➤ Rest in between the starting position and the ending position.

The following is a list of do's:

➤ Keep your abdomen tight.

➤ Keep your head facing the floor without arching your neck.

Flying Solo

Dumbbell flyes are an extremely challenging exercise for your chest since they emphasize the pec major without assistance from the anterior delts and the triceps. It's important to concentrate on your form and keep a smooth and continuous flow to the exercise. Any herky-jerkiness in this exercise is likely to result in injury. If you find yourself cheating, use less weight.

Chest flye start/finish position.

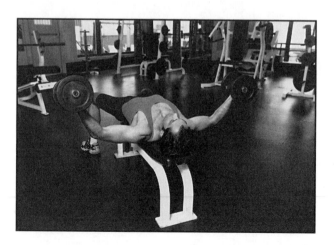

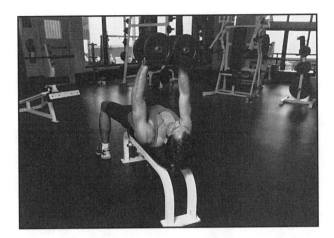

Chest flye midposition.

Here is how you properly perform a chest flye:

1. Lie down on the bench with your feet either flat on the floor, or knees bent and feet on the bench.
2. Arms are outstretched with one dumbbell in each hand.
3. Slightly bend your elbows.
4. Slowly bring your arms together until the dumbbells almost touch; then return to the initial starting position. Picture the wings of a soaring bird and you've got the right idea.

The following is a list of don'ts:

➤ Use too much weight with this exercise. You can cause serious injury to your *rotator cuff* muscles in your shoulder.
➤ Straighten your elbows—you can put excessive stress on the joint.
➤ Arch your back.

The following is a list of do's:

➤ Get a good stretch at the starting position.
➤ Focus on form.

Machines

The following are machines that can be used instead of freeweights. These are good for a little variety and a slightly different muscle engagement, as well as when the sweaty guy using the bench you had your eye on has 15 more sets to do.

Chest Press

This machine is the rough equivalent of the flat bench press. Some machines place you flat on your back, while others put you in a seated position. In either case, the machine works the same muscles as the bench press.

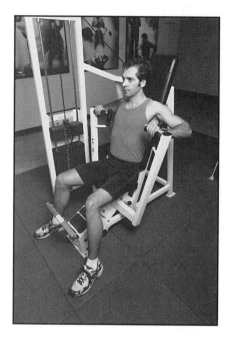

Chest press start/finish position.

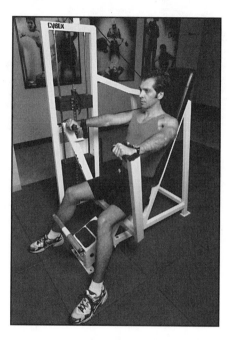

Chest press midposition.

Here is how you properly perform a chest press:

1. Position yourself on the machine.

2. Feet should be flat on the floor or on the footrest, if there is one to use. Remember: Posture counts.

3. Place your hands on the handles.

4. Push the handles forward, focusing attention on your pecs.

5. Finish the forward push just short of full extension and then slowly return to the starting position without relaxing completely.

The following is a list of don'ts:

➤ Snap or lock out your elbow as you press forward.

➤ Arch your back.

➤ Lift your upper body or head from the back pad.

➤ Lift your buttocks from the seat pad.

The following is a list of do's:

➤ Keep your feet flat on the floor or on the footrest.

➤ Keep your abdomen tight.

Pec Deck

The pec deck is a terrific machine for isolating the pec muscles. It's analogous to the dumbbell flyes, and allows you to isolate your pecs without using the muscles in your arms.

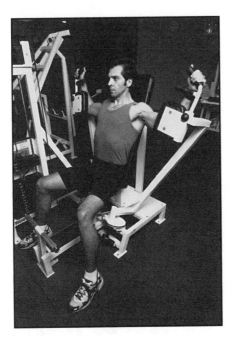

Pec deck start/finish position.

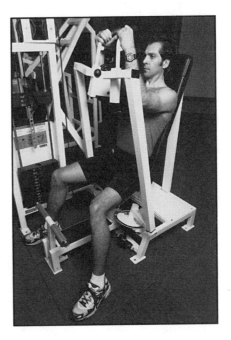

Pec deck midposition.

213

Here is how you properly perform a pec deck:

1. Position yourself on the machine.
2. Feet should be flat on the floor or on the footrest.
3. Place your hands on either side of the pads.
4. Without moving your upper body or lifting your head from the back pad, bring your elbows as close together as possible by pushing against the arm pads.
5. Resist the temptation to twist, squirm, or otherwise recruit any other body parts. Remember that the focus is on form and elegance.
6. Return to the initial starting position.

The following is a list of don'ts:

➤ Lift the elbows off the arm pads.

➤ Lift the upper body or head from the back pad.

➤ Lift your buttocks from the seat pad.

➤ Slam the stack weights in between repetitions.

➤ Arch your back.

The following is a list of do's:

➤ Keep your feet flat on the floor or on the footrest.

➤ Keep your abdomen tight.

If you have a shoulder impingement, refrain from doing this exercise.

The Least You Need to Know

➤ Well-developed chest muscles look good and perform better on the playing field.

➤ Pressing movements use lots of muscle in one exercise, while exercises like the pec deck and flyes isolate the pecs.

➤ Using machines adds variety to freeweights.

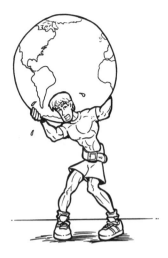

Chapter 18

The World on Your Shoulders

In This Chapter

➤ Remembering the small and oft-neglected shoulders

➤ Learning the anatomy of a shoulder

➤ Performing delt exercises

Atlas carried the world on his shoulders. Often you hear people say, "That must be a load off your shoulders!" Or, "You've been shouldering a huge burden the last few weeks." In other words, the shoulders are known to bear the brunt of hard work and mental stress. While most people relish training their chest, arms, back, and even their legs, the shoulders are one of the most neglected body parts.

Why? The shoulders (the *deltoids* or "delts") are the muscles located at the top of your arm. (If you have any questions about what the deltoid is supposed to look like, check out San Antonio Spurs star center David Robinson, though Utah Jazz power forward Karl Malone has a worthy set as well.) There are actually three parts to this muscle: the *anterior deltoid,* which raises the arm upward from the front; the *medial deltoid,* which raises the arm upward from the side; and the *posterior deltoid,* which draws the arm backward. These muscles are amazingly versatile but are relatively small and therefore fatigue easily. When you start training your shoulders, you're likely to notice, first, how weak they are, and second, how quickly they respond if you train them diligently.

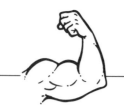

Flex Facts

Anatomy students always remember the muscles of the rotator cuff with the acronym SITS. The rotator cuff consists of four muscles—supraspinatus, infraspinatus, teres major, and subscapularis.

There's another seldom-considered set of muscles that play a large role in the health and welfare of your shoulders that you should know about: the rotator cuff. The rotator cuff muscles are located beneath the deltoids. Their function is to keep your long arm bone (the humerus) from slipping out of joint. Compared to the deltoids, these muscles are small and seldom thought about—until an injury occurs, often while straining under the load of too much weight on the bench press.

Not sure how your rotator cuff functions? Try this: Stick your arm out to the side with your elbow locked. Now twist your arm from side to side. The muscles that get the job done? The loyal rotator cuff. The supraspinatus also assists your deltoids in initiating the outward movement of your arm from the side. And it provides stability to the joint when you throw a ball, Frisbee, javelin—you get the picture. Having said all that, it should come as no surprise to hear that a thorough shoulder workout encompasses the deltoids and the rotator cuff muscles as well.

Should I?

Why strong shoulders? If you play racquet sports, baseball, or want to be the next Joe Montana, improving your shoulder strength is a must. From a cosmetic point of view, powerfully built shoulders will give your upper body more width. Add buff shoulders to a sculpted back and your waist will look significantly smaller. (And women take notice: Train your shoulders long enough, and you won't need to use those shoulder pads in your clothes.)

Freeweights

It is extremely important to lay down a good foundation when you begin to work on your deltoids. This means that the last thing you need to worry about is the amount of weight that you're using. Always make sure that your form is excellent and that you're not using your whole body to initiate the exercise.

When using freeweights for your shoulders, there are several things you must keep in mind: your form, your posture, and the smoothness of your repetitions. What does that mean? First, do the weights go up and down easily on both sides or is one side much harder than the other? If the latter is the case, decrease the weight to match the weak side until you are able to move the same amount bilaterally or concentrate on the weaker side by using machines that move independently.

Military Action

The military press is a great basic compound exercise to do. It works not only deltoids but triceps as well, and can be done in both sitting and standing positions. Deidre prefers to perform it while standing because it's easier to control the position of the lower back, especially with heavier weights. No matter which position you choose, keep your back erect, your abdominals tight, and your head in neutral position. If it sounds like we're sticklers for form, that's because we are.

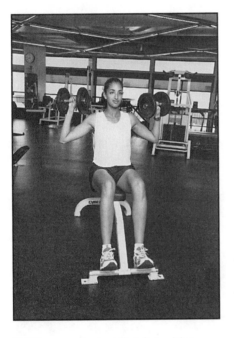

Military press start/finish position.

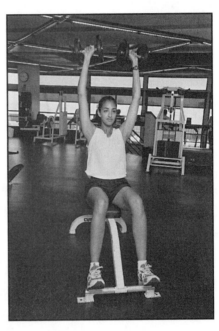

Military press midrange position.

Here is how you properly perform a military press:

1. Sit with your feet on the foot platform, if there is one, with a dumbbell in each hand.

2. Bring the dumbbells up with your palms facing forward.

3. Hold them like a driver signaling to make a right-hand turn—in a position of 90° of shoulder abduction and 90° of elbow flexion.

4. Slowly straighten your arms toward the heavens, bringing the dumbbells together.

5. While maintaining control of the weight, return to the initial starting position.

The following is a list of don'ts:

➤ Arch your back.

➤ Clang the dumbbells together.

➤ Allow your elbows to dip below the start position.

➤ Twist from the waist to nudge the weight upward.

The following is a list of do's:

➤ Keep your abs tight.

➤ Keep your head and neck straight.

➤ Pay strict attention to your form.

Literally Lateral

Lateral raises are a great exercise for isolating the middle deltoids. (They are considered one-joint exercises because the only joint flexing and extending is the shoulder joint. Military presses are two-joint exercises because there are two joints flexing and extending.) Take note that you will be doing much lighter weight with lateral raises than with the military press. Also note that you'll need to keep your elbows slightly bent to take excess pressure off of them.

Lateral raise start/finish position.

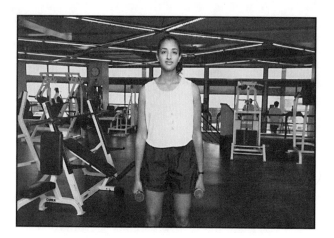

Here is how you properly perform a lateral raise:

1. Stand with your feet shoulder width apart.

2. Hold a dumbbell in each hand at your side with your palms facing the legs.

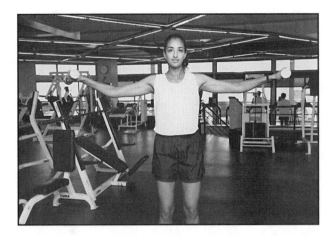

Lateral raise midrange position.

3. With a slight bend in the elbows, raise the dumbbells away from the sides of the body until the arms are parallel to the floor.

4. Return to the starting position under control.

The following is a list of don'ts:

➤ Raise your arms much above the parallel position.

➤ Dip your body downward as you lift the weights up.

➤ Lean forward.

➤ Relax completely between repetitions.

The following is a list of do's:

➤ Keep your abdominals tight.

➤ Keep your weight evenly distributed on your feet.

➤ Maintain good posture.

Front Raises

If you're wondering why we're listing so many exercises for the shoulder, keep in mind that it is a three-part muscle and that each muscle must be worked to get stronger as a whole. Front raises are another one-joint exercise, meaning that they isolate the anterior deltoid, which is the muscle that you use to reach up to grab an apple off of a tree.

Though you will see people exercise both arms at the same time, we prefer that you don't. Doing both at the same time will make it easier for you to cheat by dipping your body down as your raise both your arms up.

219

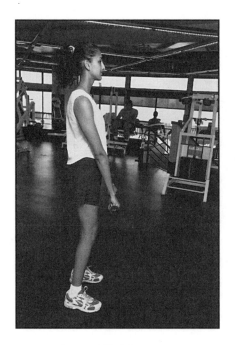

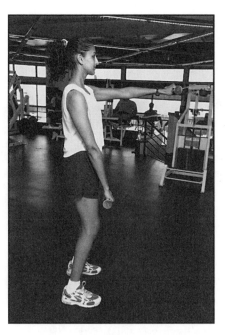

Front raise start/finish position.   *Front raise midrange position.*

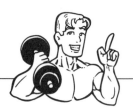

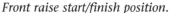

Spot Me

Although we have shown the front raise exercise with palms facing downward, people who have shoulder impingement syndrome should not perform it in this fashion since it can worsen the condition. Instead begin with your palms facing inward and keep them facing inward throughout the exercise.

Here is how you properly perform a front raise:

1. Stand with your feet shoulder width apart.

2. Hold a dumbbell in each hand at your sides with palms facing the legs.

3. Slowly raise one dumbbell up in front of the body until your arm is parallel to the floor.

4. Slowly return to the initial starting position.

5. Do a complete set with one arm before beginning the next arm.

The following is a list of don'ts:

➤ Rock your body back and forth.

➤ Raise your arms above the parallel position.

The following is a list of do's:

➤ Keep your abs tight.

➤ Maintain good posture.

Reverse Flyes

Reverse flyes are another one-joint exercise that isolates the posterior deltoid. Again, for the whole muscle to get strong, all of its parts must be worked.

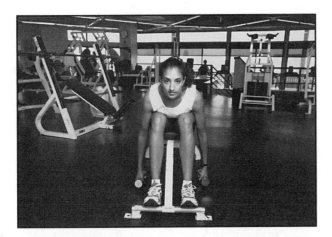

Reverse flye start/finish position.

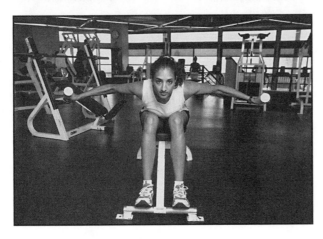

Reverse flye midrange position.

Here is how you properly perform a reverse flye:

1. Sit on a flat bench and bend forward at the waist.
2. Let the dumbbells hang down at your sides.
3. With a dumbbell in each hand, bring the dumbbells together, palms facing in.
4. Bend your elbows slightly as you raise the dumbbells away from the body.
5. Focus on squeezing your shoulder blades together.
6. With control, return to the starting position.

The following is a list of don'ts:

➤ Turn your head left or right.

➤ Raise your arms quickly, forcing your body forward.

➤ Allow the dumbbells to clang as you bring them together.

The following is a list of do's:

➤ Keep your abs tight.

➤ Maintain slow, controlled movement throughout the exercise.

➤ Squeeze your shoulder blades together at the top of the movement.

Machines

We've said it before and we'll say it again. Machines and freeweights are often interchangeable. The beauty of using both is that you won't have to wait for a bench or a set of weights if they're being used. And if you can't find a spotter, using a machine ensures that you can push to your max and not worry about dropping the weight on your foot. Here are some of our favorites.

Shoulder Press Machine

This machine is the kissin' cousin of the military press; however, unlike the freeweight version, which requires copious amounts of concentration, using the shoulder press machine is safer (and easier) since you neither have to stabilize the weight nor worry about it falling against your will.

Here is how you properly perform a shoulder press:

1. Sit on the bench with feet shoulder width apart.

2. Grasp the handles slightly wider than shoulder width apart.

3. Sit up straight and start your engine.

4. Push the handles up until your arms are just short of full extension.

5. Return to a position just short of the initial starting position to keep tension on the muscles. Remember to maintain control of the downward part of the lift.

The following is a list of don'ts:

➤ Lean backward.

➤ Lift your buttocks off the bench.

➤ Allow the elbows to snap or lockout in the midrange position.

➤ Allow the weight stack being lifted to slam against the remaining weight stack between repetitions.

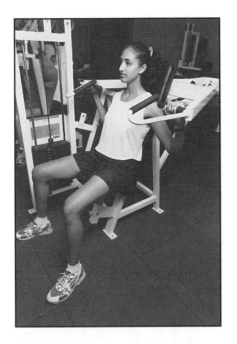

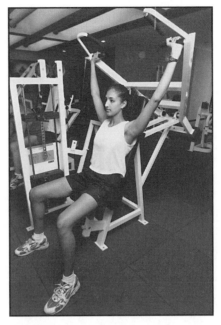

Shoulder press machine start/finish position.

Shoulder press machine midrange position.

The following is a list of do's:

➤ Keep your abdominals tight and your back erect.

➤ Keep your head on the bench.

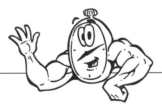

Weight a Minute

People with lower back pain or shoulder impingement syndrome should not do this exercise.

Lateral Raise Machine

This machine virtually duplicates the freeweight version of the side lateral raise. Some people prefer using a machine because it requires less concentration; others like using freeweights because it may be more comfortable for them, and they maintain a bit more control. Try both and you can make the call.

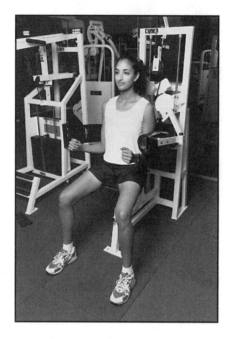

Lateral raise machine start/finish position.

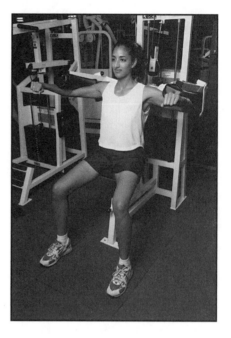

Lateral raise machine midrange position.

Here is how you properly perform a lateral raise:

1. Sit on the seat.

2. Position your upper arms against the arm pads, and lay your upper body against the back pad. The arms should extend straight down, and your elbows should be bent to 90[° with the palms facing in.

3. Keep the arms fairly straight, and raise them away from the body until they are parallel to the floor.

4. Return the weight gradually to a position just short of the initial starting position.

The following is a list of don'ts:

➤ Lift the arms to a position higher than parallel.

➤ Allow the weight stack being lifted to slam against the remaining weight stack between repetitions.

The following is a list of do's:

➤ Keep your upper body and head against the back pad to reduce the strain on your neck and back.

➤ Keep your abdominals tight and your back erect.

The Least You Need to Know

➤ The small muscles in your shoulders play a large role in your appearance and your performance on the playing field.

➤ Broad shoulders make your waist and hips look slimmer.

➤ Using a combination of isolating and pressing movements is the best way to build your delts.

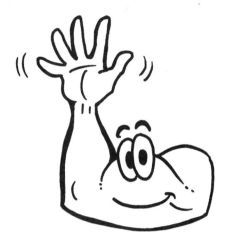

Chapter 19

Armed but Not Dangerous

In This Chapter

➤ Bulging biceps turn heads

➤ Building your biceps

➤ Boosting your triceps

Picture this: You walk into a gym for your first workout, and you're looking for a trainer. You see two trainers discussing amino acids by the office. Both have pleasing physiques but one has huge arms. Which one do you decide you want for your trainer? (Be honest.) Our practical experience says you go with Bobby Biceps.

Chew on this amusing "looks can be deceiving" tale. Jonathan used to work with a nutritionist who had enormous arms. Whenever they were together at the gym, people approached him with questions about arm exercises despite the fact that he had no real exercise background, and Jonathan, a lean endurance athlete who had a master's degree in Exercise Physiology, knew far more arm exercises than there are amino acids. Conversely, when people had questions pertaining to diet and losing weight, they came to Jonathan, assuming he was the man to ask, even though Mr. Biceps had a Ph.D. in nutrition. Go figure.

Joe's Uncle Harry, a short, jovial guy who worked for years as a paper salesman, had biceps like cannonballs from lifting stacks of paper all day. Whenever he visited, Joe insisted he make a muscle for Joe to squeeze. Even though he was only 5-feet, 5-inches, those prodigious melons on his upper arm made him feel large. The point is that bulging biceps have long been symbols of masculine strength. (Oh, Popeye, where have you gone?) Perhaps the biggest reason for this is their highly visible location. Another reason they're so identified with strength is that very often very strong men have very large arms.

As we'll discuss later, a lot of this has to do with who you picked as your parents (in other words, genetics). Regardless, big or not so big, there are lots of real-life reasons to have strong biceps.

Biceps Belong

The biceps span the front of the upper arm, beginning at the upper part of the long bone of your arm (*humerus*) and ending at the point just beyond where your elbow bends. The action of the biceps is to bend the elbow and to turn your palm up toward the ceiling. This action of flexion and supination is the way you show off when you make a muscle like Joe's lovable Uncle Harry.

Why strong biceps? Because of the following reasons:

➤ Assistance with exercises for larger body parts. If your biceps are weak, they won't be of much help when performing exercises for your back.

➤ Activities of daily living. If your biceps are weak, your arms will tire while carrying your kid from the car to the bedroom, carrying packages, or using a screwdriver.

➤ They look good. Right or wrong, big biceps are seen as a sign of strength.

Here's the skinny when it comes to your biceps. These smallish muscles are involved in virtually every pulling movement you do (lat pull downs, cable rows, and many more). As a result, you don't have to do many concentrated biceps exercises. We also recommend that you save your biceps routine for one of the last groups of exercises that you do. Why? If you exhaust your biceps first, you won't get an effective workout for your larger body parts because your biceps won't be able to withstand much more fatigue.

Bicep Freeweights

We have listed several freeweight exercises to get you started in the gym. Remember our strength-training mantra: Pay careful attention to your technique and posture. That means sitting and standing in an erect yet relaxed position, breathing deeply from your belly, and lifting the weight slowly through a full range of motion.

Standing Curls

This is the classic biceps exercise. If you have back problems, you should do this while standing against a wall. Even if you have a sound back, pay special attention to keeping your back straight and elbows close to your sides.

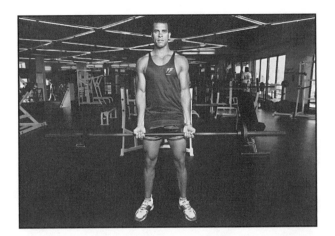

Standing curl start/finish position.

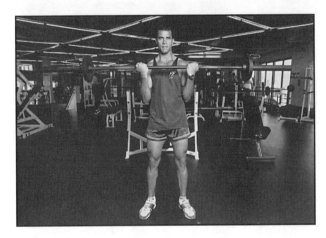

Standing curl midrange position.

Here is how you properly perform a standing curl:

1. Grip the barbell with palms facing outward, shoulder width apart.
2. Stand with your feet approximately shoulder width apart.
3. Begin with the bar resting on the front of your thighs.
4. Slowly raise the bar by bending your elbows toward your shoulders; slowly lower the bar to the front of your thighs.
5. Control the downward motion during this negative phase.

The following is a list of don'ts:

➤ Rock back and forth or bend backward in an effort to get the weight up. If you must do this you've used too much weight and should lighten the load.

➤ Let your elbows wander up as you lift.

➤ Curl the weight all the way up to your shoulders.

The following is a list of do's:

➤ Keep your knees slightly bent and your abdomen held tight; this will protect your back.

➤ Keep your elbows tucked in close to your body.

Dumbbell Curls

Dumbbell curls are similar to barbell curls except, well, you're using dumbbells, and instead of working both biceps at the same time, you have the option of lifting both simultaneously or alternately. Since alternating gives the muscle time to rest as the other arm is working, we prefer to work both arms together.

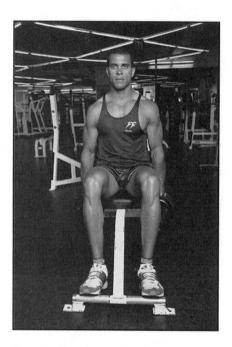

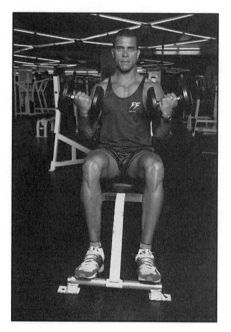

Dumbbell curl start/finish position.　　　　*Dumbbell curl midrange position.*

Here is how you properly perform a dumbbell curl:

1. Stand (or sit) with a dumbbell in each hand, palms facing inward.

2. Slowly bend your elbow. As you do, begin to twist your wrists so your palms are facing upward.

3. Stop just short of your shoulders.

4. Slowly straighten your elbow. As you do, begin to twist your wrists so that your palms are facing inward again.

5. Return to your initial starting position.

The following is a list of don'ts:

➤ Shrug your shoulders as you raise the dumbbells.

➤ Rock back and forth or arch your back. Again, decrease the weight if you find this happening.

The following is a list of do's:

➤ Keep your elbows pinned in close to your body.

➤ Keep your knees slightly bent if standing, and keep your abdomen tight whether you are standing or sitting, to protect your back.

Concentration Curls

Concentration curls are a great way to ensure that you use strict form on your curls. Because they're a little harder, you'll have to use less weight than in the previous exercise.

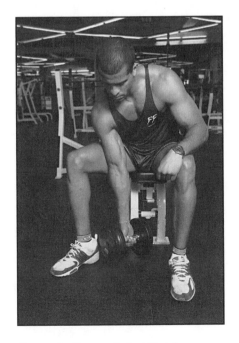

Concentration curl start/finish position.

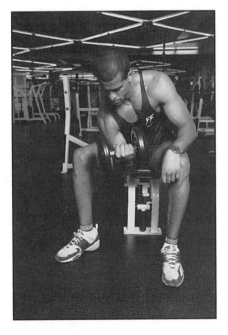

Concentration curl midrange position.

Here is how you properly perform a concentration curl:

1. With a dumbbell in your hand, sit on a bench and lean forward and rest your arm on the inner part of your thigh.

2. Your palm should be facing your opposite thigh.

3. Raise the dumbbell by slowly bending to a point just short of your shoulder.

4. Lower the dumbbell by slowly straightening your elbow to the starting position.

The following is a list of don'ts:

➤ Lean or rock backward and forward in an effort hoist the dumbbell up—you could hurt your back. If your form isn't perfect, immediately lessen the weight.

➤ Move your leg from side to side in an effort to help you lift the weight

The following is a do:

➤ Keep your abdomen tight and your back erect as you are leaning forward.

Bicep Machines

As we stated earlier, machines add variety to your workout. They're also helpful if you plan to *work heavy* (use a lot of weight during a particular session) and you don't have a spotter. The good news about training your biceps, however, is that you're not likely to hurt yourself even if you go heavy because you never have to worry about anything falling on top of you and crushing you.

The major benefit of machines versus freeweights is the constant tension placed on the muscle through every part of the movement. Typically, with freeweights you can *rest* in the up or down position, while the middle position is harder. In addition, there is less room to cheat by using your whole body to lift the weight.

Cable Curls

Cable curls are roughly equivalent to alternate dumbbell curls. They're good to do because they allow constant tension to be placed on the muscle throughout the entire range of motion. They are also good because they give you a psychological change of pace.

Here is how you properly perform a cable curl:

1. Grab hold of the handle from the bottom attachment of the Cable Crossover machine. (Different, interchangeable attachments are often used on cables. For this exercise use a square-shaped handle.)

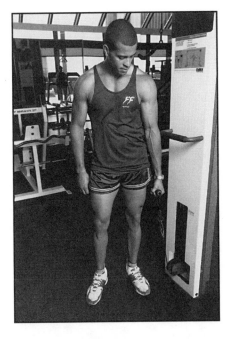

Cable curl start/finish position.

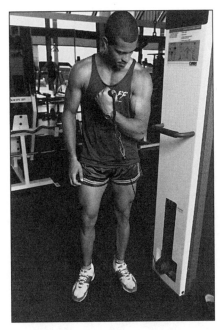

Cable curl midrange position.

2. Make sure that your palm is facing inward with your arm crossing your body slightly.

3. Stand with your feet shoulder width apart.

4. Slowly bend your elbow, stopping just short of your shoulder.

5. Slowly straighten your elbow, stopping just short of a fully straight position. The rhythm is the same here as for every other exercise, up for a three count and down for a three count.

The following is a list of don'ts:

➤ Lean backward to assist you with getting the weight up. If you need to do this before your last rep, reduce the weight instead.

➤ Allow the weight to bring your body forward as you lower it. If this happens, please lighten the load.

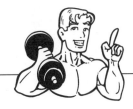

Spot Me

Although you will see people doing this exercise with both arms, we don't recommend it. Why? Because doing bilateral bicep cable curls will encourage you to arch your back. Unilateral bicep cable curls allow you to maintain proper posture during the exercise.

233

The following is a do:

➤ Keep your abdomen tight and knees slightly bent to protect your back.

Machine Curls

This exercise really isolates your biceps and makes it harder for you to cheat.

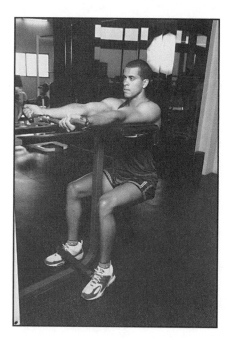
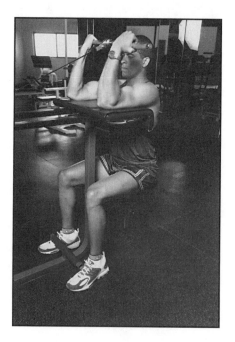

Machine curl start/finish position.   *Machine curl midrange position.*

Here is how you properly perform a machine curl:

1. Sit on the seat, and place your arms on the pad. (Make sure that a trainer has shown you how to adjust the machine for a proper fit. A poor fit will make the exercise less effective and place more stress on your elbow and shoulder joints.)

2. Grab hold of the handles.

3. Feet should be flat on the floor.

4. Slowly bend your elbows as far as you can; then slowly straighten your elbows, stopping just short of a fully straight position.

The following is a list of don'ts:

➤ Allow the weight to bring you up out of the seat as you lower the weight.

➤ Hold your breath.

The following is a do:

➤ Maintain good form, three count up and three count down.

Tricep Freeweights

You know what gives championship boxers their powerful jab? Biceps? Alas, you're wrong. It's the triceps that are responsible for that piston-like punch that will keep your opponent (or the heavy bag) at bay.

Typically, when we train biceps we do exercises to work the triceps as well. Located in the back of your upper arm, the triceps and biceps are neighbors who share a back-yard fence. The triceps are actually made of three muscles, hence the name. There are several exercises we'll describe that can be used to strengthen each of the three. This triangular-shaped set of muscles is involved whenever you use your shoulders or chest in pressing, pushing movements.

Why strong triceps? Because of the following reasons:

➤ They come in handy if you're forced to square off with Mike Tyson.

➤ Your prowess at pushing a shopping cart will improve.

➤ You'll have much stronger arms.

Tricep Kickbacks

The tricep kickback is a great way to isolate your triceps, but it requires strict form to be effective. You'll know you're doing it correctly when you feel the burn in the rear of your arm.

Here is how you properly perform a tricep kickback:

1. Place one knee and hand on the bench for support.

2. Slightly bend the standing leg.

3. The working arm should be bent 90° at the shoulder and 90° at the elbow.

4. Keep your arm close to your side. To gain the full benefit from this exercise it's important to keep your upper arm parallel to the ground. Pay strict attention to your form.

5. Slowly straighten your elbow and return to the starting position.

*Tricep kickback start/
finish position.*

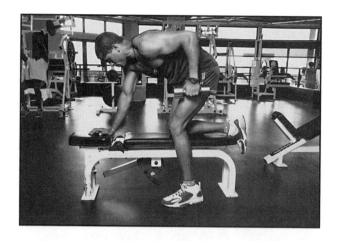

*Tricep kickback midrange
position.*

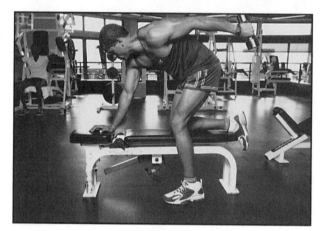

The following is a list of don'ts:

➤ Allow your back to sag.

➤ Shift your body back and forth in an effort to get the weight up.

➤ Let your upper arm drop—keep it parallel to the ground throughout the range of motion.

The following is a list of do's:

➤ Keep your back straight and your abdomen tight.

➤ Keep your eyes fixed on the bench. Looking up or sideways can put stress on your neck.

French Curls

We're not sure why this particular exercise is identified with France, but feel free to do it regardless of your nationality. The bottom line is that it's an excellent way to work your triceps.

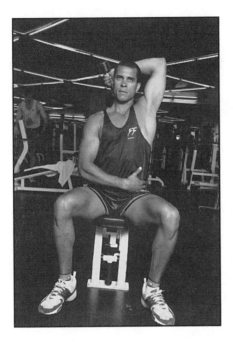

French curl start/finish position.

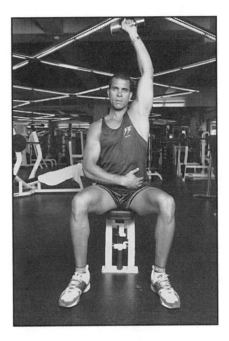

French curl midrange position.

Here is how you properly perform a French curl:

1. While standing or sitting, raise the dumbbell overhead and bend your elbow to a point where you are feeling a stretch in the tricep.

2. Begin to straighten your elbow, and slowly return to your initial starting position.

The following is a list of don'ts:

➤ Shift your body from side to side in an effort to raise the weight.

➤ Snap or lock your elbow upon straightening it.

➤ Allow the weight to fall rapidly to the starting position.

The following is a list of do's:

➤ Keep your abdomen tight whether sitting or standing.

➤ Concentrate on your triceps and move gently through a full range of motion.

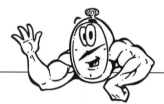

Weight a Minute

Be careful if you have been diagnosed with *shoulder impingement syndrome* (an abnormal squeezing of the structures within the shoulder joint). French curls can worsen the condition.

Tricep Machines

As we stated earlier, machines add spice to your workout and can be beneficial by forcing you to work hard throughout the entire range of motion. In fact, when working these relatively small biceps and triceps muscles, machines often provide a more complete workout since they so thoroughly isolate the muscle.

Pushdowns

It's important to push hard at the bottom of the repetition to tighten (contract) the tricep. You can use either a rope or bar attachment to perform this exercise; the rope is the harder of the two, and you will typically use less weight than with the bar.

Here is how you properly perform a pushdown:

1. Grab hold of the pushdown bar. Your elbows should be bent to 90 degrees and held close to your side.

2. Slowly straighten your elbows, and return to your initial starting position.

The following is a list of don'ts:

➤ Lean forward as you push the weight down. This reduces the isolation from the triceps and transfers it to your whole body.

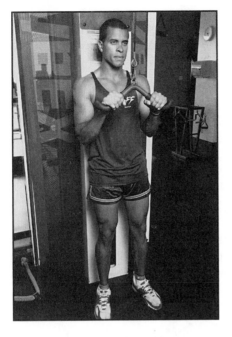 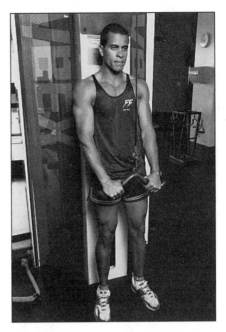

Pushdown start/finish position.   *Pushdown midrange position.*

➤ Lock your elbows in the straightened position.

➤ Allow the weight to fall rapidly.

The following is a list of do's:

➤ Keep your abdomen tight and your back erect.

➤ Keep your head facing forward, not down or sideways.

➤ Keep your elbows close to your side.

Wrist Not, Want Not

The muscles that work to bend and straighten our wrists actually originate at the elbow. In case you were curious, the muscles that bend (flex) the wrist originate on the inner part of the elbow. The muscles that straighten (extend) the wrist originate on the outer aspect of the elbow.

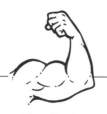

Flex Facts

If you have *carpal tunnel syndrome*, do not perform these exercises, since they're likely to aggravate it. This condition is often caused by repetitive activities done with improper body mechanics such as typing with your wrists in an extended position (they should be neutral) or repetitive squeezing activities (such as what a cake decorator would do when decorating a cake). The median nerve swells and is unable to pass comfortably through the small bones in your wrist (carpals). Symptoms of carpal tunnel syndrome are numbness, tingling, or a sharp, shooting pain into your hand.

Why strong wrists? Because of the following reasons:

➤ Weak wrist muscles can lead to golfer's elbow (*medial epicondylitis*) or tennis elbow (*lateral epicondylitis*). These injuries affect the pros as well as weekend warriors like you and me.

➤ Everyday activities like carrying heavy grocery bags or luggage can put strain on these muscles. In fact, people who use a screwdriver frequently suffer from tendinitis.

➤ If you care to embark on a career as a professional arm wrestler, you'll need strong wrists.

The best medicine is the preventive kind, which is why strengthening your wrists is important. A good way to avoid this condition is to do the following exercises.

Wrist Flexion

Here is how you properly perform wrist flexion:

1. Lean forward.

2. Place your forearms on your thighs. The dumbbell should be held in a position past your knees with your palm up.

3. Allow your wrist to bend as far back as you comfortably can.

4. Slowly bend your wrist up as far as you can; return to the initial starting position.

Wrist Extension

Perform this exercise the same as you would the wrist flexion, except your palms should be facing down (instead of up).

Here is a don't for wrist flexion and extension:

➤ Perform the movements rapidly in either direction.

And a do:

➤ Keep your abdomen tight and your back erect.

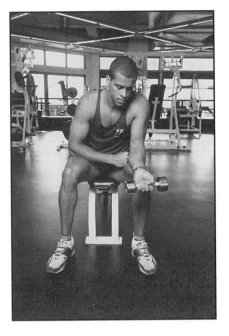 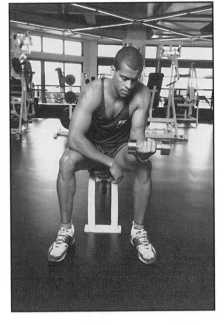

Wrist flexion start/finish position.   *Wrist flexion midrange position.*

The Least You Need to Know

➤ Strong biceps look good and help in a variety of sports.

➤ Triceps get less attention than biceps, but are actually bigger and equally important.

➤ Strong wrists will help prevent injuries.

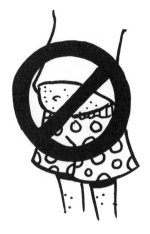

Gut Buster

Here's a bit of abdominal irony to ponder: As a nation we seem to loathe fat people even though we're the most overweight nation in the Western world. A portly belly might have been a sign of prosperity in the Far East, but in our culture a flat stomach is a prized possession, despite the fact that most people refuse to do what it takes to get there.

Socioeconomic implications aside, there are several solid reasons to build a washboard stomach: 1) it looks good; 2) it will make you feel better, especially if you have an ailing back; 3) you'll be stronger in the weight room and on the playing field; 4) you may become a famous underwear model.

Before we give you the lowdown on building up your midsection, let's review our anatomy. The first, and most common mistake, is referring to the abdominals (the "abs") as "the stomach." The abs are the muscles in your midsection; your stomach is the organ that processes the food you consume. Ab exercises have traditionally included sit-ups and leg lifts; stomach exercises include dining in a French restaurant.

Your abdominals consist of four muscles:

➤ The *rectus abdominis,* the largest muscle in the abs, is a wide, flat sheet of muscle that runs from just under the lower part of your chest to just below your belly button. When you do abdominal crunches, the old rectus abdominis muscle is hard at work. (For more on crunches, read on.) It also keeps your spine from slip-sliding around when you're exercising other body parts.

➤ The *internal obliques* and *external obliques,* which run diagonally along your sides, not only assist the rectus in curling the spine, but also twist and bend your upper body. These muscles are central in any sport involving upper body rotation—golf, baseball, kayaking, and many more—and they are integral in a strengthening program, especially if you have a bad back. Why? These muscles wrap around your waist and, when properly conditioned, provide much-needed support for your lower back. In essence, the obliques are the world's most comfortable, form-fitting girdle.

➤ The *transversus abdominis,* which sounds like a phrase from a Latin Mass, is the deepest of all the muscles in your abs. Located directly below the rectus abdominis, it is called into action when you sneeze, cough, or exhale forcefully. There are no specific exercises you can do to target this muscle, but you can strengthen the transversus abdominis by forcefully exhaling during the positive phase of your ab exercises.

Feel the Burn

As we have mentioned, having strong abs will significantly help you get rid of lower back pain. Try this: Sit in a chair. Hold your abs tight. Now let them go. Did you note a difference in your posture? You see, your abs are what keep your pelvis in a neutral position. When they are weak, your pelvis has a tendency to tilt forward, increasing the inward curve of your lumbar spine. This, of course, will throw the rest of your spine out of whack as well. All you have to do to see what we're talking about is check out the exaggerated curve of someone with a sizeable beer belly. Contrast that, say, with the posture of an athlete like an Olympic gymnast and you can begin to see the relationship between strong abs, good posture, and improved athletic performance.

Perhaps because there's so much discussion and even obsession with our bulging waistlines, there's a lot of misinformation surrounding the abs that we'd like to clear up.

Here are a few of the most common midsection myths:

1. *If I work my abs, I'll get rid of my love handles.* This is the one we hear most often. However, the bottom line is that you can do 5,000 sit-ups a day and if you still

have excess adipose tissue (a fancy medical term for *fat*), you'll have really strong abs to accompany your love handles. Since the muscle lies beneath the fat, if you consume more calories than you burn, these powerful muscles will function efficiently but not be revealed to the public at large. In other words, strong abs and love handles have nothing to do with each other. Want to lose the excess baggage? Eat less, and do more cardiovascular exercise.

2. *I need to do 500 crunches a day to get my abs in really great shape.* In fact, if you can do 500 crunches a day, you're either a Navy SEAL in training or doing something quite wrong. Done correctly, 10 to 25 repetitions for three sets is more than enough to get the job done. Why waste your time by doing so many, especially if you do them incorrectly?

3. *I do my abs every day for maximum benefit.* This is another line we hear a lot in the gym. While the abs can be worked more than your chest or biceps, for example, you should treat your abs as you treat any other muscles. Remember that they need rest just like any other stressed body part.

Freeweights

When we talk about freeweights in this chapter, we're referring to floor exercises as opposed to the various apparatus you will find in the gym. You may remember that a few years back, the Ab Roller entered the market and advertised itself as the next best thing to sliced bread. In fact, every gym this side of Istanbul had one and many frustrated people who'd been doing ab work for many a moon thought that this simple contraption was the knight in shining armor they'd been looking for. Well, the bottom line with the Ab Roller, and similar contraptions that resemble an upside-down rocking chair, is that the floor works just as well. And it's not nearly as expensive. Having said that, the machine is good for people who have neck pain, as well as those unable to keep their neck muscles relaxed throughout the exercise. So while you might want to start out using the Ab Roller in order to learn the proper position, once you learn the technique there's no reason you can't do crunches on the floor.

Crunches

If you're stuck on a dessert island with just one ab exercise, crunches are the one. Done properly, you're bound to feel a nice burn in no time flat.

Here is how you properly perform a crunch:

1. Lie on a mat with your knees bent and feet on the floor. Depending on your level of fitness, you can place your arms in any of the three following positions:

   Beginner: With your arms straight at your sides and your fingers pointing toward your knees.

Crunch start/finish.

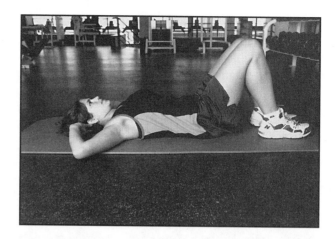

Crunch midrange.

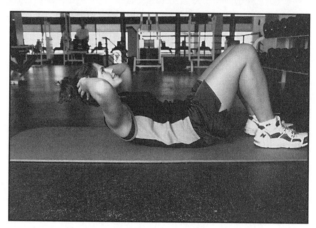

Intermediate: With your arms crossed over your chest.

Advanced: With your elbows bent and your fingers overlapping behind your neck.

2. Tighten your stomach muscles and slowly curl your torso up until your shoulder blades are off the floor.

3. Slowly return to your starting position without completely relaxing on the floor.

Initially the exercise may feel rather easy; however, after several reps you should begin to feel a burn in the upper third of your abs.

The following is a list of don'ts:

➤ Bend your neck as you curl into the crunch position. This is the biggest reason that people who do a lot of ab work complain. Imagine having a softball between your chin and your chest.

➤ Draw your elbows in. You're trying to lift your torso, not flap your elbows.

➤ Bring your torso up past 30°.

The following is a list of do's:

➤ Keep your head and neck in a neutral position; the less stress on your neck, the better.

➤ Make sure that you curl as you lift.

➤ Focus your attention on the top section of your abdominals. Let them do the work and not any other part of your upper body.

➤ Keep your lower back pressed against the floor at all times.

Reverse Crunches

Here's a tricky one that takes some time to get used to. It's not nearly as impressive-looking as some of the crazy leg lifts and other things you'll see people doing in an effort to strengthen their lower abs, but it's far more safe and effective.

Here is how you properly perform a reverse crunch:

1. Lie on a mat with your legs up and knees slightly bent. In the starting position you'll look like a big letter *L*.
2. Rest your arms on the floor at your sides.
3. Keep your head on the mat and tighten your abdominals.
4. Lift your butt off the floor so that your legs go up and slightly backward toward your head.
5. Hold this position for a second and slowly return to the starting position.

The following is a list of don'ts:

➤ Roll your hips so your back comes off the mat.

➤ Tighten your shoulders or involve any upper body movement.

➤ Hold your breath (people always seem to on this exercise).

Reverse crunch start/ finish.

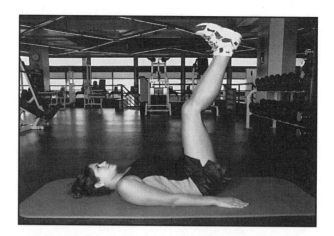

Reverse crunch midrange.

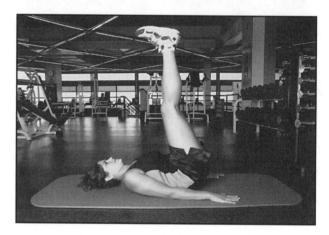

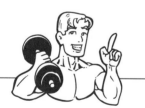

Spot Me

To help you visualize this exercise, think of a bee curling its bottom section to position its stinger. Not partial to bees? Think of a dog curling its tail.

The following is a list of do's:

➤ Keep the movement small—no need to roll back, too.

➤ Keep the movement smooth.

➤ Isolate the muscle by concentrating on the lower section of your abs.

Oblique Crunches

Here's another one that's commonly abused in the gym. Focus on moving your shoulder toward your opposite knee. Avoid the temptation to move your elbow in or your knee back.

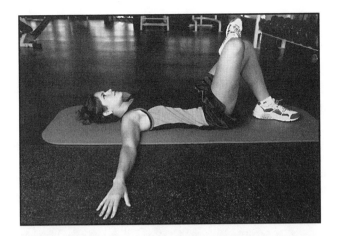

Oblique crunch start/ finish.

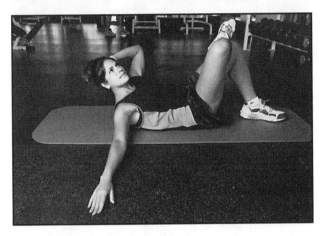

Oblique crunch midrange.

Here is how you properly perform an oblique crunch:

1. Lie on a mat with your left leg bent and your foot flat on the floor.
2. Place your right ankle so that it rests on top of your left knee.
3. Position your left hand behind your neck and keep your right arm outstretched.
4. Slowly curl up and twist toward your right knee.
5. Hold that position for a second and then slowly return to the starting position.
6. Switch legs and arms and repeat on the other side.

The following is a list of don'ts:

➤ Bend your head with your hand.
➤ Merely move your elbow to your knee.

The following is a list of do's:

➤ Curl and twist your shoulder toward your opposite knee.

➤ Keep the movement slow and controlled.

Side Obliques

Here's an alternative to the previous exercise. Use it to break up the monotony whenever you please. If you choose them, make sure to keep your knees over to the side to keep the focus on the obliques.

Side oblique start/finish.

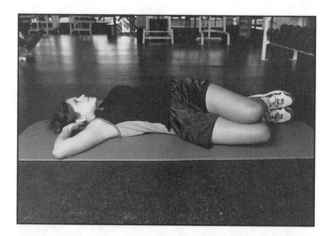

Side oblique midrange.

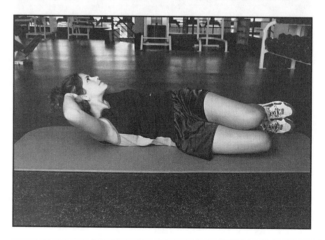

Here is how you properly perform a side oblique:

1. Lie on a mat on your right side with your knees bent.
2. Place both hands behind your neck and keep your head looking straight at the ceiling.
3. Use your oblique muscles to lift your upper body slightly off the mat.
4. Hold yourself off the mat for a second and then return to your starting position.

The following is a don't:

➤ Bend your neck to the side as you lift your torso off the mat.

The following is a list of do's:

➤ Keep your shoulder and head going straight toward the ceiling.
➤ Make sure your knees stay over to the side.

Machines

Generally speaking, we prefer floor exercises to weight machines for your abs. The design of many machines allows you to cheat by using your hip flexors to assist in the movement, taking the emphasis away from the abs. Still, machines do have some advantages, most notably the ability to easily change the resistance.

Machine Crunches

If you've ever seen an Orthodox Jew praying (or dovening) in synagogue, it looks a lot like a seated crunch. To isolate your abdomen, slowly move the arm pad toward your knees using the muscles in your upper abs. Pause for a second at the bottom of the repetition and return to the starting position without completely releasing the tension in your abs.

Here is how you properly perform a machine crunch:

1. Sit on the seat and fasten the belt.
2. Place your arms on top of the arm pad.
3. Slowly tighten your abdominal muscles, curling your torso forward. As you do this, you'll be bringing the arm pad toward your thighs.

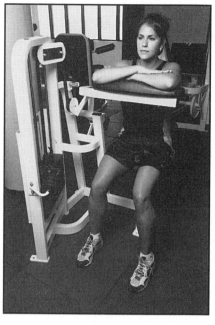 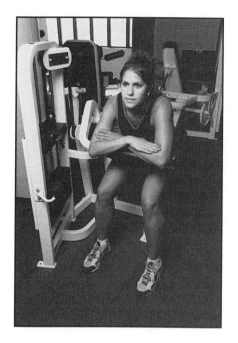

Machine crunch start/finish.   *Machine crunch midrange.*

The following is a list of don'ts:

➤ Use too much weight so that your hips are lifted off the seat.

➤ Let the weights that you're lifting slam down on the stack.

➤ Arch your back as you return to the starting position.

➤ Focus on pushing the arm pad down; rather, concentrate on curling your abdomen.

The following is a do:

➤ Keep constant tension on your abdominals as you perform the exercise.

Rotary Torso

This machine does a great job of isolating the obliques. Still, we're not big fans of this machine unless you're careful to use strict form. Do it smoothly and you'll be fine; however, constant, weighted, and uncontrolled rotation can cause your back more harm than the good it will do for your abs.

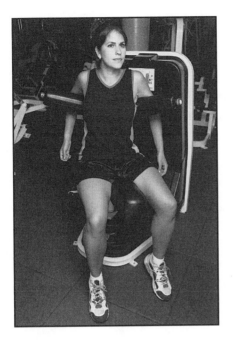 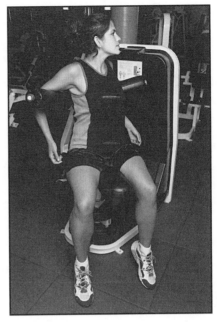

Rotary torso start/finish. *Rotary torso midrange.*

Here is how you properly perform a rotary torso:

1. Sit on the seat.
2. Position your arms behind each arm pad. Get ready to twist like a young Elvis.
3. Slowly twist your body until you can twist no farther.
4. Pause for a second and slowly return to the starting position.
5. Repeat on the other side.

The following is a list of don'ts:

➤ Use your arms to assist you.
➤ Let the weights you're lifting slam on the stack below.

The following is a do:

➤ Maintain a slow, controlled movement throughout the rotation.

People with back problems shouldn't use this machine. Instead, stick with floor exercises where you have greater control. The twisting motion can aggravate a back condition.

The Least You Need to Know

➤ A strong set of abs will improve your looks, health, and athletic performance.

➤ Abdominal exercises won't reduce fat in your mid-section, but they will strengthen your muscles.

➤ There's no need to do hundreds of reps. Use the same form for ab exercises as for any other muscles.

➤ Strong abdominal muscles support and stabilize you for other exercises and activities.

Part 5

Leaner and Meaner

Now that you've learned the nuances of the equipment, the exercises, and the philosophy behind working out, we're going to show you how to put it all together. Chapter 21 gives you guidelines on which exercises to include in your routine depending on your goals and time constraints, and what to do if things aren't working out the way you expected.

In Chapters 22 and 23 we introduce you to a variety of advanced techniques to help you take that next significant step.

In Chapter 24, you'll get a primer on the basics of bodybuilding, powerlifting, and Olympic lifting, the three pillars in the pantheon of weight-lifting sports. And in Chapter 25, we'll give the serious athlete and the weekend warrior suggested workouts to help elevate your game. Finally, in Chapter 26 you'll find everything you'll need to know about cardiovascular exercise.

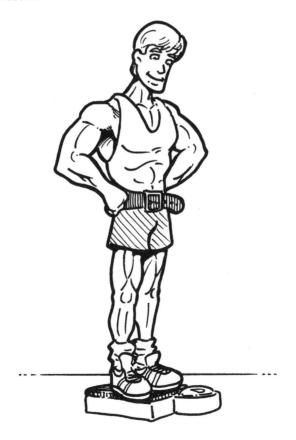

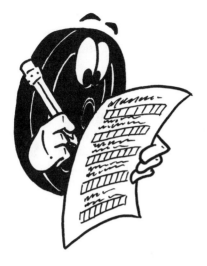

Chapter 21

Get With the Program

In This Chapter

➤ Putting it all together

➤ Knowing when sore is good

➤ Understanding when too much is bad

➤ Being bored no more

Now that you've read this far, you no doubt know more than you ever wanted to know about form, safety, sets, and reps, as well as a slew of Latin words that ensure that you know the difference between your lats and your pecs. In addition, you're now familiar with the mechanics of a host of exercises to keep you busy into the next millennium. What you may not know, however, is how to put it all together. Having all the ingredients for a soufflé is one thing; knowing how to assemble them is another. In this and in the ensuing chapters, we'll show you how to take the information we've discussed thus far in order to build a workout routine fit for a hungry king.

As we've mentioned before, talk to a dozen fitness experts, and you're liable to get half a dozen or more opinions on how much to lift, how often, and more. While virtually everyone will tell you to progress from larger muscles to smaller muscles, the wide variety of opinions can be quite confusing. While we can't say that anyone who disagrees with us is full of iron, we can tell you that if you follow what we say in this and the chapters that follow, you'll get stronger as well as look and feel better. If you're skeptical, try one of the following routines and see for yourself.

Finally, we realize that all gyms are not created equal. As a result, you may not have all the equipment that we demonstrated at your disposal. To account for this athletic inequity, we've included a few different basic workout plans to get you started.

What to Do

When you look over the programs listed below, your first reaction may be that there are not a whole lot of exercises included. There's a reason for this. Since we're asking you to work hard and exhibit perfect form on each, the trade-off is that we won't ask you to do a lot of exercises. After all, it's only human that your concentration and willpower will falter if you have to do an endless series of exercises each time out. As we promised way back in Chapter 2, "Hurry Up and Weight," working out won't take you all day, and we meant it.

These basic routines shouldn't take more than 45 minutes each. That includes about one minute for each of the exercises and two minutes off between each set. While that's not a significant investment in time, if you do these routines faithfully—with effort and concentration—you'll get stronger. As you can see from the chart below, we've imitated a Chinese menu (one from column A; one from column B) and tried to give you the option of deciding between free weights or machine exercises whenever possible. Depending on your preference and the availability of any one machine or free weight apparatus, there's no need to stick with one or the other exclusively.

Whenever you see an exercise highlighted that means we want you to do a light warm-up set with about half your normal weight before moving on to your regular set of these exercises. Remember to aim for sets of 10 to 12 reps with a three-second positive and three-second negative, with a one-second pause between. In other words, lifting the weight will take three seconds, the downward phase will take three seconds, and so on until the set is done. Take two minutes between exercises. You can take less time if you care to, but try hard not to take more. If you do, that 45-minute figure will creep over the one-hour mark.

Here's the chart to help you pick one of the following exercises from the machine column and/or freeweight column. As we said, feel free to mix it up—use some free-weight exercises and some machines if you like. Work your way from the top of the list down to the bottom.

Mix and Match Machines and Freeweights

Muscles	Machine Exercise	Freeweight Exercise
Glutes, quads, hamstrings	Leg press	Lunges
Quads	Leg extension	
Hamstrings	Leg curl	

Muscles	Machine Exercise	Freeweight Exercise
Gastroc (calves)	Standing toe raise	
Lats	Lat pull down	Pull-ups (assisted if necessary)
Traps		Shrug
Pecs	Chest press	Bench press
	Flye	Pec deck
Delts	Shoulder press	Dumbbell military press
	Lateral raise	Lateral raise
Biceps	Biceps machine	Seated dumbbell curl
Triceps	Triceps pushdown	French curl
Abs	Abdominal machine	Crunches
Obliques	Rotary torso	Oblique crunches
Lower back	Back raise	

Keeping Track

Your main goal during the first few weeks is to learn to do the exercises properly. At the same time, it's important that you keep track of what you're doing. That's where a workout log comes in. We don't want to make this seem like preparing your income tax; however, keeping accurate records of your workouts not only will help you track your progress, it's also a great way to figure out what to do when you hit a plateau. Getting stronger requires that you overload your muscles; as a result it's key that you know what you've done in previous workouts. If you're anything like us, you'll actually find it fun to see how much progress you've made in a relatively short amount of time.

Your workout log should list everything you've done that day in the gym—your choice of exercises, how much weight, how many reps—as well as the height of the seat on the machines you're using. It's also a good idea to note how you were feeling on that day; your body weight, and any other relevant facts. In time, you'll see that this physical record is a diary that will accurately reflect the relationship between your mental, physical, and emotional life. In fact, the more carefully you note the impact of outside factors on your lifting, the more you're likely to see a powerful relationship between how all facets of your life affect your weight training.

I'm Late, I'm Late

Of course, in this busy world where time is often money, even 45 minutes can seem like too much time to spare. If that's the case, don't worry. It's far better to work out just a little than not at all. Let's say you want to squeeze in a workout at lunch and

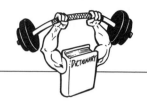

Bar Talk

Multijoint or **compound movements** are exercises that involve two or more joints. Single-joint or **isolation movements** use only one. Compound movements like the bench press or squat use more musculature and generally result in the weight moving in a fairly straight line; whereas isolation moves like the flye or leg extension focus on a specific muscle and usually have a rotary movement.

still have time to shower and grab a bite. Or perhaps you want to run a couple of miles and have just 20 minutes or so to lift afterward. No matter; we'll give you a condensed workout to keep you on track. These shorter workouts are not as thorough as the longer version, and they're better suited to maintaining strength rather than getting you stronger, but it takes care of the basics. Just as important, it ensures that you won't lose fitness.

The shorter workout is essentially the same as the longer one. The biggest difference is that each of these exercises is a *multijoint* or *compound movement*, meaning that you'll be working at least two joints. That means you'll be working more muscles during any one lift. *Single-joint* or *isolation movements* like the flye (chest) or lateral raise (shoulder) are great, but you don't cover as much ground with each exercise.

Again, do a light warm-up set of the highlighted exercises. Reduce your recovery time between sets from two minutes to one. Done correctly, you're in and out in less than 15 minutes. Remember that just because you're in a hurry, it doesn't mean that your reps should be performed quickly. Focus on proper form, and get as much out of each and every rep that you can. The key here is intensity.

The following table can be your quickie guide to a great 15-minute workout.

15-Minute Workout

Muscle	Exercise
Glutes, hamstrings, quads	Leg press
Lats	**Lat pull down or pull-ups**
Pecs	**Bench press or dips**
Traps	Upright rows
Delts	Shoulder press
Abs	Crunches

If you've got a little more time and desire, check out Chapters 22 through 25 where we give you a variety of advanced techniques built to accommodate a wide variety of goals and aspirations. In Chapters 28 through 31, we'll address issues that affect specific groups like teens and the elderly. For now, these will get you started and allow you to build a good foundation of strength.

Progress Report

Let's say you've done every rep of every set with perfect form. Let's also assume that you warm up and stretch religiously, and your nutrition is as pure as a field of soy beans. What you will discover, no doubt, is that no matter how slowly you started your program, you've had your share of aches and pains. If you're wondering if this is normal, the answer is "yes." The bottom line is that while we'll do everything we can to help you avoid injuries, muscle soreness is a natural consequence of a new weight-lifting program.

Whenever you introduce a new activity to your body, you experience what we will call growing pains. This is a natural consequence as your muscles, tendons, and ligaments adapt to the new stresses and strains of muscular overload. In fact, even someone who is ridiculously fit will be sore if they do a new routine with any intensity. What we want you to be able to do is differentiate between *good* hurt and *bad* hurt. Good hurt you can work through; bad hurt is a sure signal to stop immediately.

There are two types of soreness that you're likely to experience during weight training: acute soreness—the discomfort you feel during and right after a set—and a more gradual, duller ache that comes on in the days after you lift.

The Burn

In gym parlance, acute soreness is referred to as the "burn." Typically, it occurs during and immediately following exercise. When you're completing the last few reps of a set, your muscles are working hard. As the muscle is taxed, it actually presses against your arteries and cuts off blood flow. (This is the rough equivalent of having an inflated cuff on when you're having your blood pressure taken.) As a result, lactic acid, a by-product of anaerobic activity, accumulates. This combination of lactic acid and blood flow occlusion is what is thought to cause momentary muscle failure. Got that? The miracle of the human body is that within a few seconds of the end of the set, the burn dissipates as the muscle is engorged with even more blood than usual to compensate for what was lost during the set. This process is what causes the temporary (but ego-boosting) "pump" phenomenon.

The DOMS

Delayed onset muscle soreness (DOMS) refers to pain and soreness that occurs 24 to 48 hours after exercise. DOMS is due to the microscopic muscle damage that takes place when you lift. The eccentric or negative phase of the exercise contributes more than its fair share to this soreness—especially if you use extra weight for the negatives (a technique we'll describe in the next chapter). Usually, you'll feel the beginning of DOMS the day after you lift; however, it often reaches its peak at about 48 hours after the fact. Putting ice on the affected area can help reduce some of the edema at the site and help alleviate the pain. The soreness should start to ease after that and last no more than three to four days. If the pain lasts significantly longer or becomes worse, we suggest you see a physician.

That Hurts!

A *burn* during a set and soreness afterwards is as common as a pigeon in a park. While the term *good pain* may be a classic oxymoron, there certainly are normal pains associated with the weight-lifting game. Of course, some types of pain are not normal and shouldn't be taken lightly. In fact, unless you've been doing it a long while, the old bromide of "No pain, no gain" is generally considered passé and counterproductive.

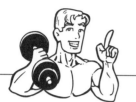

Spot Me

Though we've given you a number reasons why you should stretch, alleviating delayed onset muscle soreness is not one of them. Despite gym lore, stretching doesn't speed your recovery from DOMS. Studies have shown that while increased flexibility may help prevent or decrease the incidence of soreness in the first place, once you're sore stretching isn't going to help.

Here's the bottom line: Any sharp and shooting pain is bad, no matter where it occurs. Such an acute sensation is indicative of nerve pain and should send a warning that's attended to immediately. Pain that occurs in any of your joints (shoulder, elbow, wrist, hip, knee, or ankle) is also a red flag. As we've stressed all along, be mindful of your form and of the amount of weight that you are lifting.

If your form is not sound, you are putting additional stress on your joints simply because you are putting your body in a position that it doesn't want to be in. This means that even if you were performing the exercise with just your body weight, you would experience some pain and discomfort. Add a 15- to 45-pound barbell to the equation, and you're bound to aggravate the situation. It sounds so simple, but time and time again we see people lifting heavy weights with chronically injured joints. Determination clearly has a place in the gym, but when it's misapplied it's a sure way to court serious injury.

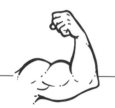

Flex Facts

While lactic acid is usually to blame when you feel a burning sensation during your lift or while sprinting to catch a bus, it's just an innocent bystander when it comes to DOMS. Even after a brutal workout, your lactic acid levels are back to normal within a couple of hours of a workout.

When Deidre was a competitive powerlifter, she hurt her left knee while squatting. It was swollen and painful for a few weeks. Not only did she have to stop squatting, she was forced to decrease the weight that she deadlifted. Her coach, John Gengo, couldn't figure out what happened until he watched videotape of her squatting. What he discovered was that her knees jutted out way beyond her toes instead of tracking directly over her toes as we advise in Chapter 15, "Below the Waist." This misalignment put significant stress on the knee joint. Once they changed her stance, she was able to return to squatting pain-free without a recurrence of the problem.

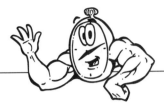

Weight a Minute

A burning sensation is normal during a challenging set of weight lifting, and soreness over the next couple of days is not unusual. However, any sharp or shooting pain while lifting is a red flag to stop immediately. If this occurs, never try to *fight through* such pain. Review your form to make sure you're not doing anything wrong. If your form isn't at fault, try another exercise that works the same body part.

In Chapter 32, "Injuries Nag," we'll outline the most common injuries that you'll find in the gym. For now, let's look at a couple of broad categories and discuss how to best treat them.

Pulls and Strains

Minor muscle pulls or muscle *strains* are a common injury associated with weight lifting. With careful attention to proper technique and caution against using too much weight, they can usually be avoided.

Sprains are another common injury, though they are usually avoidable. Moderate strains and sprains are usually treated in the same way, with rest, ice, compression, and elevation, or RICE. Here are the specifics:

➤ *Rest.* Eliminates the demands on the affected area. If you can't rest it entirely, at least modify it as much as possible. (That would be MICE.)

➤ *Ice.* Decreases swelling, pain, and circulation.

➤ *Compression.* Limits swelling with the pressure of a bandage.

➤ *Elevation.* Reduces or limits swelling by reducing blood flow to injured area.

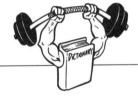

Bar Talk

A muscle **strain** or pull is a trauma to the muscle or tendon, caused by excessive contraction or stretching. **Sprains** are damage to ligaments (ligaments are the connective tissue between bones) accompanied by swelling and sometimes by discoloration.

Overtraining

Overtraining can be another source of aches and pains. It's also a factor that may inhibit muscular strength gains. Symptoms of overtraining are:

➤ Chronic fatigue

➤ Appetite disorders

➤ Sleeplessness

➤ Depression

➤ Anger

➤ Substantial weight gain or loss

➤ Protracted muscle soreness

➤ Elevated resting heart rate (we'll teach you how to measure your heart rate in Chapter 26, "Mix It Up")

➤ Lack of progress in muscular strength

If you are experiencing any of the above with your weight-lifting program, perhaps you began too ambitiously. In our experience, the two most common symptoms of overtraining are an uncomfortable night's sleep and moodiness. Listen to your body, rest, and begin again at a more modest pace.

If you've been lifting consistently, don't worry that a few extra days off will hurt your strength. Many of Jonathan's most dedicated clients travel quite a bit—either for work or for pleasure. Oftentimes, he'll tell them to relax and not work out on the road. Much to their surprise, they actually benefit from the short break, and they're stronger than ever when they return.

When she was competing as a powerlifter, our sage expert Deidre was a poster child for overtraining. Not only didn't she stretch, Deidre also worked out *every single day,* whether it was lifting weights or doing aerobics. She looked great, but she was an achy mess most of the time, especially in the morning when she struggled to get out of bed with a chronically sore lower back. During her last year of competition in 1997, she was hurt more often than not and was frequently depressed and disagreeable. If her coach said the sky was up, she'd argue otherwise. Such is the nature of a compulsive world champion. Perhaps if she had done what we are now telling you to do, she would still be competing.

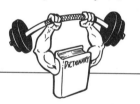

Bar Talk

Overtraining occurs when you train without allowing sufficient recovery between workouts or do too much too fast. Sometimes it rears its ugly head with physical symptoms and sometimes it's mental. Usually a couple of extra days off will help remedy the situation.

This Isn't Working

When it comes to weight training, it takes at least six weeks of consistent training to begin to notice physical changes in your body. That's six weeks of *consistent* training. Oftentimes people think they're training intensely when in fact they're pushing themselves while they lift but taking a ton of time between sets. In other words, make sure you're following our guidelines before you assume that you're making little or no progress. However, if after six weeks of diligent gym work you don't notice a change—even if it's slight—you may consider tinkering with your routine. A few ways you may alter your routine are as follows:

➤ Vary the number of reps. Generally speaking we like a range of 10 to 12, but that's not written in stone. Try decreasing the weight by 5 percent to 10 percent and bump up your rep range to 12 to 15.

➤ Decrease the amount of rest between sets. If you are resting for two minutes, decrease it to one minute. You'll probably have to decrease the weight by a few pounds, but you'll find it really challenging.

➤ Change the exercises. Most freeweight exercises we showed you have machine equivalents and vice versa. Try mixing it up for a while. Remember that the more you keep your muscles guessing, the better off you are.

To make gains in strength and in your appearance, you must continue to put stress on your muscles. If you are constantly doing sets of 10 reps with 10-pound biceps curls when you could clearly do an eleventh repetition, you're not going to see much of a change. Getting strong means using as many muscle fibers as possible during your exercise. The last few reps should be difficult. Once it becomes *easy,* you must increase the stress on the muscle by upping the weight you lift—that is, if you want to get stronger.

I'm Bored

No matter what the activity, weight training can get pretty boring if you are doing the same thing every time you hit the gym. Even if you increase the weight/reps or decrease your rest, if the basis of your routine is the same, you can become mentally tired. This is when you need to play around with some special techniques that can add a much-needed jolt to your program.

In Chapter 22, "Getting Fancy," and Chapter 23, "High Tech," we will go into great detail about the various special techniques that you can use in your training to combat boredom. From SuperSlow (an exercise technique described in Chapter 22) to break-downs, we'll show you a number of ways to alter and change your exercise program around to continue to make gains without getting bored. If you find that despite hard efforts, you don't appear to be getting stronger over the course of three to four weeks, it may be time for a rest, or a change in your program. If you're exhibiting any of the signs of overtraining that we outlined, try taking a few extra days off. If you feel good, but have just hit a plateau, you can try varying the program.

Changing a program every few months helps avoid mental boredom, but also helps keep your muscles challenged. By varying the exercises from time to time, you ensure that you present new challenges for your muscles. Even the subtle change in angle from a freeweight exercise to its machine equivalent, or switching from a barbell to dumbbells can give a muscle a little *surprise* and help push you through plateaus.

There are countless ways to tinker with your exercise plan. In the next chapter, we'll show you some advanced techniques that can be used to spice up your program.

The Least You Need to Know

➤ Now that you've learned the basics, it's time to assemble a solid routine.

➤ You can make tremendous gains in only 45 minutes a day.

➤ No matter how good your form, stiff and sore muscles are par for the course.

➤ Being enthusiastic is great; doing too much, too often can be bad.

➤ Changing your routine is great for your muscles and ensures that you won't be bored.

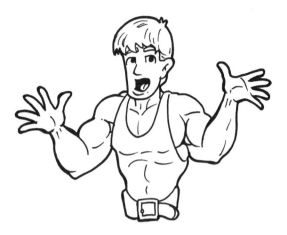

Chapter 22

Getting Fancy

In This Chapter

➤ Using SuperSlow and plyometrics

➤ Performing supersets

➤ Getting negative

➤ Lending a hand

Like a good love affair, your initial foray in the gym will be filled with grand expectations and great enthusiasm. After a while, that puppy love stage simmers down to a nice solid routine—until at some point you need another spark of enthusiasm to keep you enthralled. People who keep plodding along with the same old routine are likely to experience gains in strength, but after a while what we call the-same-old-thing syndrome is likely to bring them to a grinding plateau, physically and mentally.

Like death and taxes, this familiarity-breeds-contempt syndrome happens to the best of us. Sometimes just taking a short break from the gym is enough to get you back into the swing of things; sometimes more drastic means are necessary.

To spice up your workout we have detailed several techniques that you can work into your routine. While it seems too obvious to mention, many people—especially newcomers to the gym—assume that they need to do the same workout day after day, year after year. Nothing could be further from the truth. Initially, it's important that you learn how to perform the variety of exercises available to you. However, once you've built a solid base, one of the really fun and challenging aspects of weight training is

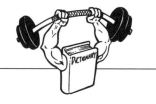

Bar Talk

SuperSlow is a protocol that, as the name suggests, involves extremely slow movement—10 seconds for the positive phase and 5 seconds for the negative. SuperSlow is a very challenging but safe method of strength training.

designing new routines to improve your fitness. Think of training as a journey in which you're traveling on your own unique route. As fitness guru Steve Ilg says, "A fitness program is not punishment for an imperfect body, but a sign of care. Love your body as it is. Then act to keep it well suited to the life tasks to which you are called."

SuperSlow

The *SuperSlow* Protocol is an exercise technique that was developed in the early 1980s by Ken Hutchins. The basis of the technique is to perform a single repetition for 15 seconds: 10 seconds up and 5 seconds down. Because each repetition takes so long, a set may consist of only three to five repetitions. By slowing things down so much, momentum is all but eliminated and orthopedic stress is minimized. Of course, curious bystanders may think you've suffered a stroke. No matter; lifting like this requires great effort and powers of concentration.

SuperSlow definitely works, but many people find it tedious to adhere to this slow-mo approach. However, many SuperSlow devotees take a hard line approach to their training, insisting that it is the only way to go. This, of course, is myopic and should-n't concern you. What is relevant is that by moving faster in the eccentric or negative phase than in the concentric or positive phase, you reduce the amount of recovery for the concentric phase. (Unless we overload with accentuated negatives, the value of moving slowly during the negatives is questionable.) Finally, while the 10-5 speed accomplishes what it says—limiting momentum and orthopedic stress while keeping muscular tension high—the 10-5 speed is not the only option. Movement cadences of 5-10, 10-10, 3-1-3 or other combinations which minimize momentum may be just as effective.

Let's consider the advantages of the SuperSlow system:

➤ You will get stronger.

➤ No use of momentum to propel the weight.

➤ No orthopedic injuries from using too much weight.

➤ It's safe.

Now consider the following disadvantages:

➤ Since the technique is so slow and the weight is so much lighter, some people may be turned off of using it.

➤ You have to pay attention to how long each repetition is by using a clock with a second hand, metronome or timer—your concentration is split between counting and lifting unless you work with a partner.

Having warned you about the boredom factor, we certainly think that SuperSlow is worth trying. It is demanding, but once you get into it, you'll find that the focused concentration required brings a new energy that your workout may be sorely lacking. No, we're not in agreement with the SuperSlow people who claim it's the only way to lift. Nor do we agree that you need to do all your workouts that way. But if you're looking for a new workout wrinkle, it's a fine way to increase the intensity of some of your workouts.

Plyometrics: Goofy Hopping

Back in the days of the Berlin Wall, East German athletes supposedly gained some of their potent athleticism from a funky method of training known as *plyometrics*. Since that dreaded wall has crumbled, this dynamic method of strength training has gained considerable popularity. So what in the name of Uta Pippig is plyometrics? Basically, it's exercises that emphasize bounding and explosive movements. In theory, doing exercises that emphasize a particular movement, say jumping on and off a platform as quickly as possible, will elicit great gains when you ask your body to perform the less exaggerated version. According to advocates of plyometrics, this type of training helps build explosive power, jumping ability, and quickness.

Let's take a look at what's behind this hop, skip, and jump craze. Plyometrics attempts to take advantage of the elasticity of the muscle by prestretching it before contraction. In other words, plyometrics uses your body's natural defense mechanisms to help produce a more forceful muscle action.

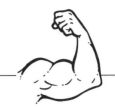

Flex Facts

While Dr. Wayne Westcott has found that SuperSlow can be an effective means of making strength gains, participants in the training program reported that they found the method particularly tedious. While having a riotous good time isn't necessarily the goal of a weight-lifting program, odds are you have a chance of sticking with it if it's enjoyable.

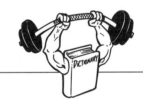

Bar Talk

Plyometrics is a method of strength training that involves bounding and jumping exercises. Both the safety and effectiveness of plyometrics are questionable, and we caution against the use of most plyometric exercises.

Let us explain. We told you about muscle spindles, the sensors in your muscles that respond to excessive stretching in an attempt to protect the muscles. As you may recall, when you stretch too far or too fast, muscle spindles try to contract the muscle before it gets injured or overstretched. Plyometric exercises intentionally and forcefully prestretch the muscle. This means the muscle spindles are excited, and that helps lead to a more forceful contraction.

Here's an example of how it works. Assuming you're sitting right now, stand up and jump as high as you can. If you're like the rest of us, you probably bent down into a coiled position just before you jumped. That's prestretching the muscle. You do the same kind of thing before swinging a baseball bat or kicking a soccer ball.

Common plyometrics exercises include throwing a medicine ball (a soft, weighted ball), as well as a variety of difficult drills in which you jump, hop, or bound—often off of or over boxes. Sounds good, and it is if you can ward off injuries. However, we have some serious concerns about the effectiveness and more importantly, the safety of plyometrics for both beginners and elite athletes.

When doing the plyometric exercises, there is significant stress on the musculoskeletal system, especially when using added weight such as a bar or a weighted vest, or when jumping from a platform. Even if the risk of injury is acceptable—and we don't think it is—there is little evidence that plyometrics are worth the risk.

Back in Chapter 3, "What Goes Where and Why," we touched on two elements that are key to an effective strength-training program: range of motion and muscle tension. When executing a plyometric movement, you often do not work the muscle through a full range of motion (ROM). Even if you do, while there is tremendous tension on the muscle at the beginning of the movement, the momentum produced by the fast speed of the movement decreases muscle tension throughout most of the ROM.

Having said that, many fitness experts swear by plyometrics. And the number of world-class athletes who use these techniques is too large to mention. Even our trusty writing companion Joe uses various plyometric exercises in his strength-training routine. The important thing to keep in mind if you're going to try some of these exercises is to make sure your technique is impeccable, and always do a thorough warm-up. Hopping around like a kangaroo on speed when you're cold is a certain way to court injury.

The following are advantages of plyometric training:

➤ Minimal equipment requirements

➤ Some simpler exercises may benefit agility

The following are disadvantages of plyometric training:

➤ High potential for injury to connective tissue (tendons and ligaments)

➤ Risk of hip, knee, and ankle strains and sprains

➤ Danger of stress fractures

Earlier we mentioned that plyometrics have gained considerable attention in the past few years. As we said, some experts swear by them; some swear against them. Even though the all-pro wide receiver for your favorite football team says that doing plyometrics has added two inches to his vertical leap, it's safe to assume that he could jump a lot higher than most mere mortals before he started bounding off of boxes. As we've said before, elite athletes sometimes reach elite status despite their training rather than because of it.

Back in 1985, the New York Giants used plyometrics extensively in their training en route to winning the Super Bowl. That year advocates of explosive movements were in their glory, pointing to the Giants as an example of the superiority of plyometrics over conventional strength-training methods. The wrinkle in the equation came the next year when the Washington Redskins won the whole enchilada. You see, Dan Riley, the strength and conditioning coach for the Redskins and one of the most respected men in the business, is an outspoken critic of plyometrics. Under Riley's watchful eye, the Redskins use only slow, controlled movements in the weight room because he sees no reason to jeopardize the safety of his multimillion-dollar players.

Would these same teams have won if they had traded strength coaches? Who knows? The bottom line is that anecdotal evidence supplied by individuals, even great ones, does not mean that you should follow their training plans. For every story of an athlete who excels using plyometrics, there's another who does just as well with safer methods, or worse, one who got hurt using plyometrics.

Certain simple agility drills such as a football player running through tires or even rope-jumping can be classified as low-level plyometric exercises, and we'd be hard-pressed to argue against them as a means of improving skill and dexterity. Still, due to the increased risk of injury as well as the lack of proof that most plyometric exercises are more effective than conventional means of strength training, it seems that they should be used with extreme caution, if at all.

Supersets

Now here's a technique we like. *Supersets* are an advanced technique that involves performing two different exercises with little rest in between.

Sometimes you work opposing muscle groups without rest. For example, a biceps curl immediately followed by a triceps extension. The more common method is to do a set of a single-joint movement like a bench flye, which isolates your pecs, and then go right into a bench press without any rest. By prefatiguing your pecs with the flye, you have now made the bench press more challenging. Why? Normally, when you do a hard set on the bench press, your triceps, which straighten your elbow, are prone to

271

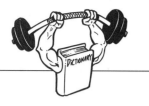

tiring out before you've fully exhausted your pecs. However, during the flye your triceps don't do any work; your pecs do. When you then move to the bench press, the pecs get an extra-hard workout without worrying about the tri's being the weak link.

To effectively perform a superset you must make sure that you have access to each machine or bench that you will be using. For instance, if you want to get a good shoulder workout, you might do a lateral raise right before a shoulder press. However, before starting either you'll need to have a light set of dumbbells for the lateral raises and a heavier one waiting for you for the presses. Any time lost fumbling around on a rack for the weights takes away from the effectiveness of the exercise. This doesn't mean that you should race around between sets. But it is important to segue from one to the other as smoothly and efficiently as possible. Another thing to keep in mind is that since your muscle is prefatigued before the second exercise, you'll need to decrease the weight you use by about 25 percent.

Since supersets are so demanding, we don't advocate using them too often. Rather, it's a way to tweak your routine when it gets stale or when you're unable to make any progress in the strength department. When Jonathan worked as a personal trainer, he liked to surprise his clients every two weeks or so by throwing in one superset per body part. Often they grumbled and groaned since it requires extra effort to combat the prefatigued muscles. However, the clients who really wanted to make progress enjoyed the extra challenge.

Remember, however, that supersets should be used judiciously. Done too often, you run the risk of overdoing it. In the next chapter, we'll give you more examples of specific ways to use supersets in your workouts.

The following are advantages of superset training:

➤ It saves time.

➤ It allows extra focus on certain muscles.

The following are disadvantages of superset training:

➤ You may not be able to use the machine that you want immediately if someone else is on it.

➤ You run the risk of overtraining.

Be Negative

No, we are not suggesting that you should develop a lousy attitude. We mean do *negatives*. The negative portion of the exercise is the lowering phase of the exercise. Physiologically, you can lower about 40 percent more weight than you can lift. In the course of a normal set, you're obviously lifting and lowering the same amount of weight, but there are ways to add extra stress to the negative.

When you stress the negative phase, you also increase the amount of delayed-onset muscle soreness that can occur, so it must be used judiciously and in a controlled manner.

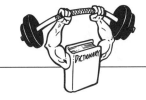

Bar Talk

Negatives are an advanced technique in which you stress the negative or eccentric phase of an exercise. They're a great way to get your body acclimated to a new weight when you've reached a strength plateau.

Negatives are a great way to get used to handling a little extra weight and help push you through a plateau. When Deidre first started competing, her bench press was stuck at 135 pounds for an eternity. Not bad for a 122-pound woman, but still not good enough if she wanted to beat the best. To get her acclimated to the extra weight, her coach had her do negatives with 145 pounds for a couple of workouts. Before you could say *pectoralis major,* she was benching up a storm. (For the record, Deidre's best bench press in competition is 176 pounds.)

There are two types of negative work that you can do:

➤ The first requires a spotter who will lift the weight and stand by as you slowly lower it—no faster than a three-second count on the way down. Do each rep like this until you have completed your set. Even though your muscles can handle an extra 40 percent for this type of training, you should start out with only 15 to 20 percent above your normal training weight. Because you're using more weight than you can move on your own, a trusted spotter is crucial, especially if you're doing a freeweight exercise.

➤ The second type involves body-weight exercises such as pull-ups and dips. If your gym doesn't have an assisted chin/dip machine, negatives are a good way to work up to full-body-weight chins and dips. Use a small platform to bring yourself to the top position for either of these exercises, step off the platform, and slowly lower yourself. Repeat this for a set of 10 or 12 or until you can no longer control the speed of the movement.

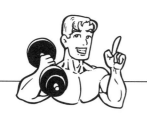

Spot Me

Here's a tip to keep in mind when you try negatives. Rather than thinking of lowering the weight, focus on resisting it, as if you were still trying to lift it. For instance, if you're using 15-pound dumbbells, think of pushing up with 14 pounds worth of force. This way the weight will slowly overcome your effort, and you'll be sure to move nice and slowly.

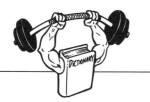

Bar Talk

With **breakdowns,** once you fatigue, you decrease the weight being used and do a few extra reps. This method allows you to reach failure twice on the same set and may promote even better strength gains than more conventional techniques.

The following are advantages of negatives:

➤ Good strength gains.

➤ Helps you break through plateaus.

The following are disadvantages of negatives:

➤ For most of the exercises, you need a spotter.

➤ Possibility of increased muscle soreness.

Breakdowns

Breakdown training is another high-intensity technique that we highly endorse. Breakdowns require reducing the amount of resistance at the point when you reach muscular failure. Usually, a 20 percent decrease in resistance will allow you to eke out three to four additional repetitions.

For example, let's say you are bench pressing 75 pounds 10 times. When you try another rep, your muscles resist and the spotter has to help you with the lift. At that point, the spotter strips the bar down to 60 pounds, and you then try to squeeze out another three or four reps. If you're really ambitious, you can strip the bar down to 50 pounds and try for two or three more reps. Try not to exceed 15 or 16 reps for the total set.

While breakdowns using a bar require a spotter, when doing dumbbell exercises all you have to do is have an extra pair waiting for you when you reach failure with the original weight. It's an even smoother transition when using a machine; all you have to do is move the pin to a lighter weight and get back to work.

The following are advantages of breakdown training:

➤ It's a great wake-up call to stalled muscle/strength gains.

➤ When using machines, you can work extra hard without the need of a spotter.

➤ Your workout will become more aerobic since your heart rate will be doing the Conga.

➤ It builds concentration and mental tenacity.

The following is a disadvantage of breakdown training:

> ➤ Spotters are needed for most freeweight exercises.

Help Me

Assisted training—a fancy name for having a spotter help you eke out a few more reps—is similar to breakdown training in the sense that it allows you to do a few extra repetitions after you have reached failure. In assisted training, rather than decreasing the resistance by stripping the bar, switching dumbbells or moving the pin, your spotter helps you to do two to four extra reps.

The key to successful assisted training is a good spotter. To get the most effective bang for your buck, you need a spotter who helps you along just enough but not so much as to make the extra repetitions useless. As the lifter, your job is to do your best to keep the weight moving. This requires maximum effort as well as good concentration. In addition to allowing you to do a few extra positive reps, assisted training gives you a great workout in the negative phase. This means you control the weight on the way down to the count of four. On the negative phase the spotter merely is there so that you don't drop the bar on your head.

Don't overdo assisted reps. If you try for more than four postfatigue reps, you're likely to give your spotter a great workout because it's doubtful that you'll have anything left in the tank. Again, the key thing to keep in mind when you're lifting is to push to momentary failure without compromising technique. Remember: form, form, form.

The following are advantages of assisted training:

> ➤ It's a great way to work harder than usual.
> ➤ It stresses negative phase.
> ➤ You don't need to switch equipment or change weights.
> ➤ It's a good way to offer and receive encouragement from your fellow lifters.

The following is one disadvantage of assisted training:

> ➤ It requires a good spotter.

Any of the methods we've described are well suited to jump-starting your training if you've found yourself in a bit of a rut. Regardless of which of these techniques you employ, pay careful attention to form, and remember that you'll need extra recovery time after any of these workouts. That's why we keep stressing that you don't try to use them too often. However, when you find yourself in a rut, any of these techniques are a great way to break through.

The Least You Need to Know

➤ When you find yourself stuck on a physical or mental plateau, it's time to vary your routine.

➤ SuperSlow is a protocol that, as the name suggests, involves extremely slow movement—10 seconds for the positive phase and 5 seconds for the negative.

➤ Plyometrics is a method of strength training that involves bounding and jumping exercises.

➤ Supersets are an advanced strength-training method that involves doing two exercises with no rest between.

➤ Negatives are an advanced technique in which you stress the negative or eccentric phase of an exercise.

➤ Advanced training techniques are excellent, but beware—they're difficult and shouldn't be overused.

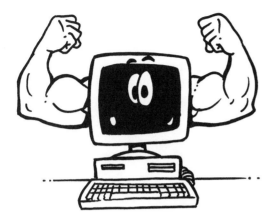

High Tech

In the August 1999 issue of *Men's Health* magazine, Chris Ballard wrote an amusing article about how your average caveman was as fit as today's Olympic athlete. Goofy, yes, but quirky enough to consider. In order to survive, your handy primitive had to have the endurance of a marathon runner to track game and a sprinter's speed to close in on a tiring elk. In the normal course of a day, a caveman lifted stones and tree trunks the way your typical NFL lineman pumps iron. Okay, their posture and table manners left something to be desired, but the point remains that their lofty feats of strength and endurance stemmed from the endless variety of ever-changing physical demands required of them.

Despite our fast-paced, sophisticated lives, we are physical beings genetically programmed to do vigorous exercise. Lifting weights is a modern means of filling this need. But as we said, if you stick to the same old routine week after week you are likely to get bored.

The willingness to change your routine regularly will not only keep you mentally challenged, but will ensure that your body adapts to the new stress as well. Meeting these constantly changing demands will help push you to higher level of fitness. In this chapter, we'll give you a variety of examples of how to use some of the techniques we described in the last chapter.

Each is more physically challenging than the basic training we've described up until now, and each will have added benefits. They're not techniques that you need to try early on in your lifting life, but they may come in handy if you want to give your workouts some extra oomph or if you ever have to flee from a woolly mammoth.

Split Routines

While we generally prefer that you work all your muscles on the same day, it's not the only way to go. Many strength experts like to use a *split routine*. These routines combine muscle groups or body parts to be worked out on alternating days. For example, on Monday you may work your chest, shoulders, and triceps; Tuesday, back and biceps. Wednesday, legs and abs. When you're doing a fairly high volume of exercises, split routines allow you to avoid spending all day in the gym. And because you're not working your entire body, you're able to do more exercises per body part as well as work out more intensely. The more focus you bring to your workout, the better.

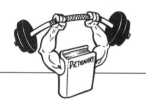

Bar Talk

A **split routine** is a regimen in which you divide your workout over two (or more) days. Split routines are particularly useful if you want to do more than two or three exercises per body part.

In a split routine, you usually work each body part twice per week. The key to a successful *split* is to avoid using the same muscles on consecutive days. So if you did a chest/shoulders/triceps workout on Monday, you'd let those body parts recover until Wednesday or Thursday.

The beginning routines we described for you in Chapter 21, "Get With the Program," include about 15 exercises that should take you about 45 minutes—a manageable load for your mind and body. You can add a few extra exercises and still be able to finish in under an hour. However, if you want to get stronger faster or to refine the look of your body, doing multiple exercises for each body part is probably the way to go. If you find yourself upping the number of exercises you're doing on any one day (say 20 or more), it's probably time to think about a split routine.

The following are advantages to a split routine:

➤ It allows you to incorporate more exercises than in a full body routine.

➤ It lets you place more focus on specific body parts.

➤ If it's done correctly, you'll get stronger faster.

The following are disadvantages of a split routine:

➤ It requires more days per week in the gym.

➤ It allows fewer rest/recovery days.

Okay, let's assume that you're a split-routine kind of person. Let's look at some of the best split routines that we've designed for you.

Push-Pull

One popular and logical way to break up your exercises for a split routine is the push-pull split. Pushing exercises are those like the bench press or military press where the resistance is moved away from your body during the positive phase. Pulling exercises like rowing and pull downs bring the resistance toward the body. Pushing exercises stress the muscles of your chest, shoulders, and triceps. Pulling movements work your back muscles and biceps. The key feature of the push-pull split routine, or any other good split, is that the same muscles are not stressed on consecutive days. If you do that, you don't allow your muscles enough recovery time, and they're too weak to do the job.

The push-pull split routine refers to working all muscle groups that push on one day followed by working all muscles that pull on the other day. For example:

Monday/Thursday	Tuesday/Friday
Legs	Chest
Back	Shoulders
Biceps	Triceps

For the sake of balance, we've included all leg exercises on the pull day. Here's a solid sample routine using the push-pull split. This routine is probably our favorite way to split things up; it allows a nice balance between muscle groups and works well for most people.

Day 1 and 4

Body Part	Exercises
Legs	Leg press
	Leg extension
	Leg curl
	Standing calf raise
	Seated calf raise

continues

Day 1 and 4   continued

Body Part	Exercises
Back	Lat pull down
	Machine row
	Upright row
	Back extension
Biceps	Seated biceps curl
	Concentration curl
Abs	Reverse crunch
	Crunch
	Oblique crunch

Day 2 and 5

Body Part	Exercises
Chest	Bench press
	Incline press
	Decline press
	Dips
	Pec deck
Shoulders	Shoulder press
	Front raise
	Reverse flye
Triceps	Triceps pushdown
	Triceps kickback

This configuration groups the pushing exercises, like all the pressing movements, together and keeps the pulling exercises together. The advantage that the split routine offers is that all the muscles that are performing a similar routine are getting a good workout throughout the entire routine. When you work your pecs as in a bench press, you are also working your deltoids and your triceps. Move on to the shoulder press, and you're using your deltoids and triceps again. When you do a typical back exercise like a lat pull down, your biceps are also doing a lot of work.

Upper–Lower

The upper-lower split routine is basically exactly what it says: upper body one day, lower body the next. Once again, it avoids using the same muscles on consecutive days. The upper-lower body split is especially effective if you want to emphasize your legs. On your lower body day, you get to concentrate heavily on your legs without worrying about having energy left for other body parts. Here's a sample program:

Monday/Thursday	Tuesday/Friday
Chest	Legs
Back	Abs
Shoulders	Lower back
Biceps	
Triceps	

Days 1 and 4

Body Part	Exercises
Legs	Leg press
	Leg extension
	Leg curl
	Standing calf raise
	Seated calf raise
	Abduction
	Adduction
Abs	Reverse crunch
	Crunch
	Oblique crunch
Lower Back	Back extension

Days 2 and 5

Body Part	Exercises
Back	Lat pull down
	Machine row
	Upright row
Chest	Bench press
	Incline press
	Decline press

continues

Days 2 and 5   continued

Body Part	Exercises
Shoulders	Military press
	Lateral raise
Biceps	Seated biceps curl
	Concentration curl
Triceps	Triceps pushdown
	Triceps kickback

As we said, a split routine makes sense if you're doing a lot of sets or, say, training for a power-oriented sport like football. Trying to do too much in one day is bound to lead to a lack of concentration and enthusiasm. While breaking up your routine allows your muscles ample recovery time between workouts, keep in mind that your body recovers as a unit, not just as individual muscles. A split routine guarantees that you'll be in the gym on consecutive days during the week, which puts an extra demand on your body. While it's wise to eat well and get plenty of rest no matter how hard you work out, once you start training, more rest and nutrition becomes even more important.

Remember our checklist of symptoms of overtraining in Chapter 21? Often, the drive that prompts people to go to a split routine is the same impulse that leads to chronic fatigue. Recognizing the signs of overtraining—irritability, sleeplessness, loss of appetite, and so on—before you smack into the dreaded wall is key if you hope to stay healthy.

Superset Routines

In Chapter 22, "Getting Fancy," we told you that a superset is a pair of exercises performed with no rest in between. (Again, you can superset opposing muscle groups or the same muscle groups.) We also told you that we really like supersets as a way of pushing your muscles real hard.

We'll now describe superset routines for the same muscle groups. One of the best reasons for performing supersets is that you can get an extremely effective workout without the increased risk of orthopedic injuries from using too much weight. In fact, because your muscles are taxed harder, you usually use less weight when doing a superset.

Yes, it's an ego-buster if you get hung up on how much is *enough,* but unless you decrease the weight for the second set by about 25 percent, you'll never manage to do more than a couple of reps on the second exercise.

Way back in Chapter 1, "Let's Get Physical!" we told you that you'd benefit from the countless mistakes the three of us have already made. Here's one for you. The first time Jonathan tried doing a superset years ago, he did a good hard set of flyes to exhaust his pecs and jumped right to a bench press. Ambitious lad that he was, his plan was to use the same amount for the bench press as he usually did. Halfway through his first rep, painful visions of a mouse in a trap came to mind. He struggled to finish one rep with his normal weight, checked his ego at the door, and graphically learned how effective preexhaustion can be.

Nice Legs

As we mentioned in Chapter 15, "Below the Waist," squats and/or leg presses will be the key exercises for most leg routines. One of the major pluses of either exercise is the fact that they work lots of large muscles in one shot: glutes, hamstrings, and quads. While this is generally considered a positive, the exercises don't allow you to place specific emphasis on one particular part of your legs. Supersets are a great tool that can be used to selectively stress a certain muscle of your legs.

A good quad superset routine requires that you have immediate access to whatever machines you'll be using in your routine. Since compound leg movements like the squat or lunge work both your quadriceps and your hamstrings, doing a set of leg curls (hamstrings) or leg extensions (quads) before one of those exercises lets you choose which muscle you want to emphasize. Remember, moving from one routine into the other without rest means you'll need to decrease the weight of the second exercise by about 25 percent.

Quad supersets:

leg extension/leg press

or

leg extension/squat

or

leg extension/lunge

Of the three, we prefer the first combination because the leg press allows you to work hard without the same safety concerns of a squat. If you choose the squat, be sure to use a spotter and be conservative with the weight. Lunges are a distant third place for our favorite quad superset combinations because you only use one leg at a time. Since the idea of a superset is to prefatigue the muscle and work it while it's tired, the rest you get between working each of your legs reduces the desired effect of the exercise.

Hamstring supersets:

> leg curls/leg press
>
> or
>
> leg curls/squats
>
> or
>
> leg curls/lunges

By throwing in a hamstring exercise before the compound movement, you shift the emphasis of the squat, leg press, or lunge to your hamstrings rather than your quads. Again, we prefer to use the leg press as the second exercise, but the others can work if necessary. (In Chapter 13, "Gluteus What?" we told you that the primary function of the hamstrings is to bend your knees. While this is true, they also work in conjunction with the glutes to extend, or straighten, your hips as in the squat, leg press, or lunge.)

Just about everybody, from mountain bikers to senior citizens, can benefit from strong legs. Put simply: Supersets are a guaranteed way to improve your leg strength.

Nice Pecs

Since most chest exercises also involve the smaller and weaker muscles of the shoulders and triceps, it is the perfect body part for supersetting. This will ensure that your pecs get a good workout without worrying about smaller muscles cutting your workout short. While the bench press is often considered the single best pec exercise—and it is a very good one—your triceps, which are smaller and weaker than your pecs, are more likely to give out before your pecs. By prefatiguing your pecs in the first part of a superset, they get that extra oomph that will pay obvious dividends.

Pectoral supersets:

> dumbbell flyes/bench press or dumbbell press
>
> or
>
> dumbbell flyes/chest press machine
>
> or
>
> pec deck/chest press machine

Any of the above will do the trick nicely and really overload your pecs. The key to a successful pec superset is to make sure you really burn them out with the isolation exercise (pec deck or flyes) before moving on to the pressing exercise. Many experienced lifters complain that while they've gotten stronger and their arms have gotten bigger, the cosmetic changes in their pecs lag behind. That's usually due to an over-dependence on pressing movements, where your triceps give out before your pecs are fully used. Supersets may be just the trick for such people.

Nice Delts

The deltoids respond nicely to a superset routine. The muscles are small enough that you don't have to use significant weight, especially when using this technique. As with other supersets, the key is to work as hard as possible on the first set. Done properly, your delts will be well on their way to exhaustion before you even begin the second set.

Deltoid supersets:

lateral raises/military press

or

lateral raises/shoulder press machine

or

lateral raise machine/shoulder press machine

Again, the pattern is an isolation exercise followed by a compound movement. Don't plan on hailing a cab, fanning a campfire, or waving to a friend soon after a good deltoid superset—your shoulders should be too tired to raise your arms.

Nice Lats

Because the lats are so large, they tend to be very strong. Because they're so strong, the biceps are usually the weak link in an exercise like a lat pull down or a chin-up. Without a machine like the Nautilus Super Pullover, it's hard to isolate your lats. Unfortunately, this great machine has become a rarity in most gyms. (The Super Pullover was the first machine sold by Nautilus inventor Arthur Jones.) In its absence, the reverse flye is a decent way to prefatigue the muscles of your back, as well as your rear deltoids.

Lat/rear deltoid supersets:

reverse flyes/cable rows

or

reverse flyes/bent rows

Nice Traps

Supersets are also an excellent way to strengthen and fill out your traps. The best way to isolate them is with shrugs, so we'll include them. As we mentioned in Chapter 16, "Flip Side," upright rows are a great exercise that work your deltoids and biceps in addition to your traps.

In order to place the concentration on your traps, we'll prefatigue them with shrugs followed immediately by upright rows. Strong traps are essential for everything from carrying shopping bags to rowing.

Trap superset:

> Shrugs/upright rows

While we prefer prefatigue supersets to those that work opposing muscle groups, the latter is a good way to speed up a workout on days when you're pressed for time.

Here's an example of exercises that you can put back to back. In each case, the movement is in the same plane—what varies is the direction of the resistance. For instance, a lat pull down and a military press are essentially the same movement. In one case (military press) the resistance is pushing you down and in the other (lat pull down) it's pulling you up.

Here are a few examples of opposing supersets:

➤ Leg extensions/leg curls

➤ Abduction/adduction

➤ Lat pull downs/shoulder presses

➤ Machine rows/chest press machine or bench presses

➤ Upright rows/dips

➤ Crunches/back extensions

Circuit City

Circuit training is defined as a series of resistance exercises performed one after the other with minimal rest between exercises. By minimal we mean approximately 30 seconds or less. This fast-paced, aerobically based routine has also become increasingly popular in class settings. Many fitness experts consider circuit training a *compromise* between strength training and cardiovascular exercise. Strictly speaking, it is; however, it's a good compromise. So while you're neither maximizing your muscular payoff nor getting as good a cardiovascular workout as if you went for a run in the park, you are building strength and burning calories.

In circuit training, the amount of weight you use is considerably less than you would normally use—usually 40 percent to 60 percent of your usual weight for the same exercise. One of the advantages to this type of training is that it can increase local muscular endurance due to the low rest period between exercises. Another advantage is that it saves significant time, making it ideal for people who have limited time to commit to the gym.

Here's our take on circuit training: The continuous, or near continuous, activity of circuit training does raise your heart rate, leading some to believe that your cardiovascular system will benefit from such exercise. The problem with that reasoning is that the physiology behind raising your heart rate while lifting is different than during traditional cardiovascular training such as jogging, cycling, and swimming.

Why? Follow this short physiology lesson. When you run, swim, or bike, your heart rate quickens, as does the amount of blood that your heart pumps with each beat. On the other hand, when you lift, your heart rate increases, but the volume of blood pumped with each beat remains about the same and sometimes actually decreases. The point of the lesson? An elevated heart rate is not always an indicator that your heart is getting stronger. If that were the case, you could start a fitness movement by telling people to shelve their running shoes and bicycles and replace those workouts with a steady diet of scary movies. I can hear the infomercial now: "Hey man, how'd you run such a good marathon? Hill work?" "No, *Silence of the Lambs!*" "You?" "*Blair Witch!*"

The bottom line on circuit training is that while it may be a compromise between traditional strength and cardiovascular exercise, it's not nearly as effective as either one separately. Still, done from time to time, it can be another effective way to add pizzazz to your gym life.

The Least You Need to Know

➤ Diversifying your routine will challenge your mind and body.

➤ The split routine is a way to train each body part more intensely.

➤ Supersets are a super way to bump up the intensity

➤ Circuit training gives you some cardiovascular benefit along with strength gains.

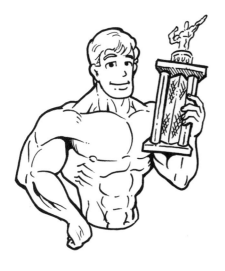

And the Winner Is ...

The competitive aspect of strength training is a relatively esoteric part of the sports tapestry in this country. (Okay, try to name one Olympic weight lifter, powerlifter, or Mr. Universe in the last three years.) However, knowing about the folks who are pushing the proverbial pedal to the metal can be both inspiring and just plain interesting. The relatively obscure competitive outlets available to weight lifters who just can't get enough of a good thing are bodybuilding, powerlifting, and Olympic weight lifting. Despite the immense differences found in these sports, each requires tremendous strength, technique, and discipline.

Most of you probably feel no need to compete. And many of the techniques employed by athletes in these disciplines contradict much of what we've taught you so far. Before this chapter, we've stressed that your goal in the weight room is to get as strong as possible and not show off for those around you. Well, guess what? For competitive lifters, showing off is what it's all about.

Sometimes, challenging yourself to enter one of the above contests will be the added incentive you need to push you to achieve a personal goal. But even if you have no interest in competing, it is interesting and informative to see how the muscleheads live.

Here's more than a bit about the rudiments of each sport.

Arnold's World

Who isn't familiar with Arnold Schwarzenegger, the six-time Mr. Olympia–turned-movie-mogul? In his prime, the Austrian Oak was one of the most imposing and muscular humans (at least we think he's human) to walk the planet. He certainly is the most well-known bodybuilder to ever strike a pose, and was as instrumental as anyone in popularizing this oft-misunderstood sport. Arnold had some help, however, from legends of the sport like Franco Colombo, Frank Zane, Lou Ferrigno, and Lee Haney, to name a few.

What made Schwarzenegger so popular? Aside from his enormous personality, his physique was extraordinary. At 6 feet 2 inches, and 235 pounds, his measurements were the stuff that sculptors pine for:

Arms: 22"

Chest: 57"

Waist: 34"

Thighs: 28.5"

Calves: 20"

It is very difficult for a man of that height to pack on that much muscularity while remaining so exquisitely proportioned. Typically, bodybuilders who are densely muscled and symmetrically proportioned tend to be shorter, since it is easier for a smaller frame to give the appearance of greater muscle mass. In fact, one of Arnold's chief rivals during his heyday was Franco Columbo, a man so strong he was able to blow up a hot water bottle like a balloon until it exploded. This Italian dynamo had similar measurements, but he was nearly a foot shorter. Since Arnold was so statuesque, he won easily.

To excel at bodybuilding one needs to have an incredible work ethic as well as an extraordinary genetic predisposition toward muscular growth. Simply put, without Mom and Dad's generous DNA, Arnold might still be in Austria doing who knows what. (He certainly would not be married to a Kennedy and one of the richest men in Hollywood—not that there's anything wrong with that.) While a strong work ethic and favorable genetics are prerequisites for hitting the big time, there's plenty of room in the sport for regular (lesser) oaks like you and me.

The goal of the sport is simple: to sculpt your body, giving it as much size and definition as possible. Perhaps more than any other sport, in bodybuilding, diet is given as much attention as training, especially near competition time. Why? People can win or lose based upon whether or not they were on target with their diets.

A typical bodybuilding routine consists of three to six sets of 12 to 15 repetitions. Rest in between sets is usually no more than 60 to 90 seconds. Many of the advanced techniques that we wrote about in Chapter 21, "Get with the Program," and Chapter 22, "Getting Fancy"—supersets, breakdowns, preexhaustion, and negatives—are standard fare here to achieve maximum results.

Due to the high volume of exercises and short rest sets used, bodybuilders cause an increase in muscle size through hypertrophy of existing muscle fibers. Muscle enlargement may also be attributed to an increase in capillaries, the smallest blood vessels. It appears that an increase in capillaries is associated with the high intensity and higher volume of strength training common among bodybuilders but not found in powerlifters and Olympic weight lifters.

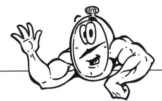

Weight a Minute

Strength training increases the size and strength of not only muscle tissue, but of tendons and ligaments as well. Without this adaptation, damage to ligaments and tendons would be more likely to occur. The use (or abuse) of steroids, which unfortunately is common among professional bodybuilders, causes rapid increases in size and strength of skeletal tissue without the requisite strength in tendons and ligaments. As a result, tendon tears are common in athletes who abuse steroids.

Competition Anyone?

A bodybuilding contest is a little like a Miss America pageant. Although instead of the swimsuit and evening gown parade, athletes clad in little more than a cocktail napkin display their physical wares. The show itself consists of two phases: prejudging and the actual competition. Prejudging, which takes place first, is the weeding out process. Competitors are lined up and instructed to strike several standard poses. The competitors who cut the mustard are asked to come back to go head to head during the next phase. The prime-time event has participants in light-, middle-, and heavyweight classes.

Each competitor performs a five-minute routine that he feels highlights his physique. Once each competitor has performed his individual routine, they all come out for a face-off or *pose down,* which consists of freestyle posing. With the bright lights blazing and music blaring, it's rather a surreal scene. Judges choose the winner using a point system based on muscle size, definition, *symmetry,* and the skill demonstrated during the posing routine.

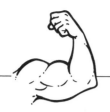

Flex Facts

At 6 feet, 2 inches, 204 pounds, Nicole Bass, a popular Ms. Olympia competitor, is one of the largest female competitors ever officially weighed for a show. By contrast, Carla Dunlap—a far more accomplished bodybuilder, measured 5 feet, 3 inches, 126 pounds, proving that shape and symmetry are more important than size alone.

While men's bodybuilding has been popular since Arnold came on the scene in 1970s, women's bodybuilding reached its zenith in the early 1980s when a handful of charismatic competitors like Carla Dunlap, Rachel McLish, Gladys Portuguese, Mary Roberts, Laura Creavalle, and Cory Everson hit the scene. Not only were these woman strong and full of well-defined muscles (also known as being "ripped"), they were gorgeous, a marketing fact which made the mainstream press more eager to feature them on their pages.

During the 1980s, female bodybuilding (particularly American female bodybuilding) emphasized a muscular yet *feminine* aesthetic—broad shoulders and back; narrow waist and hips. That all changed when the Americans and Europeans began competing against each other on a more regular basis. The Europeans tended to be bigger and more muscular—much more muscular!—and before you could say *latissimus dorsi* the face of female bodybuilding had changed.

Since that change, female bodybuilding has lost much of its appeal and popularity. Said simply: Many of the top professional female bodybuilders look like hyperdeveloped men in bikinis. More common now are what's called "fitness shows." These women are muscular, but not grotesque. However, these shows are more like watching a Miss America pageant since competitors wear high heels with their competition suits and perform routines heavy on dancing and gymnastics rather than on posing.

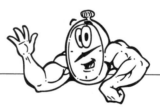

Weight a Minute

One of the reasons that bodybuilding is so intimidating to aspiring competitors is the cartoonlike proportions of some of the high-profile names in the sport. While it's something that people don't like to talk about, many bodybuilders' physiques have been affected by the abuse of anabolic steroids and/or plastic surgery. For those whose aspirations are a little different than the pro's, *natural* bodybuilding contests are available. Drug testing is far stricter in such competitions.

Deidre's World

Powerlifting, a sport that became popular in the '70s, was for a long time the ugly stepchild of bodybuilding. Oftentimes, powerlifting events were held late in the evening only after bodybuilding competitions were over.

Early in Deidre's weight-lifting career, she seriously considered competing as a bodybuilder. However, as she learned more about the two sports, she decided powerlifting was the more pure sport because, unlike bodybuilding, it was not subjective. The goal in powerlifting is quite simple: The one who lifts the most wins.

Just as bodybuilding is a display of muscularity, powerlifting is a demonstration of strength. The disciplines in a powerlifting meet are the squat, the bench press, and the deadlift. A powerlifting competition consists of nine rounds of lifting for each competitor—three attempts at each event. Since the highest successful lifts are added together, the winner is the one who totals the most weight.

If you're a 122-pound woman interested in competing at the world-class levels, here's what you're up against. When Deidre won her first world championship in 1995, her totals were: squat, 303 pounds; bench press, 159 pounds; and dead lift, 336 pounds. By her peak, those numbers were up to 336, 187, and 370 pounds. If your aspirations are more along the line of local meets, half that will do just fine.

How It's Done

All three of these lifts are familiar to you by now, but the technique used in competition is very different than what we've recommended you do for your training. Here are the main differences:

➤ Whenever possible, lifts are made *explosively.* Momentum can make the difference between a successful lift and a miss.

➤ You hold your breath. The increased pressure caused by a valsalva maneuver (holding your breath while lifting) makes the lift easier. Unless you have learned this from a good coach, don't try this at home since there is a tremendous increase in blood pressure generated when you hold your breath.

➤ You squat below parallel. When we described the squat in Chapter 15, "Below the Waist," we advocated bending your knees until they're parallel to the floor. Stop there in a powerlifting meet and the lift is considered a no-go.

➤ You arch your back while bench pressing. In Chapter 17, "Chest or Bust," we told you to always keep your back pressed into the bench when lifting in order to protect your lower back. Powerlifters arch their backs as much as possible to bring their chest up higher and shorten the range of motion of the lift. Again, their sole aim is to hoist as much weight as possible.

The mistake that most lifters make in competitions is selecting a weight that they can't manage on their opening attempt. This is potentially disastrous because if you miss your opener, you can't change the weight. The rules dictate that you must stay with that same weight for your next two attempts. If you miss all three, it's all over. Deidre's openers were always a weight that she could do for two repetitions in the gym.

What Is Done

There are two types of powerlifting events: those with equipment and those without. The equipment involved in powerlifting is nearly as restrictive as medieval armor. Once a lifter actually manages to wriggle into it, the lifting is the easy part. For the equipment-aided event, you'll need:

➤ **Squat suit** This is a tight, stiff outfit that is made to give the lifter support during the squat. A good suit makes the squatting difficult, but it shoots you back to a standing position with comparative ease.

➤ **Belt** Some belts offer the barest of support; others are so big they look like they could hoist a train wreck. Deidre first wore a belt called a lever belt that was fortified with hooks and a latch that looked like a harness for an ox. This sucker was so tight that she could barely bend to get underneath the bar to squat.

➤ **Knee wraps** These wraps are made of semi-elastic material that grudgingly gives an inch when you bend your knees. Along with the suit, the wraps are what give the lifter bounce when coming out of the squat. If you are eager to walk like a mummy, powerlifting knee wraps are for you.

➤ **Squat shoes** These hard-soled shoes give the lifter support while squatting. The stiffness of the shoe restricts forward and backward sway as the lifter sets up with the weight on his/her back. The less sway, the more balance and control the lifter has.

➤ **Bench press shirt** Made of either the same material as the squat suit or denim, these shirts are so tight that it is virtually impossible to hold your arms at your side. Claustrophobics need not apply. An old powerlifting joke is that a good bench shirt can lift 40 or 50 pounds if you just lay it on the bench.

➤ **Unitard** This is a one-piece wrestling singlet worn on top of the bench press shirt.

➤ **Wrist wraps** Made from the same semi-elastic material as the knee wraps, these provide support during the bench press.

➤ **Deadlift suit** Similar to a squat suit, the deadlift suit differs in that it's usually looser in the hips (so that you can get down to the starting position).

➤ **Deadlift shoes** These are flat, soft-soled shoes that bring the lifter closer to the ground to decrease the distance the bar travels from the floor to the lifter's midthigh. Wrestling shoes or even ballet slippers are often used as well. (You haven't lived until you've seen a 275-pound bruiser wearing ballet slippers.)

If you ever want to get the normally animated Deidre really hot and bothered, ask her about the joys of donning a squat suit. This tortuous garment took two people 20 minutes to pull on and off. She's likely to wax poetic about the cuts in her legs where the suit dug in so tightly. (This is the hallmark of a good suit. If it slides up the legs it decreases the amount of support through the quads and hips.) And she's sure to mention how the squat suit fit so well that her legs went numb. If any of these sounds like fun, you're probably ready to launch your career as a powerlifter.

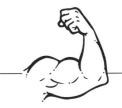

Flex Facts

Those of you who paid attention in high school physics class will recognize that powerlifting is a misnomer. By definition, power is the rate at which work is done—the faster the movement, the greater the power. In the sport of powerlifting, all that matters is how much weight you lift—not how fast you lift it.

Of course, if powerlifting intrigues you but the equipment doesn't, then you'd be a candidate for a *raw* meet where the only equipment required is a unitard and the only other paraphernalia allowed is a standard weight-lifting belt. The good thing about raw meets is that lifters tend to be far more careful in their selection of attempts. Wearing a squat suit or a bench press shirt often gives lifters a false sense of security, and they often choose weights that are not within their capabilities. This, of course, is a great way to get injured.

Let's look at the three disciplines a bit more carefully.

The Squat

The squat is the first event in a powerlifting meet and the most nerve racking, primarily because you wear the most equipment and feel the most vulnerable standing under all that weight. It is also the lift that requires the lifter to be almost perfect in terms of form and technique—especially when the weight approaches double or triple body weight. As we mentioned, for the squat attempt to be deemed good, you must lower your body until your hip joint is below your knee joint. In other words, below 90°. Such a maneuver is what keeps orthopedists in business.

Deidre squatting in competition—start.

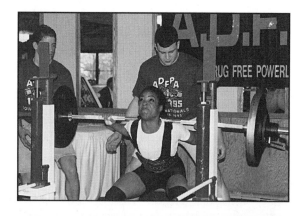

Deidre squatting in competition—finish.

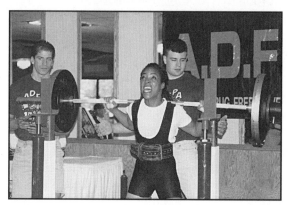

Here are the elements required for a near-perfect squat during a competition:

➤ *The setup.* How the lifter approaches and gets underneath the bar is probably the most psychological aspect of the lift. Approach with fear and more often than not you're likely to miss. Approach with a mixture of nervousness and confidence, and you'll nail it almost every time.

➤ *The walk out.* Once you have come under the bar, you must stand with the weight on your back and walk backward so you don't hit the squat racks. The best way to walk out is to use the least number of steps possible. The more steps you take, the more the weight bounces on your back, throwing off your balance and rhythm. It also gives you too much time to think about just how much weight you're carrying on your back. The best walk out is to take one step back and stop.

➤ *The squat.* Once you've stopped moving your feet and are focused and steady, you are given the signal to squat. The best way to begin the descent is to hear the signal, take a deep breath, and squat. (Some people take several quick, shallow breaths before squatting, which just wastes time and energy.) One breath and squat is all you need. Basically, the more time you have the weight on your back, the heavier it begins to feel.

The Bench

The bench press is the second event and, like the squat, requires a substantial bit of technical precision. Here are the basics:

➤ The lifter brings her feet as far back toward her head as possible in order to arch the back.

➤ A spotter lifts the bar off the rack and hands it to the lifter.

➤ The lifter takes a deep breath and lowers the bar until it touches her chest. Only after it comes to a complete stop can the grunting competitor press the weight off her chest. Any bouncing of the bar or uneven extension of the arms and the lift is disallowed.

The Deadlift

There's an old powerlifting adage that says, "The meet doesn't start till the bar hits the floor." This sage piece of lifting wisdom means that meets are often won and lost with the deadlift—the final lift of the day.

Deidre won many meets where she trailed after the squat and bench press, only to pull it out at the end. In fact, her lifting partner and friend, four-time national champion Jacqueline Davis, once won a national meet by outlifting her competitor by 75 pounds in the dead lift!

Here's what to expect during the dead lift:

➤ First your hands will be covered in chalk to help you grip the bar. Your shins and thighs will be similarly covered in baby powder to help the bar slide up your legs more easily. (Mix up the two and expect the bar to slip out of your hands or stick to your thighs.)

➤ Grip the bar as described in Chapter 16, "Flip Side" or in a variation known as the sumo position.

➤ Take a deep breath and pull like an ox plowing a hard field. The lifter is required to stand fully erect before receiving the "down" call from the head official.

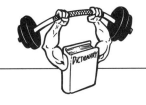

Bar Talk

The **sumo deadlift,** which Deidre used in competition, is when the lifter takes a wide stance and places her hands inside her legs.

So there you have it: familiar lifts done with unfamiliar technique. With all their hooting and hollering, chalk-smattered and often bulky bodies, powerlifting meets can be an intimidating place. (Although the raw meets are generally a bit more laid-back, we hesitate to call them civilized.) In either case, many meets have a novice division, which is a great way to check out this little-known sport.

USA Powerlifting is the largest sanctioning organization in the sport, though many others exist. *Powerlifting USA* magazine is the bible of powerlifting and a good resource for information on upcoming meets and coverage of the sport.

The Big Boys

The sport of Olympic weight lifting, sometimes known simply as weight lifting, is better known to the general public than powerlifting due to the exposure it receives every four years during the Olympics. The fact that very few Americans distinguish themselves on the international level tends to keep it in the athletic closet. (The Eastern Europeans dominate the sport.) Compared to powerlifting, there's a minimum of equipment—only a belt and knee and wrist wraps. The competitor wears a singlet and hard-soled shoes.

Though it will still be only a *demonstration* sport, in the 2000 Olympics women will be allowed to compete in the weightlifting events for the first time.

The two lifts used in competition are known as the snatch and the clean and jerk. Each competitor is allowed three attempts in each lift. The sum of the lifter's best snatches and best clean and jerks is the lifter's total.

The reason we've not described these lifts in previous chapters is because there's little justification for anyone but a competitive lifter to do them. If you're inspired to try to learn these lifts, a knowledgeable coach is a must. These lifts are performed explosively, and since they require you to hoist the weight over your head, there's a substantial risk of injury. In fact, one of the exciting aspects of this sport—other than the incredible totals these lifters put up—is the explosive speed and power a lifter must possess in order to leap under the weight. Even the superheavyweights, men who resemble rhinos more than athletes, possess a startling grace once they grasp these seemingly immovable pounds of iron.

To find out more, you should contact USA Weightlifting. They list everything from equipment to meets to coaches for the sport.

So that you know what's going on in Sydney at the 2000 Olympics, here's a description of both lifts.

The Snatch

The more technical and more explosive of the two lifts, the snatch looks like a great way to dislocate both of your shoulders. Done correctly, it's a picture book demonstration of grace, speed, and power. How is it done?

The snatch is performed in one continuous movement. The bar is brought from the platform to a position overhead using one fluid motion. The lifter pulls the bar up from the platform. When the bar reaches the lifter's chest, he or she then leaps into a squat position under the bar, securing it overhead with arms held straight. Once the lifter has accomplished that impracticable move, he or she must stand upright. Sounds impossible. It almost is.

The Clean and Jerk

While this lift sounds like one of those goofy Jim Carey movies, in fact this is a deadly serious lift where competitors hoist far more weight than the snatch. As the name implies, the clean and jerk is a two-part movement. For the clean, the lifter must yank the weight from the platform to the shoulders in one motion and stand erect. The jerk part is where the lifter thrusts the bar from his shoulders to a position overhead in one motion while splitting his legs. If he's made it that far, the lifter must put his wobbly legs together and stand motionless. After he gets the okay sign, it's time to send the weight crashing back to earth where it belongs.

The Least You Need to Know

➤ If you love to lift as well as compete, you should check out one (or all) of the three: bodybuilding, powerlifting, or Olympic-style weight lifting.

➤ Bodybuilding requires countless hours in the gym to build a muscular, symmetrical, and lean body.

➤ Powerlifting involves three common exercises, but with uncommonly heavy weight.

➤ Olympic weight lifting uses two technically challenging lifts in competition.

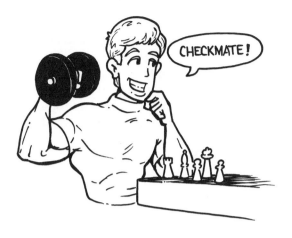

Chapter 25

Lift Well, Play Hard

In This Chapter

➤ Lifting will improve your game

➤ Injury prevention is as important as anything else

➤ Pick the sport, and we've got the exercises

Whether you're a jockey, synchronized swimmer, or badminton player, virtually every athlete can benefit from increased strength. In this chapter, we'll help you design strength-training routines aimed at helping your performance in a variety of sports, from golf to football. What may surprise you is the similarities in how we train athletes for such diverse sports. Certainly the demands of these sports are very different, and the muscles that need to be trained vary from sport to sport, but surprisingly the techniques used in the weight room will not.

Specificity of training, the concept that exercises should be based on the physiological demands encountered during the performance of a sport, is one of the most misunderstood items in exercise science. Some strength coaches advocate using sports-specific exercises in the weight room that mimic the movement used in your sport. The theory seems sound: By copying such movements, you will help develop strength in that particular movement. While that seems like a logical line of reasoning, many experts think that it may in fact be counterproductive.

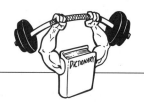

Can You Be More Specific?

Specificity is much like pregnancy—it either is or it isn't. For example, specific training for a basketball player could be practicing his jump shot, not shooting a weighted medicine ball. In fact, by attempting to mimic a precise sports movement such as swinging a baseball bat or golf club, you can undo countless hours of skill training. You see, the neuromuscular pathways that allow your brain to tell your muscles exactly what to do—and how to do it—take countless hours of practice. In turn, the use of added resistance (for example, the medicine ball) when copying such movements can disturb that motor memory.

Princeton University's Matt Brzycki is one of the most outspoken strength critics of copying sports movements in the weight room. Says Mr. Brzycki, "Strength training should not be done in a manner that mimics or apes a particular movement pattern. A stronger muscle can produce more force; if you can produce more force, you'll require less effort and be able to perform the skill more quickly, more accurately, and more efficiently. But again, that is provided that you've practiced enough in a correct manner so that you'll be more skillful in applying that force."

> **Bar Talk**
>
> **Specificity of training** is a well-accepted physiological theory that suggests that adaptations made during training depend on the type of training used. For instance, if you want to become a faster runner, the most appropriate way to accomplish this is by running, not by walking in the park and not by riding a bike.

Just as we don't advocate different training techniques in the weight room for men and women or the young and the old (more on that in the next few chapters), there's no reason to train athletes from different sports using different techniques. Good form for a cyclist is good form for a tennis player. What should, and will, vary is the selection of exercises since the muscles that are used will differ from sport to sport. That's where we'll *customize* the programs. For example, a kayaker will do more upper body work than a runner, but the upper body work that they perform they'll do exactly the same.

A few years ago, Jonathan attended a seminar held by John Philbin, an assistant strength and conditioning coach with the NFL Washington Redskins. What surprised many in attendance was that while the Redskins vary their exercises from position to position (no sense in worrying about the throwing arm of the free safety), the form used is exactly the same for any and all of the athletes. Typically, a lithe cornerback can bench press far less than a burly linebacker, but the exercise is executed exactly the same way.

While improved performance is an obvious reason for an athlete—weekend warrior or professional—to hit the weight room, it may not be the most important one. In fact, injury prevention is probably the biggest benefit from a solid off-season training regimen. After all, it doesn't matter how talented you are if you're on the sidelines nursing an injury. Barry Chait, former assistant strength and conditioning coach with the NFL New York Jets, stresses that, "Though we obviously try everything possible to make the players bigger, faster, and stronger, our primary goal is to ensure they make it through the game in one piece. That means never taking any chances in the weight room, and it means working on less glamorous muscles like those in the neck."

As we mentioned in Chapter 1, "Let's Get Physical!" many athletes used to resist weight lifting for fear of becoming muscle-bound. (One can only imagine how many more homers Mickey Mantle would have hit had he touched a weight during his career. Even if he didn't hit any more dingers, he would have hit them much farther, and he may have avoided the debilitating leg injuries that curtailed his career.) Now that the muscle-bound myth has gone the way of the eight-track tape, many athletes still shy away from the weight room fearing that they'll lose valuable training time that would be better spent practicing their sport.

Certainly we agree that all the strength in the world can't make up for the lack of a sport-specific skill; however, there's no reason to choose between the two. By now, we hope we've convinced you that a sensible lifting program doesn't need to take more than 30 to 45 minutes per gym visit. (Look back at Chapter 2, "Hurry Up and Weight," for some valuable tips on how to find time in your hectic day to make it to the gym.)

Since very few athletes compete year-round—Steffi Graf where have you gone?—there's no reason to have the same program in-season as you do out of season.

Here's how it works. In the off-season your primary goal is to get as strong as possible. During the season, however, you should aim to maintain your strength. If you try to keep up the same schedule while you compete as you did in the off-season, you're begging for overtraining injuries. Of course, if you lay off your lifting completely, you'll quickly undo all the good you've done. Aim for two or three lifting sessions in the off-season and once a week for maintenance in-season. Try to keep your in-season workout on a different day than a hard sports workout, and at least a few days away from a race.

Stick Your Neck Out

Strong neck muscles (primarily the sternocleidomastoid, scalenes, splenius capitus, and splenius cervicis) may not be of any particular use to a golfer, but they can be invaluable for anyone whose sport has a risk of head and neck injuries. This, of course, is invaluable for a football player or a wrestler, but even a cyclist will benefit from added neck strength. (If you don't believe us, check out Jonathan's collection of cracked helmets from bicycle crashes he's been in.) On the other hand, a golfer or kayaker would be wise to focus on grip strength far more than a swimmer or runner.

Some gyms have specially designed neck machines, and others have a harness that you can wear on your head to do various exercises. We've described the simplest way of doing them, which is with manual resistance—you press against your head with your hand. Not very high-tech, but reliable and effective.

Here is how to properly perform neck flexion:

1. Sit in a chair with back support.

2. While looking forward, place the palm of your dominant hand on your forehead.

3. Bend your head forward, chin toward your chest. Resist the movement of your head by applying backward pressure to your forehead with your hand.

4. Slowly return to the starting position.

Neck flexion—begin/end position.

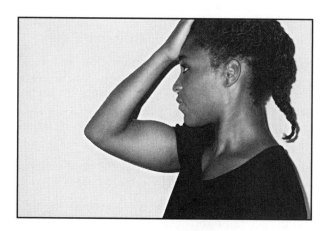

Neck flexion—middle position.

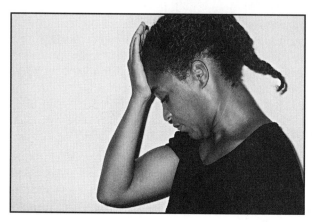

Here is how to properly perform neck extension:

1. Sit in a chair with back support.

2. While looking forward, place the palm of your dominant hand on the back of your head.

3. Bend your head backward so that you are looking up toward the ceiling. As you do so, resist the movement by applying forward pressure to the back of your head with your hand.

4. Slowly return to the starting position.

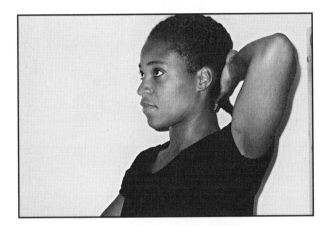

Neck extension—begin/end position.

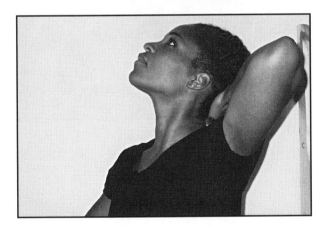

Neck extension—middle position.

Here is how to properly perform a neck lateral flexion:

1. Sit in a chair with back support.

2. While looking forward, place the palm of your hand on the side of you head.

3. Bend your head sideways, making sure to keep your nose facing straight (not toward the ceiling). As you do so, resist the movement by applying pressure to the side of your head in the opposite direction.

4. Slowly return to the starting position. Repeat on the other side.

*Neck lateral flexion—
begin/end position.*

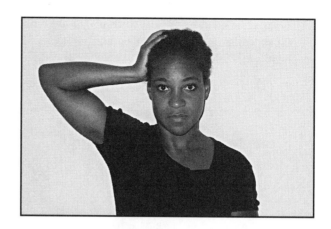

*Neck lateral flexion—
middle position.*

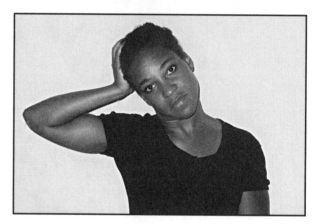

What follows is a list of exercises based on the demands of a particular sport. Remember that selection of the exercises we choose is specific to the sport, but the form used is the same regardless of the sport.

Running

While running over a half-mile or so is primarily an aerobic activity, even long-distance runners can benefit from improved muscular strength. The added strength will help you to power up hills, but the main reason for runners to lift is injury prevention. For example:

➤ Patellar tendinitis, an inflammation of the connective tissue around the knee-cap, is a common running injury that can be prevented or minimized with improved quadriceps strength.

➤ Hamstring strains, which are as common to veteran runners as Gatorade at road races, can be prevented with a sound strength-training program as well.

➤ Trochanteric bursitis is another condition common in runners, cross-country skiers, and ballet dancers that can be kept at bay with weight training. When the bursa becomes inflamed, the result is a deep, burning pain on the *trochanter* itself or, less often, down the side of the thigh. Treatment of this condition, aside from rest, ice, stretching, and anti-inflammatories, involves strengthening all of the gluteal muscles.

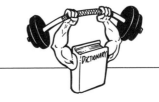

Bar Talk

The **trochanter** is the prominent bone found on either side of the hip; a bursa is a sac found between muscle and bone or bone and tendon that helps decrease friction.

Another concern of distance runners that can be improved with a sound weight program is the imbalance between the hamstrings and the quadriceps. Most distance runners have well-developed hamstrings but weak quadriceps. Strengthening the quads can help prevent running injuries and will help restore the proper balance.

Finally, while running is obviously primarily a lower body activity, you'd be surprised at how much your upper body contributes. If you don't believe us try running up a hill with your hands behind your back. Large muscles are a hindrance; strong muscles will help you run faster.

The following table lists specific body parts and exercises that are good to perform together if you are a runner.

Body Part	Exercises
Legs and hips	Squat or leg press
	Leg curl
	Abduction
	Adduction
	Standing calf raise
	Seated calf raise
Back	Pull-ups (assisted if necessary)
Chest	Dips (assisted if necessary)
Shoulders	Shoulder press
Arms	Seated biceps curl
	Triceps pushdown
Midsection	Reverse crunches
	Crunches
	Oblique crunches
	Back raises

Cycling

Many of the injuries among cyclists are a result of improper mechanics rather than muscular weakness. Some of these injures include patellar tendinitis, quadriceps tendinitis, pes anserinus bursitis, chondromalacia patella, and iliotibial band syndrome.

Jonathan hard at work.

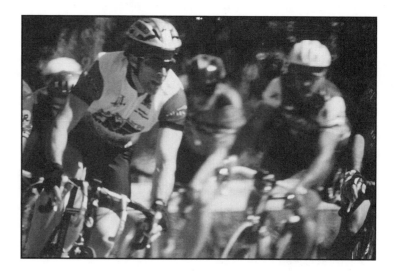

Just as with runners, cyclists often suffer from muscular imbalances, though their imbalance is the opposite of what runners encounter. While Jonathan's quads have served him well through hundreds of bicycle races (as well as a few races up the Empire State Building), by comparison, his hamstrings are woefully weak. A good dose of leg curls could help remedy his problem. (We hope he'll read this chapter and act accordingly.)

As in the case of runners, added extra body bulk can be detrimental, but upper body strength is necessary when sprinting and riding out of the saddle while you're powering your way up a steep hill. In addition, midsection strength can help give you a good, solid base for all those miles in the saddle. Back exercises can help reverse the hunched posture caused by all those hours of riding. Finally, don't forget those neck exercises we mentioned earlier.

The following table is a sample program for the cycling fans.

Body Part	Exercises
Legs and hips	Squat or leg press
	Leg extension
	Leg curl
	Standing calf raise
	Seated calf raise

Body Part	Exercises
Back	Pull-ups (assisted if necessary)
	Upright row
Chest	Dips
Shoulders	Military press
Arms	Seated biceps curl
	Triceps push down
Midsection	Reverse crunches
	Crunches
	Oblique crunches
	Back raises
Neck	Extension
	Flexion
	Lateral flexion

Notice the neck exercises listed here specifically.

Tennis

If you have any questions whether strength can help a tennis player, you need look no further than the Williams sisters, Venus and Serena, the 1999 U.S. Open Doubles. These tall, powerfully built young women regularly serve at speeds comparable to men on the pro tour. Equally as impressive is their all-court athleticism. This combination of speed and power has propelled them to the top of their sport.

Tennis and other racquet sports require good upper body strength for hitting the ball; abdominal and oblique strength for twisting of the torso; and leg strength to help get you to the ball. When Andre Agassi rededicated himself to tennis en route to winning the 1999 French Open, he credited his rigorous weight program for giving him that extra "oomph" on the ball.

The most common injuries associated with tennis are lateral epicondylitis (known as tennis elbow) and to a much lesser extent, medial epicondylitis (known as golfer's elbow but also seen in tennis players). The best way to prevent and/or resolve these injuries is to strengthen the muscles of the forearm with wrist flexion and extension exercises.

These exercises should keep you on the court and hitting hard. You still might not be able to give either of the Williams sisters much to worry about, but you'll certainly look impressive on the way to and from the court.

Body Part	Exercises
Legs and hips	Lunges
	Abduction
	Adduction
	Standing calf raise
Back	Bent row
	Lat pull down
Chest	Pec deck
	Bench press
Shoulders	Lateral raise
	Military press
	Internal rotation
	External rotation
Arms	Seated biceps curl
	Triceps kickback
	Wrist curls
Midsection	Reverse crunch
	Crunch
	Rotary torso
	Back raise

Golf

Okay, so you don't need to be the world's greatest athlete to excel in golf, and you're not likely to see the paunchy Fuzzy Zoeller on the cover of *Ironman* magazine any time soon. On the other hand, we've already told you that increased strength increases club head speed and drive distance, so golfers certainly can benefit from a strength-training program. And one has to look no further than the game's greatest player today, Tiger Woods, who has lifted weights for years. Is there any correlation between his mammoth drives and his whippetlike strength? We certainly think there is.

Muscles of particular importance to golfers include the gripping muscles of the hands and forearms, the obliques for twisting during the shot, and the muscles of the arms and shoulders to help power the ball. In the routine that follows we pay particular attention to these body parts as well as a thorough midsection routine to power your torso through your stroke.

As for injuries, medial epicondylitis is much more common in golfers than it is in tennis players. Again, the best way to prevent and/or resolve it is by strengthening the forearm muscles with wrist flexion and extension exercises. In addition, back pain among golfers is common due to the fast, twisting motion. Strengthening your abs, obliques, and lower back can keep you on course. (Bad pun, but it's true.)

Here's a solid lifting program for golfers. By the way, ditch the cart and walk instead—you'll up your fitness quotient considerably.

Body Part	Exercises
Legs and hips	Leg press
	Leg curl
Back	Lat pull down
Chest	Bench press
Shoulders	Lateral raise
	Military press
Arms	Seated biceps curl
	Tricep pushdown
	Wrist curls
Midsection	Reverse crunches
	Crunches
	Rotary torso
	Back raise

Baseball

John Kruk, the portly former all-star first baseman for the Philadelphia Phillies, once said, "I'm not an athlete, I'm a baseball player." Certainly he wasn't the first player to prove that you don't need be a stud athlete to make it on the diamond. Flash forward to Mark McGwire, the Paul Bunyonesque St. Louis first baseman who has clearly demonstrated that a little (or in his case, a lot of) strength doesn't hurt.

In fact, one of the biggest changes in professional baseball in the last 15 years is the number of athletes who lift weights during the off-season. Take fleet-footed shortstops like Derek Jeter, Nomar Garciapara, and Alex Rodriguez and you can see the benefit of weight training on their overall play. Don't get us wrong, these guys are superior athletes who would be perennial all-stars even if they didn't lift, but their long-ball power is no doubt aided considerably by all their time in the weight room.

Power aside, baseball is a game of spurts and starts with a healthy dose of arm strain thrown in. Arm injuries such as rotator cuff tendinitis and shoulder dislocations can be prevented or improved with a proper strengthening program. Midsection strength can help avoid back injuries from the repetitive motion of swinging a bat. And both upper and lower body strength can improve one's arm and bat speed. Remember that if the bat moves faster, the ball goes farther.

These exercises should keep you on the field. And if you "got no game," they'll at least have you looking more athletic than the hard-hitting yet portly Mr. Kruk.

Body Part	Exercises
Legs and hips	Squat or leg press
	Leg curl
	Abduction
	Adduction
Back	Pull-ups (assisted if necessary)
	Bent row
Chest	Bench press
Shoulders	Military press
	Internal rotation
	External rotation
Arms	Seated biceps curl
	Tricep push down
	Wrist curls
Midsection	Reverse crunches
	Crunches
	Rotary torso
	Back raise

Basketball

Ever know a guy who could shoot the lights out during warm-ups, or win any game of HORSE, but could barely score a point during the game? How about the player who excels early in the game, but whose jump shot always hits the front of the rim as the game goes on? Sure you need to be able to shoot the ball, but if you don't have the physical ability to run up and down the court, and establish your position in the paint, all the skill in the world won't do you any good.

Watch an NBA basketball game, and you can't help but marvel at the incredible athleticism exhibited on the court. Speed, strength, and flexibility are all necessary physical attributes of a successful player. You may not be playing in the pros any time soon, but to excel at the weekend pickup game at the Y requires those same physical abilities.

Strong legs are essential to establishing position in the low post and jumping. Upper body strength can help your jumping as well, and is necessary when shooting and boxing out for a rebound.

In the injury prevention realm, anterior cruciate ligament tears are an all too common injury among basketball players (especially women, in part due to the width of their hips) Once again, increased quadriceps strength can help prevent or minimize such injuries.

These exercises should help fortify you on and off the court.

Body Part	Exercises
Legs and hips	Squat or leg press
	Leg extension
	Leg curl
	Standing calf raise
	Seated calf raise
Back	Lat pull down
Chest	Bench press
Shoulders	Military press
Arms	Seated biceps curl
	Triceps push down
Midsection	Reverse crunches
	Crunches
	Oblique crunches
	Back raise

Swimming

Swimming fast requires a tremendous amount of skill and strength. The chiseled physique and V-shaped taper of an elite swimmer should leave little doubt about that. The muscles used vary from stroke to stroke, but it's safe to say that swimmers need good chest, shoulder, and back strength as well as abdominal strength for stability when rotating to breathe. Leg strength for the kick is also essential.

Swimmers, especially elite swimmers, are extremely flexible, which affords them enormous range of motion (ROM) while they propel themselves through the water. This flexibility, coupled with overdevelopment of the muscles of the front of their upper body (pecs and anterior delts), puts swimmers at risk for rotator cuff injuries, tendinitis, muscle tears, and shoulder dislocations. A weight-training routine that emphasizes strengthening the upper back muscles and the posterior deltoid muscles will decrease the muscle imbalance often associated with these aquatic types. Strengthening the rotator cuff muscles will decrease the risk of the shoulder injuries so common to hard-core swimmers.

The thing that all athletes should keep in mind—especially those whose sport depends on a greater-than-average range of motion—is that strength training does not inhibit flexibility as long as you lift through a full range of motion. Strength training will decrease that risk without decreasing your flexibility.

Here's a regimen that should make Summer Sanders proud.

Body Part	Exercises
Legs and hips	Leg press
	Leg curl
Back	Lat pull down
	Upright row
Chest	Bench press
Shoulders	Military press
	Lateral raise
	Reverse flye
	Front raise
	Internal rotation
	External rotation
Arms	Seated biceps curl
	Triceps kickback
Midsection	Reverse crunch
	Crunch
	Rotary torso
	Back raise

Skiing and Snowboarding

A successful downhill or slalom skier needs strong quads and glutes in order to hold the tucked position. In addition, upper body strength is helpful when you're working your poles through bumpy terrain.

Just as with cyclists, there are two types of skiers, those who have crashed, and those who haven't crashed yet. For that reason alone, the greater stability that stronger muscles give you can help minimize injuries in the event of a crash. Quadriceps strength is also important in the prevention of knee injuries that can be brought on by the twisting and pivoting motion of hammering downhill.

Here's a list of exercises that will get you ready.

Body Part	Exercises
Legs and hips	Squat or leg press
	Lunges
	Leg curl
	Leg extension

Body Part	Exercises
	Abduction
	Adduction
Back	Lat pull down
Chest	Bench press
Shoulders	Military press
Arms	Seated biceps curl
	Triceps push down
Midsection	Reverse crunch
	Crunch
	Oblique crunch
	Back raise

Skating

Both ice-skating and its newfangled dry-land cousin, in-line skating (commonly known as rollerblading), require quite a bit of leg strength, as well as more upper body and midsection strength than you might realize.

Obviously, the muscles of your legs are the engine that propels you forward; however, strength in your lower back and abs will allow you to stay in a tight tuck as you work your arms to help keep you rolling along. Several elite bicycle racers have made the transition from cycling to speed skating because of the similarities between the physical demands of the two sports. Another thing that cyclists and skaters have in common is that they both inevitably hit the ground sooner or later. That's our way of reminding you not to skip the wrist and neck exercises that we recommend.

Here's a program catered to keeping you swift, fit, and healthy.

Body Part	Exercises
Legs and hips	Squat or leg press
	Lunge
	Abduction
	Adduction
Back	Lat pull down
Chest	Bench press
Shoulders	Military press
Arms	Seated biceps curl
	Triceps push down
	Wrist curls

continued

continued

Body Part	Exercises
Midsection	Reverse crunch
	Crunch
	Oblique crunch
	Back raise
Neck	Flexion
	Extension
	Lateral flexion

Kayaking

Line up the competition at a kayak race and you're bound to see lots of broad, muscular, V-shaped torsos atop spindly legs. That's because paddlers spend hours at a time working away with their backs, shoulders, and arms while their legs remain safely tucked away. (Your legs actually are instrumental in a sound stroke, but they act mostly as stabilizers instead of sources of speed.)

There's no need for a paddler to spend a lot of time on his or her legs, as you'll see from the program we've designed. On the other hand, hours of twisting the torso are facilitated by strong obliques, abs, and lower back muscles. The muscles of the back and shoulders provide most of the power in the stroke, so that's where we'll place our primary emphasis.

The most common injuries among paddlers involve the rotator cuff, so don't forget those internal and external rotation exercises.

The following exercises may not float your boat, but they'll definitely get it moving through the water faster.

Body Part	Exercises
Legs and hips	Leg extension
	Leg curl
Back	Pull-ups (assisted if necessary)
	Dumbbell rows
Chest	Bench press
	Dips (assisted if necessary)
Shoulders	Military press
	Lateral raise
	Internal rotation
	External rotation

Body Part	Exercises
Arms	Seated biceps curl
	Triceps push down
Midsection	Reverse crunch
	Crunch
	Oblique crunch
	Back raise

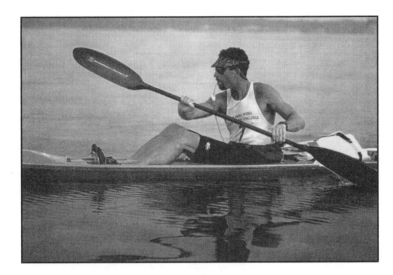

Joe, somewhere between Chicago and New York.

Martial Arts and Boxing

Mention training for boxing to most people, and they'll probably think of a regimen of countless sit-ups and hard roadwork, as well as punching slabs of beef. All of the above are fine, but we prefer you pound blocks of tofu since overgrazing is a big problem in our country.

Martial arts? With more and more people getting involved in these Asian arts, boxing and kickboxing, there's still room for some more conventional training methods. Whether it's the real thing or classes, strengthening your body can help you perform better.

While we are all in favor of you waxing hundreds of cars a week (see *The Karate Kid*) or meditating under frigid waterfalls, our workout regimen has you building strong legs (for fancy footwork), strong shoulders (for packing a punch), and a strong midsection and neck (in case you're on the receiving end of one of those blows).

Here's a workout strategy that should keep you in fighting shape.

Body Part	Exercises
Legs and hips	Squat or leg press
	Leg curl
	Abduction
	Adduction
Back	Pull-ups (assisted if necessary)
	Dumbbell rows
Chest	Bench press
	Dips (assisted if necessary)
Shoulders	Military press
	Lateral raise
Arms	Seated biceps curl
	Triceps kickback
Midsection	Reverse crunch
	Crunch
	Oblique crunch
	Back raise
Neck	Flexion
	Extension
	Lateral flexion

The Least You Need to Know

➤ No matter what the sport, improving your strength will help you on and off the court.

➤ All the talent in the world won't help if you're sidelined with an injury.

➤ Neck exercises may not sound exciting, but they're important for sports that involve crashes or contact.

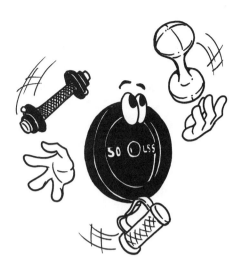

Chapter 26

Mix It Up

In This Chapter

➤ Lifting, running, and being merry

➤ Calculating your pace

➤ Spinning, stepping, and dancing

If you haven't guessed by now, we're kind of keen on weight training as a way to improve your health and fitness. While we've extolled the virtues of weight training for the better part of 25 chapters, we would be remiss if we didn't stress that aerobic exercise is a necessary complement to weight training. In other words, if you want to get strong, lift weights; if you want to be truly fit, add cardiovascular (CV) exercise into the mix.

While it may come as a revelation to most of you, it's a misconception that aerobic exercise tones and firms muscle. Aerobic exercise helps you to decrease your level of body fat, which helps improve the muscle definition by thinning out the layer of fat that obscures the muscles, but weight training is what makes the muscles worth looking at. Theoretically, you can be thin from doing tons of aerobic exercises, yet still be flabby and/or weak. In order to achieve a balanced physique, you must include both aerobics and weight training in your routine.

Take Deidre's early foray into the world of endorphins. She started off doing aerobics without weight training; then weight training without aerobics. Next she did both,

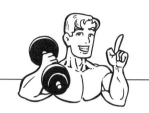

Spot Me

During the first 20 minutes of cardiovascular activity, carbohydrates are the primary energy source. Aerobic activity that lasts longer than 20 minutes begins to metabolize fat for energy. While short, intense bursts of exercise can help your cardiovascular system, moderately paced (not slow), longer workouts are preferable if your goal is to burn fat.

though she paid no attention to nutrition. Finally, she hit pay dirt when she combined aerobic exercise, weight training, and proper nutrition. Not only did she look strong, lean, and muscular, she felt great as well. (It was only after she'd been competing as a powerlifter for several years that her body said, "No more!")

Unlike weight lifting, there are an infinite number of aerobic activities that one can choose from: cross-country skiing, swimming, in-line skating, hiking, running, cycling (on- or off-road), stair climbing, and walking. Given this wide range of activities, almost anyone who enjoys working up a sweat can find something he or she derives joy from.

This isn't to suggest you have to become a marathon man like Joe or Jonathan. Consider one of Deidre's friends who would rather have rusty tacks driven under her fingernails than exercise aerobically indoors. Instead of making it a dreaded chore, she cycles or blades from her apartment in Brooklyn to her office in Manhattan and back several times a week. Integrating her working out into her workday leaves her feeling fit, virtuous, and on time. She's lucky enough to have access to a shower at her job, and brings a stack of work clothes in every Monday.

Deidre, on the other hand, prefers doing her aerobic workouts indoors rather than dealing with traffic, unruly dogs, and/or the aggressive cyclists one often finds in Brooklyn's Prospect Park. (It's bad enough that she lives with an aggressive cyclist.) Since she is basically a fast-twitch muscle person—no genetic predisposition to endurance in that muscular body—long periods of aerobic activity are not her idea of fun. In turn, unless she's jogging through a flowery meadow to soothe her urban soul, she'd just as soon escape to a treadmill in the gym and grind away as she listens to her Walkman. While writing this book, Deidre was training for her first New York City Marathon.

Jonathan is another case study. He'll exercise wherever he can find pavement, a treadmill, or virtually any piece of aerobic exercise equipment. Tell him you have a new machine that works your anterior hip abductors called a floppy-loop, and he's sure to give it a try. He'll train in any kind of weather and at any time of the day or night. He loves it when it's 90 degrees; he loves it when it's raining. Call him noble, call him maladjusted, or just call him a true exercise junkie.

Joe is in the Jonathan camp. However, unlike Jonathan, who sinks even looking at water, you'll find Joe wherever kayaks lurk. He also has a penchant for climbing mountains and/or running or biking on trails. By the way, did we mention snowshoe marathons and winter triathlons? In fact, pick a cardio exercise that is long, hard, or stupid and he's generally game. (In fact, on Jonathan's insistence he trained for and competed on the Concept II rowing machine in an indoor regatta known as The St. Valentine's Day Massacre.)

Before we continue, let's define what me mean by aerobic exercise for adequate cardiovascular fitness and weight loss. This is any activity that sustains an elevated heart rate for at least 20 minutes, preferably at least three or four times per week. Once you are comfortably able to sustain 20 to 30 minutes of a CV activity, try to extend your aerobic exercise session to 45 minutes. Of course, don't try to do this all at once. Rather, up the ante 5 minutes per week. What we really hope to avoid is your attempting more than you can handle at one time. That's one way people get frustrated and stop.

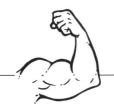

Flex Facts

In Chapter 8, "To Supplement or Not?" we told you that caffeine releases fat into the bloodstream, where it can be more easily used during aerobic activity. If you're already a coffee or tea drinker, you may want to experiment with a cup about an hour before a workout. If you're not, don't start.

Lub Dub: Heart Rates

To get a good cardiovascular workout, it's helpful to know how hard to push yourself. (Going too slow loses the training benefit; training too hard is often unnecessary or even counterproductive.) As a result, the best way to monitor your pace is by figuring out your heart rate and knowing at what level of exertion to train.

Although it initially may seem complicated, figuring out your heart rate while you exercise is quite easy. In fact, before you know it, you'll be monitoring your heart rate like Jonathan. A number cruncher at heart, he often checks his heart rate after a shower, while watching a scary movie, or when waiting in line at the bank. (Please don't ask why he does this. While he's extremely knowledgeable on all aspects of fitness, he is rather, how shall we say, unique.)

To make the heart rate number crunching game worth your while, you'll need to know a few basic things.

To maximize weight loss, you want to exercise at 60 to 75 percent of your maximal heart rate (MHR).

For cardiovascular fitness, you want to increase this to about 85 percent of your MHR. Elite athletes, like Olympic sprinters, often push the envelope and exercise at nearly 100 percent of their MHR.

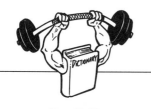

Figure It Out

The simplest way to determine whether you're exercising aerobically or *anaerobically* is the talk test. If you can carry on a conversation with your training mate while you're jogging around the park, you're training aerobically; you may be huffing and puffing, but you can be understood and respond without gasping for breath. If your partner asks, "How ya doin'?" and you reply like a breathless mugger wearing a ski mask, well, you're in the anaerobic range.

You can also use what is called your rate of perceived exertion (RPE). This is a chart that attempts to quantify for you how hard you're working when you're exercising. This is very often used with patients who are participating in cardiac rehabilitation after suffering a heart attack or cardiovascular surgery. The RPE scale is imperfect because it's so subjective, but it can be a useful tool to go along with monitoring your heart rate.

The following is the scale for rate of perceived exertion (RPE):

0	Nothing at all
0.5	Very, very weak
1	Very weak
2	Weak
3	Moderate
4	Somewhat strong
5	Strong
6	Strong
7	Very strong
8	Very strong
9	Very strong
10	Very, very strong
•	Maximal

If you don't have anyone by your side to talk to and fear being considered a nut job carrying on a one-sided conversation, there are two formulas that you can use to figure out what your target heart rate should be during your workout.

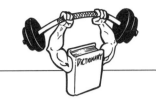

The first formula to figure out your MHR is as follows:

1. 220 minus your age.
2. Take that figure and multiply it by 60 percent. This represents the low end of your target heart rate.
3. Multiply your predicted maximum heart rate by 85 percent. This is the high end of your target heart rate.

Bar Talk

Your **target heart rate** is the most efficient zone within which you gain a significant cardiovascular benefit from your aerobic exercise.

The second, more accurate way to figure your *target heart rate* during aerobic activity is called the Karvonen formula. First we need to record your resting heart rate (RHR). To get an accurate reading, take your pulse first thing in the morning before you get out of bed on three consecutive days. Average the three, and take that to be your resting heart rate. Here's the rest of the equation:

1. 220 minus your age is your predicted maximum heart rate (MHR).
2. MHR minus your resting heart rate (RHR).
3. Multiply that number by 60 percent and 85 percent.
4. Add your RHR to each of these values for the low end and high end of your target heart rate zone.

Sounds complicated but it's not. For example: Deidre Johnson-Cane, age 36. Resting heart rate, 72. Here's how she would figure out her target heart rate:

1. $220 - 36 = 184$
2. $184 - 72 = 112$
3. $112 \times .60 = 67.2$
4. $72 + 67.2 = \mathbf{139}$

How to Measure

There are two places that you can use to take your pulse: your radial pulse, which is on the thumb side of your wrist, or your carotid pulse, which is located on your neck on either side of your throat. Use your index and middle finger to check your pulse at either site.

323

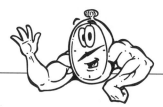

Weight a Minute

If you take your pulse at your carotid artery, be sure not to press too hard. Just a light touch is all it takes. Too much pressure on the artery can result in a sudden decrease in blood pressure. We don't want you fainting in the middle of a workout.

Once you find your pulse, count the first beat you feel as zero, the next as one, then two, and so on, for 10 seconds. Multiplying that figure by six will tell you your heart rate in beats per minute.

If you find that your pulse is ticking along comfortably at 138 beats per minute, say five beats or so above your calculated target heart rate, keep going. If, however, you're unable to mutter your name three consecutive times, slow down until you can tell someone what you had for dinner last night. In other words, use common sense. Jonathan recently saw a new gym member running on a treadmill like a business-man sprinting for the last train home. It seemed like only a matter of minutes before he was expelled from the revolving belt like a watermelon seed squeezed from one's fingers. When Jonathan asked this ambitious but misguided chap what he was doing, the wheezing runner explained that he was five beats below his target zone. (Jonathan checked his pulse and found out that in fact he was over his target zone by a wide margin.)

The thing to note about this story is this: Check your heart rate a few times to get an accurate reading. Second, listen to your body. Target heart rates are good guides, but they're not written in stone. If, you're cruising along comfortably at the top end of your zone, that's fine. If, on the other hand, you're struggling to keep pace at the low end of the zone, it's okay to back off a little.

If you don't want to be bothered with taking your pulse, but want to be sure that you're training in your target zone, heart rate monitors are available. A wireless trans-mission is sent from a chest strap to a wristwatch receiver, and you get an accurate reading of your heart rate. Some treadmills, bikes, and stair climbers in your gym may also be able to read your heart rate directly from the transmitter. Polar is the best known and most widely used heart rate monitor manufacturer, though others, in-cluding Cardiosport, have entered the market. Models range from the simplest ver-sion, which tells you nothing but your heart rate, to ones with alarms to tell you when you're out of your training zone, to the real fancy-schmancy ones with a stop-watch, bicycle speedometer, and computer interface.

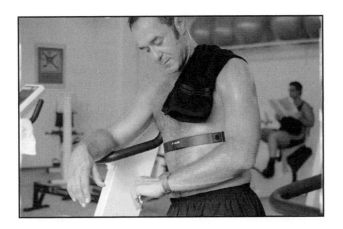

Runner with a heart rate monitor.

(Photo courtesy of Polar)

Take a Class

Within the gym, there are numerous ways to exercise aerobically. Before former martial arts standout Billy Blanks made Tae Bo a national exercise rage, the craze was spinning. Before that, there were step classes, and aerobic dance before that.

Some people look at these theme classes as gimmicky—and we suppose some of them are—but many are great ways to churn and burn in a group setting. The workouts can be quite demanding, but the group dynamic and pulsating music distracts you from the intensity of your effort. Even if you're highly motivated and work out diligently on your own, taking a class is a fun way to diversify your routine. If you're someone who needs to be motivated, these classes may be just what you need.

Below, we will discuss briefly the various forms of aerobic activities available in a majority of gyms.

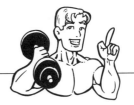

Spot Me

Exercises that use large muscle groups like your legs are usually your best bet for cardiovascular exercise. It's much easier and more comfortable to elevate your heart rate when using your legs, or legs and arms together, than when using just your arms.

Spinning Out

Spinning, which is done on an exercise bike, was developed in California by a character named Johnny G. Typically accompanied by loud funky tunes and sparkling and flashing lights, you stand and sit, spin fast and slow to the calls of your instructor. No one moves (at least not forward) but you get an incredible workout.

Jonathan and Deidre have friends who swear by spin classes. One couple, Richard and Belinda, take the spin classes together every chance they get. The reason this class is

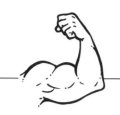

especially good for Richard is because he has gout. Since gout is exacerbated by weight-bearing exercises like running, a spin class is the best aerobic exercise for him to do. Because you adjust the tension on your bike pace in a spin class, they're well suited for a wide variety of fitness levels.

Flash Dance

Aerobic dance has been a mainstay of health club aerobics and home exercise tapes for many years. Ranging from high impact (lots of jumping) to low impact (no jumping), a good aerobics class is a fun way to work your upper and lower body. Like spin classes, the instructor cranks the tunes and tries to motivate participants to push a bit harder than they could push themselves. However, the good teachers will make sure that you're working at a pace comfortable for you.

Flex Facts

While many hardcore cyclists scoff at spinning classes, Jonathan has several teammates who take classes in the off-season and some of his competitors teach spinning classes. A couple of years back he had a teammate who took up racing for the first time after spending several months in spinning classes.

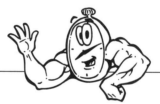

Weight a Minute

Many of the early aerobic dance tapes and classes contained countless contraindicated movements. In fact they're not perfect today either. Look for classes and tapes taught by certified instructors—not dancers.

About 10 years ago, another variation of the basic aerobics classes, called step aerobics, hit the scene. This class uses a step that you hop up and down on to get your heart rate up. There are two different step heights to choose from; the higher the step, the more intense the exercise.

One of the temptations when you first take one of these classes is to try to keep up with the Joneses. Resist that urge and go at your own pace. Often the pace of the class is just too fast, even if you've been running and working out with weights. If you find that you're huffing and puffing so hard that you're thinking about pulling the fire alarm, throttle back. Don't just stop. This will cause blood to pool in your legs. Instead, alter your movements. For example, if the instructor wants jumping, you can hop from side to side at a comfortable pace.

The second important thing to remember is hydration, hydration, and hydration! You should drink 8 to 16 ounces of water 30 to 60 minutes before exercise, 4 to 10 ounces of water every 15 minutes during your workout, and 8 to 16 ounces of water after exercise. Doing strenuous exercise in a hot, smallish room will have you sweating like you're in a sauna.

As we've pointed out many times, exercising without proper hydration is like moving lead weight. Take it from Deidre, who for some reason has shunned drinking pure water for most of her life. (She's happy to drink coffee, soda, or juice, but the pure stuff isn't her cup of tea.) Even though she drinks more water now, there are days that she forgets. When this happens, she can be on a modest five-mile run and suddenly feel as if she's slogging through mud. Her breathing becomes labored, and her concentration is shot. "Why do I feel so awful?" she wonders, until it hits her like a waterfall—drats, forgot the water.

Run, Spot, Run

Running is as pure a sport as you can get. All you need are a good pair of sneakers, shorts, and a T-shirt. (For the women, a jog bra is usually a plus.) The beauty of running is its versatility: If you're feeling solitary, boom, you're out the door alone with your thoughts. If you want company, it's easy to find a mate eager to join you. If you don't know anyone who likes to run, joining a running club is an easy way to find a partner.

When you start out, it's important to learn how to pace yourself so you can cover the distance you set out to run. To lose weight, running at a conversational pace for 30 to 40 minutes is more important than how many miles you go. For cardiovascular fitness, it's helpful to know exactly how far you're running so that you can measure your times as you continue to train. Again, for particular training tips, joining a running club is a great way to go. Typically, clubs have "speed" days at a track as well as long distance days. If there's not a club in your area, check out one of the many books dedicated to the subject. *Runner's World* magazine also is a good guide to training tips and local races in your town or city.

Step, Two, Three, Four

Step machines like the StairMaster offer another great aerobic workout. Essentially, all you're doing is walking up and down on a pair of pedals. You set the level of intensity and time and start stepping. While this is a very simple exercise, we often see people using the machine with their arms fully extended on the handrails bearing a lot of their weight. Clearly, this makes the exercise much easier to perform and much less effective—roughly the equivalent of hanging from a bar and placing your tippy-toes on a scale. If you need to lock out your elbows while you're doing your thing, lessen the intensity. *Cheating* in this fashion not only guarantees that your workout will be compromised, but you also won't burn as many calories as the machine's console says you do.

Jonathan's personal favorite step machine is the Gauntlet. The Gauntlet, made by StairMaster, is basically a set of revolving steps that allows you to actually mimic climbing stairs as opposed to the up and down movement on most other step equipment. More than anything else, it's like walking up a down escalator (a training method that once got Jonathan severely reprimanded by a perplexed guard during his college days). When training for the race up the Empire State Building, Jonathan has been known to spend two or three hours on a Gauntlet. For those of you with slightly saner aspirations, 20 to 30 minutes will suffice.

One of the good features of these machines is the feedback they offer. Almost all step equipment has a computer pad that allows you to work out to several different programs. You can do a steady climb, a hill workout, and various permutations in between. These various programs offer a good change of pace for those of you who get bored doing the same thing all of the time.

There are some pieces of equipment that also take your pulse as you hold the side rails. This is convenient because you don't have to find and hold your pulse while watching the clock. It also saves you the burdensome task of having to multiply lofty sums like 24 times 6.

The Least You Need to Know

➤ If you want to get strong, lift weights, but if you want to be truly fit, take to the treadmill.

➤ There are a number of good ways to figure out how hard to do your cardiovascular work: the talk test or monitoring your heart rate.

➤ Spinning, stair climbers, and aerobics classes are some of the best indoor cardiovascular workouts you'll find at your gym.

Part 6

When in Rome

In this section, we'll address special health issues that may be important to some of you. If you're out of town and dying to work out but don't know how or where, check out Chapter 27 for a variety of solid suggestions. Chapter 28 addresses strength-training issues specific to women, while Chapter 29 talks about the importance and viability of strength training for seniors.

The last three chapters may not apply to you specifically, but they deal with overcoming obstacles. Chapter 30 is geared toward the physically challenged, and Chapter 31 will give guidelines for a safe and effective workout for youngsters. Finally, Chapters 32 and 33 deal with working out with injuries and illness. Even if you're in perfect health, skim through these last two chapters; you'll no doubt see that common folks faced with immense obstacles routinely do the impossible.

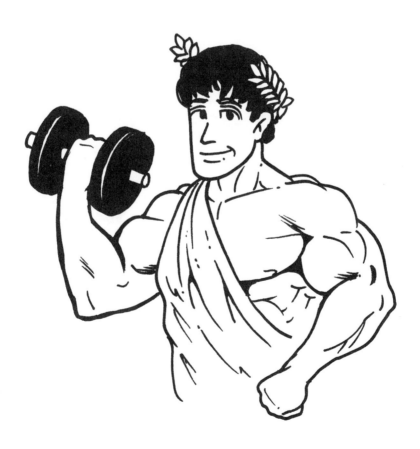

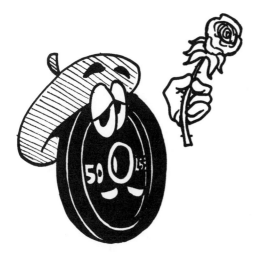

Chapter 27

On the Road Again

In This Chapter

➤ Getting a workout on the road

➤ Doing the old standby: push-ups

➤ Crunch to build a powerful midsection

➤ Weight your ankles and wrists for a good workout

➤ Rubber bands build bodies

For a busy person with a demanding job, especially someone who regularly travels for business, the hardest part of beginning and adhering to a fitness regimen is continuity. While it's certainly no big deal to miss four or five days during a business jaunt, once you skip one week it somehow becomes easier to take another week off when you get home. As we've mentioned previously, taking time off every few months is not a problem. In fact, often it's just what the doctor ordered. However, start stacking the off weeks fairly close together and you're on the slippery slope to exercise oblivion.

This might sound like the cautious words of an exercise fanatic, but we've seen it time and time again: Start skipping workouts—especially if you're going to be eating in restaurants three times a day—and it becomes much harder to get back in the swing of things. Timing a break with an out-of-town business trip is perfect if you've been training consistently and your body could use a break. However, if your training has been inconsistent, your best bet is to continue some sort of routine while you're away so that it won't be like starting all over again when you return home.

Don't get us wrong: We understand that it can be a challenge to find the time and/or motivation when you're on the road. After all, if you're on a business trip or vacation you want to work or relax, not work out. On the other hand, miss too many workouts and you're likely to return home with an extra five or 10 pounds. What to do?

In this chapter, we will outline ways for you to continue your good workout habits while away on business or pleasure.

Gym Away from Home

These days many hotels have recognized the needs of many of their fitness-oriented patrons and gotten with the program by having a gym on the premises. Virtually any travel agent worth her weight in frequent flier miles can find you a hotel with a gym. Many of the higher-end joints have swimming pools as well. Obviously, if you're staying in a place with a gym, you have no excuse not to pump iron. Often we hear people say, "I didn't like the equipment." True, not all of these facilities are state-of-the-art fitness centers, but as long as the equipment is subject to the effects of gravity you can get the job done. After all, weight is weight.

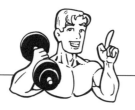

Spot Me

As we discussed in Chapter 4, "Look Before You Lift," IHRSA (International Health Racquet and Sportsclub Association) is a confederation of gyms that are either free when working out at an affiliated gym, or charge a small fee when working out at an affiliated gym. Most health clubs will have a list of member gyms.

If your hotel doesn't have a gym, they often have an affiliation with a nearby gym that allows you access for free or for a discounted fee. If not, you can try to get a day pass to go to a gym in the neighborhood. Also, find out if the gym you belong to at home is a member of IHRSA or another organization that has national affiliations. If it is, you can work out at any of the participating gyms either for free or for a slight fee.

A new gym is a great opportunity to try different strength-training and cardiovascular equipment. We all crave the security of our familiar routine, but it's good practice to break out of old patterns and try something new. Remember that when in doubt, don't be afraid to give an unfamiliar piece of equipment a try.

No Excuse Not to Push

If you don't have access to a hotel gym, or the local gyms are not so local, you can always resort to the old army standby: push-ups. Push-ups are great because they work multiple muscle groups—the pecs, triceps, and deltoids—and they ain't easy.

If you doubt the payoff of this tried-and-true exercise, you should read about the workout regimen of former Heisman Trophy winner and NFL standout Herschel Walker. This fleet-footed 6-foot, 1-inch, 222-pound athlete was built like a Greek god but insisted he never touched a weight in his life. The secret to his splendid physique? Push-ups. Admittedly, he did thousands a day, but the fact remains: You don't need to pump iron to get good results.

To make them even more effective, you can do a variety of push-ups in addition to the normal 3-1-3 shoulder-width method:

➤ Slow push-ups. Fifteen-second push-ups (try 10 seconds up, 5 seconds down) are a sure way to humble your ego and strengthen your pecs and triceps.

➤ The big ouch: Instead of locking your elbows at the top of the push-up, pause midway up and then midway down. Without *rest* during a repetition your muscles will become fatigued that much quicker.

➤ Wide width: Place your arms approximately four to six inches outside your shoulders. This will tweak the muscles in your pecs more than it will those in your triceps.

➤ Narrow: Place your hands just a couple of inches apart beneath the chest. This one is a great way to put extra emphasis on the triceps.

➤ Elevated push-ups: Place your feet on a chair or sofa and have at it. The higher your feet, the harder the pushup. Remember to take your shoes off if you're using Mom's sofa.

When Joe was climbing mountains for a book called *To The Top*, a large-format photography book on the highest mountain in each of the 50 states, he was worried that he'd lose upper body strength since he would not have access to a gym. Virtually every day he did 200 push-ups, including a few sets on the top of Mount Rainier—at 14,420 feet, the highest mountain in the state of Washington.

With each variation, make sure that your form remains sound.

Keep the following tips in mind:

➤ Keep your abdominals tight.

➤ Make sure your back doesn't sag and don't allow your body to touch the floor.

➤ Perform three sets. Whether your set has 5 or 50, go to the point where you can no longer maintain perfect form. Take anywhere from one minute to 90 seconds to rest in between sets.

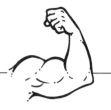

Flex Facts

According to the Guinness book of World Records, the record for the most push-ups in 24 hours is 46,000 and is held by Charles Servizio. That's a lot of push-ups to do in a lifetime, let alone all at once!

An excellent complement to the push-up that you can easily do in any hotel room is chair dips. In Chapter 17, "Chest or Bust," we introduced you to the regular way to do dips in the gym. The chair dip is a variation on that original theme:

1. Sit on the very edge of a chair with your hands gripping the chair's edge.

2. Keeping your legs straight, slide your buttocks off the chair. As you do so, keep your arms straight.

3. Slowly bend your elbows, lowering your buttocks to the floor—without touching the floor.

4. Slowly reverse the position by straightening your arms.

5. Repeat this slowly for as many repetitions as you can with good form.

If these are too easy, elevate your feet on a low bench or chair.

Chair dips—start and end position.

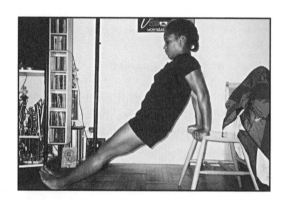

Chair dips—middle position.

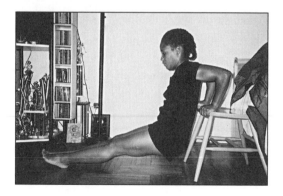

On Your Back

When it comes to no-frills exercises, there's no shortage of abdominal work you can do. In fact, most of the abdominal exercises we taught you back in Chapter 20, "Gut Buster," don't require equipment. In short, there's really no excuse not to work your abs while you're on the road.

For a thorough ab workout, do three sets of the following exercises:

➤ Crunches

➤ Reverse crunches

➤ Oblique crunches

In fact, if you have just 15 minutes to work out while you're on the road, do an abdominal routine. Building a strong center is a good way to keep your mind attuned to the act of working out. Perhaps it's because strong abs make you feel fit, but for some reason, nothing gets people motivated like the prospect of having solid, good-looking abdominals. In addition, people who routinely do ab work seem to watch what they eat. Take a vacation to the beach and you'll be doubly motivated to get that old ab routine back in gear.

Lead Shoes

If you really can't stomach push-ups and chair dips, you may want to try working out on the road with ankle and wrist weights. They come in a variety of shapes and sizes (they used to only be filled with sand) and are easy to carry in your suitcase. While they're not a perfect alternative to dumbbells and barbells, there are many exercises you can do with them to get a good workout.

The more common, sand-filled ankle and wrist weights range from one pound to as much as 15 pounds. For an effective workout, you should probably use weights ranging from 5 to 10 pounds.

Here are the advantages of sand-filled ankle weights:

➤ They are not expensive.

➤ They can be used for a variety of exercises.

Here are the disadvantages of sand-filled ankle weights:

➤ As you progress and purchase additional weights, they can take up a lot of space.

➤ They can rip and tear. When this happens, you'll be following a trail of sand that you'll be cleaning up for months, if not years.

Another type of ankle weight comes with lead columns that fit into slots. This is good because you only need to purchase more lead columns as opposed to new ankle weights when you want to increase the resistance.

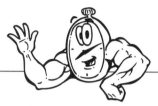

Weight a Minute

Perhaps you've seen an ambitious, but misguided fitness fanatic running with ankle weights. While it may seem like a fine way to make your run more challenging, it's an even better way to injure your knees and ankles. The best way to make a running workout harder is to run faster—or uphill—not weigh yourself down.

Here are the advantages of lead-column ankle weights:

➤ They don't take up as much space as the sand-filled variety.

➤ They're easily adjustable.

Here are the disadvantages of lead-column ankle weights:

➤ You may need to purchase many lead columns in order to get an effective workout.

➤ Lead columns can get fairly expensive.

➤ Additional lead columns can be cumbersome.

➤ They're annoying to get through security at the airport.

The following is a sample workout with ankle weights:

Body Part	Exercises
Glutes/quads/hamstrings	Lunges (weights on shoulders)
	Abduction
	Adduction
Calves	Heel raises (weights on shoulders)
Back	Dumbbell rows
Chest	Chest press
	Flyes

Body Part	Exercises
Shoulders	Military presses
	Lateral raises
	Front raises
	Reverse flyes
Biceps	Curls
	Concentration curls
Triceps	French curls
	Kickbacks

When doing these exercises, always keep proper form in mind. Just because you are not in a gym per se doesn't mean that you shouldn't adhere to proper technique.

Dyna-Band What?

Dyna-Bands are a color-coded progressive resistance program using what are essentially super-duper rubber bands made of elastic. They're most often used in a rehab setting (Deidre used them extensively with her patients when she worked in a physical therapy clinic), but they function really well in a quick workout. They come in a variety of colors, with different degrees of resistance associated with each color from pink (easiest) to silver (hardest).

Accessories are available to make the exercises more versatile, including exercise handles and door anchors. These accessories enable you to work out with the bands with greater stability.

We like Dyna-Bands for quick, easy workouts on the road. They're certainly not perfect, and we're not suggesting that you can get in great shape using them all the time, but ease of use and convenience makes them a solid choice when you're on the road.

Here are some of the pluses of Dyna-Bands:

➤ Easy to pack

➤ Variable resistance

➤ Can be used for a variety of exercises

➤ Very safe to use

Nothing (including Dyna-Bands) is perfect. Here's what we don't love about them:

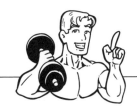

Spot Me

When you use Dyna-Bands, you can vary the resistance by changing where you hold the band. The shorter the length used, the harder it is to stretch it for the full range of motion of an exercise.

337

➤ Much like the elastic band used by the Soloflex that we described in Chapter 5, "There's No Place Like Home," the resistance is not constant throughout the range of motion (ROM). Often there is too much slack at the beginning of the movement. And if you choose a size of band that gives you tension at the beginning range, it's not large enough to allow you a full ROM.

➤ While there are some good exercises to do for the smaller body parts like shoulders and arms, there are not many effective exercises to do for larger body parts like your glutes, quads, and hamstrings.

However, using them on the road is far better than doing nothing at all. If you want to check them out, the following are a few exercises that you can perform.

Body Part	Exercises
Legs	Seated leg press: Sit on a step or bench with your knee bent. Wrap the Dyna-Band around one foot, and grasp both ends in each hand. Keep your toes pointed slightly downward. Slowly straighten your leg (don't lock your knee). Slowly return to the starting position.
Back	Seated rows: Sit on the floor and wrap the Dyna-Band around the balls of both feet. With elbows bent, pull your arms back while squeezing your shoulder blades together. Slowly return to the starting position.
Chest	Chest press: Wrap Dyna-Band around your back. Grip the band ends with both hands and press your arms forward. Slowly return to the starting position.
Shoulders	Lateral raises: Stand with feet shoulder width apart and place one end of the Dyna-Band under your foot as you hold the other end in your hand. Slowly raise your arm out to the side until you reach shoulder height. Slowly return to the starting position. Front raises: Same starting position. Slowly raise your arm upward until you reach shoulder height. Slowly return to the starting position.
Biceps	Bicep curls: Stand with your feet shoulder width apart and place one end of the Dyna-Band under your foot as you hold the other end in your hand. Slowly curl your arm by bending your elbow toward your shoulder. Slowly return to the starting position.
Triceps	Tricep extensions: Place a towel around your neck. Place the Dyna-Band along the towel. Grip both ends in each hand so that your elbows are bent at 90°. Keep your elbows close to your body as you slowly straighten your arms. Make sure to keep your wrists straight. Slowly return to the starting position.

Manual Labor

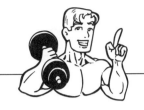

If you are an old-fashioned type and decide that nothing else will do except for dumbbells, there are portable dumbbells on the market that are made especially for people on the go. An excellent alternative to conventional weights is the water-inflatable weight system called AquaBell Ankle Weights. This portable weight-lifting system is perfect for people who travel because they are easy to carry—the thing weighs only eight ounces when collapsed and inflates to eight pounds of resistance—and can provide you with enough resistance to get a good workout.

Here are some of the pluses of the Ankle Weight Water System:

> **Spot Me**
>
> Dyna-Bands can be purchased through physical therapy catalogues or surgical supply stores in either 6-yard or 50-yard quantities, or in individual bands. The price varies depending upon the amount of resistance.

➤ It's extremely lightweight and takes up very little space.

➤ It inflates to a fairly decent amount of resistance.

➤ It's made of tough, high-tech material that will last for years.

➤ You can pack more than two ankle weights since they are so light, so you can add more weight to your workout.

Here are some of the disadvantages of the AquaBell Ankle Weight Water System:

➤ Can't think of one.

➤ Well, okay, the name is kind of cumbersome.

The AquaBell Water System also manufactures dumbbells. The AquaBell Dumbbell system weighs only 24 ounces when collapsed. When filled with water, each dumbbell can provide 16 pounds of resistance.

The great thing about these is that you are already familiar with the exercises that are available for you to do. Following is a list of them.

Body Part	Exercises
Glutes/quads/hamstrings	Lunges
Calves	Standing calf raises
Back	Dumbbell rows
Chest	Dumbbell presses

continues

continued

Body Part	Exercises
Shoulders	Military presses
	Lateral raises
	Front raises
	Reverse flyes
Biceps	Curls
	Concentration curls
Triceps	French curls
	Kickbacks

A lot of people wonder: What do I do if the amount of resistance available is not enough? Good question: Here are a few ways that you can make your workout effective.

Instead of the 2/4 count that we have been advising you to follow, you can make the repetitions even longer. For example, try using a 5/10 count. The slower the repetitions are, the harder the exercise becomes. You can also decrease the amount of rest that you take in between sets. Instead of recovering for 90 seconds, rest just a minute between sets.

The decision of whether or not to work out while on the road is up to you. You should choose an option that you enjoy and are likely to stick with for the duration of your trip. If you have the time, call ahead to find out what is available near where you'll be. If there is no gym in the hotel or if the gym is not a convenient distance away, decide whether you're going to do push-ups, sit-ups, or use ankle weights, Dyna-Bands, or water weights.

Here's another important point: It's often easier for people to continue cardiovascular exercise on the road than it is to do a strength-training routine. If you're a runner who lifts but don't have access to a gym on the road, by all means lace on your running shoes and head for the hills. If you're so inclined, do three sets of push-ups before and after your run. This will give you a modest pump and keep you primed when you return to the gym. The larger point, however, is continuity. Since it's difficult, and even unpleasant, to start working out again after a long layoff, the key is to do something, anything really, especially if you find it fun.

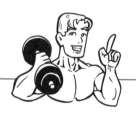

Spot Me

We know it's hard to squeeze in time for the gym while you're out of town. Keep in mind that just one good weight-lifting workout per week is enough to *maintain* the strength gains you've already made.

The Least You Need to Know

➤ Many hotels have in-house gyms, or affiliations with neighboring gyms.

➤ The most basic and effective strength-training exercise requires no special equipment. We're talking about the push-up.

➤ If you want abs of steel, find a comfortable rug and have at it.

➤ Ankle and wrist weights can be a bit cumbersome to travel with, but they are effective.

➤ Rubber bands are easy to take on the road and provide a challenging workout.

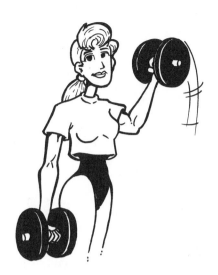

Chapter 28

Real Women Lift

> ## In This Chapter
>
> ➤ Becoming strong, not big
>
> ➤ Understanding that time of the workout
>
> ➤ Lifting for two
>
> ➤ Ironing out your diet

In many parts of the world, at many points in history, women have performed as much physical labor as men. During the nineteenth century, on the family farms that dominated much of this country, women often hauled water, plowed fields, and cut hay alongside their husbands. And *women's work*—scrubbing clothes on a washboard, churning butter, baking bread in cast-iron stoves—was probably as physically demanding as men's.

After the turn of the century, increasing urbanization, mechanization, and prosperity led to more general acceptance of the feminine ideal, a woman too delicate and too refined for physical work. Of course, the feminine ideal was also too delicate for all but the tamest sports—badminton, anyone? Now the pendulum is swinging back. In the past 25 years, women have fought for their right to become firefighters, construction workers, or soldiers. They have fought for the right to play sports in school with equipment and facilities on a par with men. (Several women are even on the rosters of NCAA Division I football programs, albeit as place kickers.) At the time of this writing, the Women's National Basketball Association is in its third season, and women's World Cup soccer played in 1999 to sell-out crowds—in the largest stadiums in the United States.

While we should be proud of reaching these milestones, it's important to remember the female sports pioneers of times past. For example, at the very first modern Olympic games held in Athens in 1896, a woman named Melpomene petitioned to compete in the marathon. Of course her petition was denied. However, this did not stop her from running the 40 kilometers from Marathon to Athens. Her finishing time? Four hours, 30 minutes. Sound like archaic discrimination? Katherine Switzer, who disguised herself as a man to run the 1968 Boston Marathon, was attacked by the race director, who tried to pull her off the course. It took nearly 100 years before women had their own Olympic Marathon to run. (The winner? Joan Benoit at the 1984 Games in Los Angeles.)

Now, while Melpomene's story has nothing to do with weight training, it does have to do with toughness, both mental and physical—characteristics found in women as often as in men. So why do some women just assume that weight lifting is beyond them, or that strength is a guy thing? The old feminine ideal, though publicly discredited, is not quite dead. She lives on in the form of the Barbie doll, society's vision of the perfect woman. And, more damaging, she lives on in women's own subconscious minds.

But the good news is that women have learned to question what society thinks. They've learned they can change the rules, and set and achieve their own goals. Badminton and croquet may be fun, but there's a whole lot more out there to do— judo or downhill mountain biking—and women can do it all.

This chapter is not meant to describe a different set of lifting rules for women. There are no different rules. Just as there is only one way to run a marathon, there is only one way to lift weights—with all you've got. What we want to do here is clear up misconceptions about women and weights and take into account situations that are clearly unique to women—menstruation, pregnancy, and osteoporosis. Let's get started.

I Don't Want to Get Too Big

One of the most common reasons women don't want to participate in a weight-training program is that they don't want to "get big." Well, we are here to tell you, unequivocally, not to worry. Bulging muscles just aren't going to sneak up on you six months into a weight-training program. Here's why: Muscle size is due to high levels of the hormone testosterone. Women do have testosterone, but not in high enough quantities to cause them to bulk up during weight training the way some men do. With weight training, a woman's muscles will become more defined, but not appreciably larger.

So, what about women like Deidre? While her lack of testosterone limits how big her muscles can get, she's obviously much more muscular than your average woman (or your average man, for that matter). However, her physique is the product of two fairly rare conditions. The first is a genetic predisposition to muscularity; specifically, higher-than-average levels of testosterone and fast-twitch muscle fibers. The second is a commitment to many years of aggressive training—harder work than most people, men or women, would want to take on. Try squatting almost triple your body weight and you'll begin to understand how strong she really is.

Some women who lift weights limit themselves to light weights/high reps routines under the misconception that this will tone and lengthen their muscles, while heavy weights and low reps will make them bulky. Wrong again! Muscles don't change length and they don't know the difference between light weights and heavy weights. They only know how hard they're working. If the weight is sufficiently difficult and you lift consistently, you will get stronger. If your DNA gave you higher-than-average levels of testosterone and your muscles are programmed to get larger with appropriate stimulation, then your muscles will get larger.

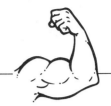

Flex Facts

At rest, men have 10 times the amount of circulating testosterone that women have. The abuse of steroids can raise testosterone levels in women to the levels in men, or higher.

Here's another caveat emptor: Don't be scared off by pictures of female bodybuilders on the covers of *Muscle & Fitness* and other muscle magazines. These professionals are genetically gifted and they work out for a living. (In addition, there is reason to speculate that a few of the *supplements* taken by these women have contributed to their tremendous muscle growth. Read: Women with 18-inch arms and mustaches have been known to take steroids.)

Deidre has the genetic gifts and work ethic necessary to gain muscle mass, and we don't know many women prouder of that fact. Interestingly, back in her power-lifting days, it was always other women who would caution her not to get any bigger. From the guys, she'd hear, "You're awfully strong for a girl." We are fairly sure that comment was meant as a compliment. Our Miss Dee would reply, "Why can't I just be strong?" and get on with her workout.

Weight training provides the following benefits for women:

➤ Increased lean body mass, which provides women with more functional strength

➤ Enhanced bone remodeling, which increases bone strength and decreases risk for osteoporosis

➤ Stronger connective tissue (ligaments and tendons), which protects joints and decreases risk of injury

➤ Increased strength for sports and activities of daily living (carrying luggage, walking up and down stairs with groceries, lifting children)

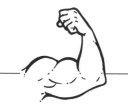

Flex Facts

Even with genetic gifts and hard work, a woman will not gain the degree of muscularity that an extremely fit man has unless she is abusing anabolic steroids, which significantly increases testosterone levels. Even then, the workouts needed to reach that level are insanely difficult. You won't get there by accident.

➤ Increased lean body mass and decreased non-functional fat

➤ Increased metabolic rate due to more active muscle

➤ Increased self-esteem

In short, women reap the same benefits from strength training that men do. Though men have greater absolute strength than women because of height, frame dimensions, and larger muscles, women can develop as much or more relative strength as men.

As we said earlier, this chapter does not offer a program tailored to women, for the simple reason that women should not train any differently than men. Strength gains are achieved by forcing the muscle to adapt to greater and greater loads. If women train with submaximal efforts, they will not reap the many benefits available to them.

Guide Me

The section that follows gives general guidelines for how women can weight lift during menstruation and pregnancy, as well as the effects of weight lifting on osteoporosis and menopause. These are extremely general; always, always check with your doctor before embarking on a program.

That Time

Gone are the days when you could get out of physical education class by letting your teacher know it was "that time of the month." Today most women feel perfectly comfortable keeping up their exercise programs during menstruation. In fact, doctors recommend exercise to relieve the symptoms of premenstrual syndrome (PMS)—fatigue, edginess, depression—as well as the muscle cramps that come later.

There's no reason not to weight train during your period, as long as you use common sense and listen to your body. If you have a day or two when you feel especially weak, it makes sense not to push it. You probably don't want to add weight to your usual routine on these days. This is especially important if you tend to be anemic. But if you're just a little tired and cranky, stock up on your feminine hygiene products and head to the gym. Keep in mind that many Olympic athletes have competed for and won medals while menstruating.

Female Trouble

Some women, particularly elite female athletes, experience variations in their menstrual cycle that can be linked to their athletic activities.

There are three types of menstrual irregularities:

➤ *Oligomenorrhea,* which is defined as an irregular menstrual cycle in women who previously had a normal one

➤ *Secondary amenorrhea,* which is defined as the absence of menstruation in women who previously periodically menstruated (*primary amenorrhea* is defined as previously regular cycles that have ceased)

➤ *Dysmenorrhea,* which is defined as pain during menstruation

Highly athletic women, particularly those who have low body fat, are more prone to irregularities with their menstrual cycles (either oligomenorrhea or secondary amenorrhea) than their sedentary counterparts. That's because adipose tissue (fat) is the site of conversion of androgens (male hormones) to estrogens (female hormones). An alteration in body composition can change the estrogen levels in the body and therefore affect the menstrual cycle. It should be noted, however, that there are athletes with low body fat who do not suffer altered menstrual cycles, and some heavier athletes who do. The women most prone to menstrual irregularities are young athletes engaged in intense daily training who have both low body weight and a low percentage of body fat.

On the other hand, dysmenorrhea—abdominal pain with menstruation—is reported to occur *less* frequently and with *less* severity in athletes than in the rest of the population.

Amenorrhea or oligomenorrhea have no detrimental effects on athletic performance. However, whenever a change in the menstrual cycle occurs, a gynecologist should always be consulted. While "the absence of menstruation" might sound more like a cause to celebrate than to worry, the problem that faces women who have irregular or no menstrual cycles is the possible early onset of bone density loss, which normally begins at menopause.

Baby Time

Being pregnant can be the most wonderful but anxiety-ridden experience that any woman can have in her adult life. So many things to think about: nutrition, weight gain, prenatal care, maternity leave, college funds, working out—hey, what about that brand-new weight-lifting fitness routine? Can I keep it up?

Exercise during pregnancy can be safe and effective.

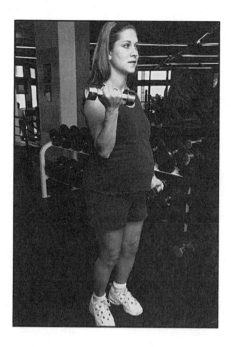

Fear not, soon-to-be mothers. Pregnancy does not preclude an exercise regimen. As a matter of fact, it can help to reduce many of the problems that can arise during pregnancy—mainly back pain and depression. In the section that follows, we will outline basic guidelines set up by the American College of Obstetricians and Gynecologists (ACOG) and tell you what to watch out for as you continue with your healthy lifestyle.

Years ago, exercise during pregnancy was completely unheard of. Pregnancy was considered a delicate condition. Women were barely allowed to pull out a chair to sit down, let alone ride a bike, run, or lift weights. Ironically, it is in childbirth that women throughout the ages have demonstrated their strength. If women can labor and bear children, they can certainly exercise.

If you began exercising before becoming pregnant, ACOG states that you can continue exercising. Again, listen to your body. Most women will naturally adjust their exercise intensity based upon how they feel as their pregnancy progresses. If you are pregnant and plan to begin an exercise program for the first time, contact your physician prior to initiating any new program. Bungee jumping and/or skydiving, while fun, should be postponed until Junior exits the womb.

While exercising, even women firmly entrenched in a routine should be aware of the competition for oxygen, blood flow, and nutrients between the mother's muscles and the developing fetus. Adjust intensity according to how difficult you find the exercise, as opposed to heart rate alone. The rate of perceived exertion (RPE) scale can be a useful tool to make sure you're not working out too hard. See Chapter 26, "Mix It Up," for a chart of this scale.

There is no proof that exercising during pregnancy will lessen labor pains—although it undoubtedly improves your physical and mental ability to handle pain. Exercising before and during pregnancy offers a multitude of benefits: improved muscular fitness and aerobic capacity; faster recovery from labor; a more rapid return to prepregnancy weight, flexibility, and strength levels; increased psychological well-being; and a decrease in episodes of depression after childbirth.

Follow the Guidelines

Following are three lists of guidelines developed by ACOG for safe exercise prescription during pregnancy, reasons to stop exercise and seek medical advice, and contraindications to exercise during pregnancy.

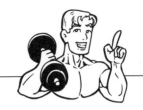

Spot Me

The old ACOG guidelines suggested a maximum heart rate during exercise of 140 beats per minute. These guidelines were revised to take into account that the mother's resting heart rate is elevated 15 to 20 beats per minute during pregnancy, which invalidated standard training heart rate formulas.

The following are ACOG recommendations for exercise in pregnancy and postpartum:

1. During pregnancy, women can continue to exercise and derive health benefits from mild to moderate exercise routines. Regular exercise (at least three times per week) is preferable to intermittent activity.

2. Women should avoid exercise in the supine position (on their back) after the first trimester. This position is associated with decreased cardiac output in most pregnant women. Prolonged periods of motionless standing should be avoided as well.

3. Women should be aware of the decreased oxygen available for aerobic exercise during pregnancy. Intensity should be modified according to maternal symptoms. Pregnant women should stop exercising when fatigued and not exercise to exhaustion. Weight-bearing exercises may under some circumstances be continued throughout pregnancy at intensities similar to those before pregnancy. Nonweight-bearing exercises (cycling, swimming) minimize the risk of injury.

4. Exercises that may contribute to the woman's loss of balance should be avoided. Any exercise involving the potential for abdominal trauma should be avoided.

5. Pregnancy requires an additional 300 calories per day in order to maintain metabolic homeostasis. Pregnant exercising women should pay close attention to maintaining an adequate diet.

6. Pregnant women who exercise in the first trimester should make sure to stay sufficiently hydrated during exercise.

7. Many of the changes related to pregnancy persist for four to six weeks postpartum. Prepregnancy exercise routines should be resumed gradually based upon the woman's physical capability.

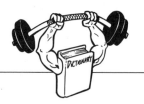

Bar Talk

Phlebitis is an inflammation of a vein. The cause is unknown but it usually occurs in acute or chronic infections or following surgery or childbirth.

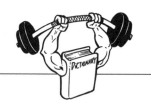

Bar Talk

Palpitations are an abnormally rapid throbbing or fluttering of the heart.

ACOG reasons to discontinue exercise and seek medical advice during pregnancy:

1. Any signs of bloody discharge from the vagina
2. Any *gush* of fluid from the vagina
3. Sudden swelling of ankles, hands, or face
4. Persistent, severe headaches and/or visual disturbance; unexplained spells of faintness or dizziness
5. Swelling, pain, and redness in the calf of one leg (*phlebitis*)
6. Elevation of pulse rate or blood pressure that persists after exercise
7. Excessive fatigue, *palpitations*, chest pain
8. Persistent contractions (from six to eight per hour) that may suggest onset of premature labor
9. Unexplained abdominal pain
10. Insufficient weight gain (less than 2.2 pounds per month during the last two trimesters)

The following are ACOG contraindications for exercising during pregnancy:

1. Pregnancy-induced hypertension
2. Preterm rupture of the membrane
3. Preterm labor during the prior or current pregnancy
4. Incompetent cervix
5. Persistent second- to third-trimester bleeding
6. Intrauterine growth retardation

Deidre has a friend, a runner, who, after the birth of two children, weighs less than her prepregnancy self. With her first pregnancy, she ran well into her seventh month. With her second, she stopped running way before that because she just didn't feel well. When you listen to your body and do what feels right, you can't go wrong.

Good Moves for Pregnant Women

Added abdominal strength can be especially helpful for pregnant women. Since we've already warned you that after your first trimester you should avoid exercising on your back, an alternative to crunches is needed.

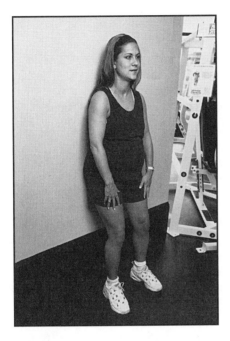

Standing crunch start/finish position.

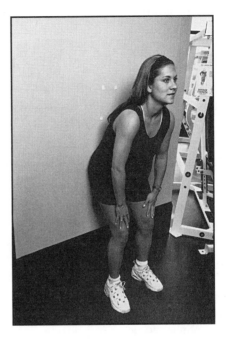

Standing crunch midrange position.

The standing abdominal crunch is a great exercise for women to do in the second and third trimester of pregnancy to continue abdominal strength.

Here is how you properly perform a standing crunch:

1. Stand against the wall with feet shoulder width apart and arms by your side.
2. Tighten your abdominals and slowly bend forward until your midback comes away from the wall.
3. Slowly return to your starting position.

The following is a list of don'ts:

➤ Hold your breath.

➤ Perform the exercise rapidly.

➤ Allow your lower back to come away from the wall.

The following is a list of do's:

➤ Blow out through your mouth as you tighten your abdominals and bend forward.

➤ Inhale through your nose as you slowly return to your starting position.

➤ Perform the exercise slowly, with control.

Osteoporosis

Osteoporosis—a softening of the bone—is a condition that develops silently over the years and is often not discovered until after a fracture has taken place. It is far easier to prevent than to treat. In this section, we'll explain what causes osteoporosis and how exercise and proper nutrition can prevent it from occurring.

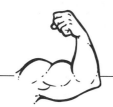

Flex Facts

Wolff's Law—accepted by some, but not all, scientists—states that bone grows or remodels in response to the stresses placed upon it. This means that you strengthen your bones by stressing them with activity.

Bones maintain their structure over the years through a process of old bone removal (*resorption*) and new bone formation. In early adulthood, the rates of loss and replacement are balanced. However, as women age and go through menopause, their estrogen levels drop and the rate of bone removal outpaces the rate of bone replacement. Twenty-five million women are affected by osteoporosis—one out of five women over the age of 45 and 4 out of 10 women over the age of 75. Although osteoporosis is thought of as a women's disease, the fact is that 3.5 million men over the age of 50 suffer from this disease due primarily to falling levels of testosterone.

You can tip the balance in your favor through weight training. When skeletal bone is subjected to strains 10 times that required for typical daily activities, it responds by creating stronger tissue. That's one reason why weight training is so valuable for older women.

The Problem with Diets

Postmenopausal women are not the only women at risk for osteoporosis. A growing number of women in their twenties, even those who exercise, are experiencing bone density loss usually associated with women in their forties or fifties. The reason is our national obsession with dieting. A young woman who limits her intake to 1,200 or 1,300 calories a day, and relies heavily on diet soda, rice cakes, and salads, is probably not getting all the calcium and vitamin D she needs. Couple this with the stress of vigorous aerobic workouts and you have a body under constant assault without the tools to rebuild itself. Injury, illness, and depression can result.

Even female athletes are at risk. Disordered eating, amenorrhea (cessation of menstruation), and osteoporosis—known collectively as "the female athletic triad"—is common in sports such as gymnastics, figure skating, and diving, where enormous emphasis is placed on being thin. Estrogen is the hormone that protects women from bone density loss. As we discussed above, estrogen is created in fat tissues. In female athletes, aggressive training coupled with misguided eating habits brings body fat levels so low that estrogen levels drop and menstruation stops. Prolonged estrogen deficiency can put women at risk for osteoporosis later in life. Any woman with this experience should be evaluated for the status of her skeletal health.

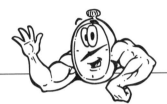

Weight a Minute

The female athletic triad is all too common in sports where shape and form are considered integral to the sport. As a young athlete matures, she adds weight. Since this can affect her ability to jump—or even just change the way she looks while jumping—she follows a strict diet while maintaining a strenuous workout routine. In the worst-case scenario, poor nutrition leads to cessation of menstruation, which leads to osteoporosis.

Menopause

Menopause is the period of time when a woman's menstrual cycle ends. According to the *Physician and Sports Medicine* journal, the many problems that may be associated with menopause are:

➤ Hot flashes

➤ Bone loss

➤ Cardiovascular disease

➤ Urogenital atrophy

➤ Depression and sleep disturbance

➤ Weight gain

➤ Muscle weakness

A few of these problems (weight gain, muscle weakness, cardiovascular disease) are a result of aging. The others are a result of decreased estrogen stores. Although active women certainly experience the symptoms and problems associated with menopause, on the whole they fare better than sedentary women.

A complete exercise program for postmenopausal women should involve aerobic exercise, resistance exercise, and stretching. Aerobics should include 20 to 60 minutes per session of cycling, brisk walking, swimming, aerobics, or rowing 7 days per week; each individual, depending upon her general level of fitness, determines the intensity. For sedentary women just beginning a routine, 15 minutes of walking at a comfortable pace 3 days per week is a good start. The goal is to gradually increase time, frequency, and intensity.

Resistance exercise should be performed 3 times per week with freeweights or machines. To prevent injury, the exercises should be done with instruction and under supervision until form and technique are perfected. A stretching program should be done following each aerobics session and resistance training session to maintain flexibility.

The benefits of exercise for postmenopausal women are many:

➤ Lowered incidence of cardiovascular disease

➤ Prevention of obesity

➤ Maintenance of muscle strength necessary for the most simple activities such as transferring from sitting to standing, walking up and down stairs, and carrying groceries

➤ Decreased risk of osteoporosis

➤ Relief from depression and sleep disturbances

Weight training and other forms of exercise do so much to improve the quality of life for all women, particularly older women. A strong woman remains independent longer and just plain feels better. These days, older women are not automatically consigned to the rocking chair and the knitting basket—they are skiing, parasailing, and running marathons alongside their daughters and granddaughters. And sometimes they come in first.

The Least You Need to Know

➤ Conforming to the feminine ideal doesn't mean you can't lift and get strong.

➤ The biggest myth about women and weights is that lifting will make them bulky.

➤ Exercise during pregnancy can be beneficial before, during, and after childbirth.

➤ Whether you're a teen or postmenopausal, eating right is crucial to your health.

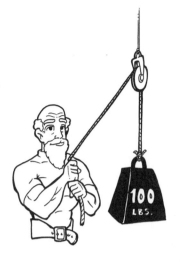

Chapter 29

With Age Comes Wisdom

In This Chapter

➤ Realizing that youth is wasted on the young

➤ Turning back Father Time

➤ Knowing how often and how hard

➤ Expecting the unexpected

Most of us complain about getting old, but when you consider the alternative, it's a welcome option. The other saying that speaks volumes is the line "Youth is wasted on the young."

It's only when you look back at your twenties and thirties that you really understand the foolishness of young people smoking cigarettes, drinking too much booze, and generally not taking advantage of (or even appreciating) the health and energy they've been granted.

That's the bad news. The good news is that there are many benefits to getting older— life experience, actual wisdom, and if you're lucky, financial security. Unfortunately, maintaining good health requires more work as we age than it did when we were mere callow youths. We see this all the time with professional athletes—their reflexes slow, they lose a step, and take longer to recover from injury than they used to. (Of course, the motto of the cagey veteran is "Age and treachery will always overcome youth and skill.")

Therefore it follows that if you compare a 40-year-old athlete to his 25-year-old team-mate, you're likely to see a fairly large difference in their physical abilities. Take the 40-year-old Rickey Henderson of the New York Mets. Considered the greatest leadoff hitter in baseball history, Henderson is still a top-flight player and still a potent base stealer; however, his acts of daring on the base paths now pale in comparison to those of his prime. However, contrast the 40-year-old Henderson with even a 30-year-old couch potato and you will find the gap between the two staggering.

The effects of aging *and* inactivity are extremely profound:

➤ Muscle atrophy

➤ Weight gain

➤ Balance impairment

➤ Decreased reaction time

➤ Hypertension

➤ Coronary artery disease

➤ Decreased physical endurance

➤ Decreased walking speed

Here's a news flash: Following a sound exercise program can reverse some of the effects of aging. While we all know this, many people are unwilling (or unable) to do something about it. There have been several studies conducted that reveal that seniors can gain muscle and lose body fat by beginning an exercise regimen without a huge investment of time.

Now just because we do enjoy lifting weights, we don't ask that you lift just for the sake of lifting. Rather, we want you to understand the importance of the saying, "If you don't use it, you lose it." Muscle is what moves your skeleton. When your muscles atrophy because of inactivity, your ability to move your skeleton through space becomes compromised. Your balance becomes poor because your muscles can't support you and you lose the ability to walk long distances, or even stand in one place for five minutes at a time, because of a lack of muscular endurance. Simple activities like standing from a sitting position and carrying bags become a chore.

Don't get us wrong. We're not saying that starting and maintaining an exercise program is easy, especially when you start collecting social security checks. (In fact, starting is very difficult.) However, the results and sense of well-being one reaps are certainly worth it. The biggest ingredient is desire. With proper supervision and instruction anyone can safely reap the benefits that exercise has to offer.

One of Joe's athletic heroes is a 77-year-old Alaskan named Yule Kitcher. When Joe met the farmer from Homer, Alaska, he was suffering from a stiff lower back. "How'd you hurt it?" Joe asked. "Skiing with a quartered moose," he replied matter-of-factly. If you're like Yule you don't need to pump iron; it is, however, much less expensive when it comes to your dry cleaning.

Benefits

Again, we can't stress enough how important it is to stick with an exercise program as you get older. To hammer home our point, let's review some of the major pluses:

➤ Increased muscular strength and endurance, which help the elderly continue to perform regular everyday activities with greater ease.

➤ Through the aging process, it is natural and quite easy to gain weight. Gaining weight can be the root of many problems associated with aging like hypertension (high blood pressure), coronary artery disease (CAD), and myocardial infarction (MI or heart attack). Cardiovascular exercise helps to keep your weight down, which controls your cholesterol levels and decreases the risk of heart disease.

➤ For older women, exercise decreases the risk of bone density loss and decreases the symptoms and problems associated with menopause.

➤ Reduced risk of muscle, tendon, and ligament injury.

➤ The ability to remain independent, run after your grandkids, and enjoy life to its fullest with continued functional strength.

We begin to lose muscle mass in the third decade of life, approximately one pound of muscle each year or about 8 percent per decade. As a result, the performance of the most mundane and ordinary activities requires close to maximum effort for the elderly as compared to younger folk. (Watch an infirm 75-year-old walk up a flight of stairs and you know what we mean.) Furthermore, once muscle function becomes impaired, any acute illness, trauma, or surgery will require extended periods of bed rest. An elderly person can enter a hospital fairly mobile and after two weeks of being inert be unable to stand without assistance.

Get Dense

Dr. Wayne Westcott conducted two interesting studies on seniors and exercise. The first consisted of 31 seniors (average age 65 years) who participated in 25 minutes of strength exercise and 25 minutes of endurance exercise, three days per week. The result? The subjects gained 3.5 pounds of lean weight and lost 5 pounds of fat weight after eight weeks of training.

The second study included 85 seniors (average age 65 years) who performed 25 minutes of strength training with 25 minutes of endurance exercise two times per week. The subjects added 2 pounds of lean weight and lost 4 pounds of fat weight after eight weeks of training.

Another study by Dr. Westcott revealed that regular weight training resulted in lower resting blood pressure in seniors, as well as, mildly hypertensive individuals.

In addition to gaining muscle and losing fat, results of several other studies showed the following:

➤ An increase in bone density for both men and women

➤ Enhanced glucose metabolism, which may decrease adult onset diabetes

➤ An increase in gastrointestinal transit speed which may result in a reduced risk of colon cancer

➤ Reduced lower back pain with properly executed exercises

➤ Alleviation of arthritic discomfort

➤ An improvement in blood cholesterol profiles

Physiological benefits are not the only gains from initiating a weight-training program. A study conducted at Harvard University in 1997 showed that after 12 weeks of strength exercise, 14 of 16 seniors no longer met the criteria for clinical depression. This should come as no surprise to people who exercise regularly, but in the West, where we're more skeptical about the mind/body connection, it often seems like a revelation.

Yet another study by Westcott in 1996 compared the results of young, middle-aged, and older adults following an eight-week training program consisting of 30 minutes of strength training and 20 minutes of endurance training.

The 1,132 participants included 238 young adults (21 to 40 years); 553 middle-aged adults (41 to 60 years); and 341 older adults (61 to 80 years). All the groups began the program with similar body weights and body fat levels. After eight weeks of exercise, the body weight and body fat changes were comparable for the three groups.

The point of the studies is to show that seniors can gain muscle and lose fat at rates comparable to young and middle-aged folk. Which proves still another old adage: "You're never too old to start acting young."

Suit Yourself

If you take nothing else from this chapter, here's what we'd like you to learn loud and clear:

> The key to adhering to an exercise program, whether you're old or young, is doing something that you enjoy.

In other words: Have fun!

In the cardio realm that means choosing an activity that you look forward to: swimming, cycling, brisk walking, hiking, jogging, in-line skating, stair climbing, or water aerobics, you name it—as long as you enjoy it. While those activities will provide enormous physical and mental benefits, none of them provides you with the benefits that weight training does. In a study conducted over a period of 10 years, the subjects, elite middle-aged runners, were shown to lose five pounds of muscle during the course of the 10 years.

Our experience, however, is that if you regularly engage in a sport that you like, you'll have the energy and eagerness to lift weights, even if you find it as interesting as watching the grass grow. Remember that we're only asking you to pump iron anywhere from 15 to 45 minutes several times a week.

You're Getting Better

All of the things that people associate with getting older—weakness, loss of motor skills, trouble with walking, osteoporosis, poor balance, dependency, and more—are not inevitabilities that one needs to automatically accept. By adhering to a consistent weight-training and cardiovascular program, most of the physical deficiencies associated with aging are reversible. In fact, one's eagerness not to accept this is one of the more important factors in insuring that you act your age and not the way you think you're supposed to act.

As we have previously stated, weight training can prevent osteoporosis, which is a major problem in postmenopausal women. As you probably know, osteoporosis is indicated in a majority of broken bones in the elderly.

Another complaint often voiced by the elderly is their inability to participate in regular, everyday activities like grocery shopping, cleaning, cooking, doing the laundry, or going out with friends. This gradual decline forces seniors to depend on others. Similarly, this loss of independence can lead to depression, which creates a vicious cycle of great dependency. This scenario, which occurs far too often in our society, need not be taken for granted. Weight training is a great way to make sure that you're able to fully participate in the simple pleasures most of us take for granted.

In our society, where the elderly are frequently shipped off to nursing homes, it's no wonder that we shun the thought of getting older. However, aging does not have to mean sitting home alone, waiting for Meals on Wheels. Staying fit and strong clearly requires work, but the alternative is sufficiently grim to inspire just about everybody. To put it simply, here are your options in a nutshell:

> Option one: Lift weights at the gym for thirty to forty-five minutes, two to three days per week.

Not only are you getting the physical benefits, but you'll be rubbing elbows with other like-minded social people. Work out enough and you can save your money for vacations instead of for home attendants.

The social aspect of working out in a gym is an extremely important but often overlooked point, especially for people who live alone. Weight training provides seniors with a place where there is exposure to people of various ages and backgrounds.

Clearly, the sad part of getting older is that you begin to lose friends you've had for a long time. Since many seniors don't often make new friends, they can often end up alone and lonely. Health clubs expose seniors to young and old alike. While you'll never be able to replace your dear old friends, you're likely to meet new people who inspire you to stay invested in living.

> Option two: Don't go to the gym and allow the natural effects of aging to take place.

The following scenario will most likely occur:

➤ You will become weaker because of natural loss of muscle.

➤ You will find carrying objects like luggage, groceries, and grandkids much more difficult.

➤ You will find walking up and down stairs much harder.

➤ You will find that your balance is not as good as it used to be. (You may come to rely on a cane.)

➤ You may give up going out unless you are with someone because you are afraid you'll fall.

➤ You may hire someone to do your shopping, laundry, and cleaning because you can't do it yourself any longer.

➤ You may fall often enough to break a bone.

➤ You may end up in an assisted living facility because you are unable to take care of yourself. If you can't afford that, you may end up with private duty care 12 to 24 hours per day.

This may sound quite harsh and depressing. And clearly it can be; however, we must not ignore the pressing fact that we all must attend to our health. So take your head out of the sand and make the necessary changes to ensure that you're not feeble before your time.

Choices, Choices

Which option would you prefer? We're not suggesting that if you work out you'll be immune to unforeseen problems that often strike the fittest among us. However, while we can't control how long we live, we certainly can control how well. Isn't it better to control what you can rather than to try to control what you can't?

Let us give you an example that illustrates just what we're preaching about.

One of Deidre's home care patients was a 95-year-old man who was referred to her for physical therapy due to the weakness he experienced after two weeks in the hospital. When Deidre first saw him, he couldn't walk without the walker that he brought home from the hospital. During their initial evaluation, Deidre learned that this plucky chap regularly used the treadmill for roughly one hour a day before being hospitalized. In addition, he lifted weights at a local gym two days per week. Once she learned this, Deidre knew his convalescence was just a matter of time.

Deidre laid out an exercise program for him and within two weeks' time this dedicated man was walking around his apartment without a walker or a cane. Soon after, he was back on the treadmill. At first it was for as little as five minutes, but within three weeks he was up to 30 minutes three days per week. After a month, he was walking outdoors alone and using the treadmill just as he had before his hospital stay. Had he not had the background of aerobic conditioning and weight lifting, we don't think he would have been able to return to a level of independent ambulation (physical therapist speak for walking alone) unless he had a cane or a walker. The key again was his prior fitness and eagerness to get back to that state of well-being, even if he was nearly a century old.

Let's take it one step further. Lifting weights will afford you far greater pleasures than doing your laundry. Gaining and maintaining strength also enables seniors to participate in strenuous activities that require balance and muscle endurance. We're talking about in-line skating, hiking, bowling, golfing, ice skating, rowing, you name it. There is no end to the possibilities; you only need to pick up a weight two or three days per week. It sounds too simple to believe, but it's true.

Not long ago, Joe participated in the World Sea Kayak Championship, a 33-mile crossing of the St. Lawrence Seaway in northern Quebec. After he had finished, a ruddy-cheeked chap from Massachusetts congratulated him on finishing so strong. "I couldn't keep up with you," he said. Joe, who was paddling a 28-pound racing kayak, seemed stunned. "Were you in the race?" he asked. "No," said the man, "but I paddled my canoe a few miles from the finish to see you guys coming in. I got so excited I tried to keep up with you." Before they parted company, the 75-year-old retired engineer said he really ought to lift weights more since he was having a bit more trouble removing his canoe from the roof rack on his car.

If that's not enough, in 1994 Joe paddled in an 800-mile-long stage race from Chicago to New York. This grueling event was billed as the world's longest and toughest race. The oldest finisher? Seventy-two-year-old Verlan Kruger from Lansing, Michigan. Five years later, Joe checked up on this retired plumber (and father of nine), and he was off in Alaska doing a 300-mile solo trip on a river above the Arctic Circle.

By the Book

According to the American College of Sports Medicine (ACSM), the following guidelines should be followed for seniors beginning a weight-training program:

➤ *Intensity.* Perform one set of 8 to 10 exercises that train all the major muscle groups (gluteals, quadriceps, hamstrings, pectorals, latissimus dorsi, deltoids, and abdominals). Each set should involve 8 to 12 repetitions that elicit a perceived exertion rating of 3. (Refer back to Chapter 26 "Mix It Up," and Chapter 28, "Real Women Lift," for a review of the RPE scale.)

➤ *Frequency.* Resistance training should be performed at least twice a week with at least 48 hours of rest between sessions. Make sure you eat a healthy dose of complex carbohydrates within 30 minutes of working out. (This helps speed muscle recovery.)

➤ *Duration.* Sessions lasting longer than 60 minutes are likely to have a detrimental effect on your body unless you're an experienced lifter. Shoot to complete a full routine in 30 to 45 minutes.

As we already mentioned, initiating an exercise program is not a guarantee that you'll escape illness—much of that is programmed into our genes. And while there's ample evidence that suggests even major diseases can be suppressed, minimized, or postponed with proper exercise and nutrition, we do know that working out will guarantee that you will have the resources for a speedier recovery and the ability to remain mobile and independent.

Following are additional guidelines set by ACSM to ensure injury-free resistance training:

➤ The first few sessions should be closely supervised and monitored by a personal trainer familiar with the special needs and abilities of senior citizens.

➤ The first eight weeks should be done with minimal resistance to allow the connective tissue to warm to the demands.

➤ Proper techniques should be taught and adhered to at all times.

➤ Maintain normal breathing patterns while exercising.

➤ To ensure strength gains, increase the number of repetitions before increasing the amount of resistance.

➤ Never use a weight so heavy that at least eight repetitions cannot be performed.

➤ Exercise within a pain-free range of motion.

➤ Perform multijoint (compound) exercises rather than single-joint (isolation) exercises.

➤ Use machines whenever possible, rather than free weights, because machines require less skill, and protect the user's back by stabilizing body position. They also allow the user to start with lower resistances, allow smaller increment increases, and allow greater control through the range of motion.

➤ Do not overtrain or overstrain. Two strength-training sessions per week are the minimum number required to produce positive physiological results.

➤ Never permit arthritic clients to participate in sessions during active periods of pain or inflammation.

➤ Engage in a year-round, resistance-training program on a regular basis. In other words, once you start, don't stop unless you have to.

➤ When returning from a layoff, start with resistances of less than 50 percent of the previous intensity. When you're ready, gradually increase the weight.

Use Your Head

Whether you're lifting weights, swimming, or cleaning your barbecue, every new task requires attention to detail as well as an understanding of what you need to do to accomplish the task. When it comes to seniors and weight training, we cannot state strongly enough the importance of getting off to a safe and smart start. Here are a few tips to make your strength-training routine safer:

➤ Never initiate a program on your own. Get clearance from your doctor to make sure that you are healthy enough to undertake this new activity. When you are scouting clubs to join, make sure you know whether there are trainers and whether they are certified in training seniors.

➤ Don't go it alone until you are absolutely positive about what you are doing. And never, ever follow the advice of some young buck who says it's cool to try and *max out*. In fact, if you don't know what maxing out is, you'll be better off. (For the record, it's lifting as much as you can in one single lift.)

➤ Use machines instead of freeweights whenever necessary; they require less skill and there is less risk of injury. You can concentrate on posture, breathing, and technique with much more ease. Done correctly, weight training is a safe and healthy way to improve your health. However, you need to remember that there's always the possibility of hurting yourself if you're not careful.

When in Doubt

If you are working out in the gym and come across a piece of equipment that you can't operate, always ask for assistance. Remember that if you are not properly set up on the equipment, you can pinch a nerve or pull a muscle.

If you begin to feel tired during your routine, chances are you have overworked. Here's where your wisdom should kick in: Take a rest. Once you return, reduce the amount of weight you're lifting or the number of repetitions in each set. Take it slow and steady. If you continue to feel tired and overworked, see your physician.

Variations

While there are no substitutes for weight training, there are variations in where you do your weight training—at home or in the gym.

In Chapter 5, "There's No Place Like Home," we reviewed various pieces of home equipment, including dumbbells. If you have the space and the money, this can be a good investment for you. However, we would urge you to talk to the equipment manufacturer about whether a senior can handle the equipment you're thinking about buying. If so, ask the representative if he or she would be able to give you a demonstration to make sure you're able to use the stuff safely.

Of course, you can also have a trainer come to your home to train you. If you have dumbbells, trainers can create various safe routines for you. If you don't have weights at home, there are many trainers who are good at working you through a routine of manual resistance exercises that could be useful.

The problem with manual resistance is that you can't quantify the amount of pressure the trainer is using and therefore you can't chart your progress. The other issue is that you can't reproduce this type of exercise on your own. As a result, you're dependent upon someone coming to your home and paying him or her for the privilege.

Lucky Strike in the Third

If you're thinking that no one can stop the march of time, then the Hawaii Ironman triathlon is a great event to show you otherwise. This ultratriathlon is a world-famous event that draws dedicated athletes who are well into their seventies and eighties. While it's one thing to enter, most of these senior triathletes finish this incredibly demanding event.

In case you don't remember, the Ironman consists of three back-to-back events: a 2.4-mile ocean swim, a 112-mile bicycle ride, and a 26.2-mile marathon run. Contrast these vivacious seniors to some of the older sedentary patients that Deidre sees—many of whom can barely stand up without assistance. What do you think the difference is? Attitude, mostly. The active 75-year-old refuses to give up participating in sports just because of his age while the other senior relents and lets nature take its course. As we've said, the essential difference takes place between the ears and in the heart. Willpower and enthusiasm are hard characteristics to define but quite easy to measure.

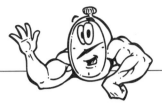

Weight a Minute

The September 1999 issue of *Runner's World* magazine featured a story on world-record holder Erwin Jaskulski. Name doesn't ring a bell? In Honolulu, Mr. Jaskulski set a record by running the 100-meter dash in 24.01 seconds, shattering the previous best for the 95-plus age group by 14 seconds!

We are not expecting you to enter the Ironman. Heck, we would be hard-pressed to finish this event without months of diligent training. What we do want you to understand is that with minimal investment, you can enjoy continued independence and reduce potentially harmful health risks. We are all going to age. What we can and should do is remain independent as well as psychologically and physically healthy by participating in a well-structured cardiovascular and weight-training program. The choice is yours. However, if you've read this far, we're certain that you're eager to have at it.

The Least You Need to Know

➤ Far too often we fail to realize that our health is not to be taken for granted.

➤ Despite what many senior citizens think, a sound exercise program can retard the ravages of time.

➤ Get help from a certified trainer and use light weights as you get started.

➤ Acting your age has more to do with your attitude than it does with your chronological age.

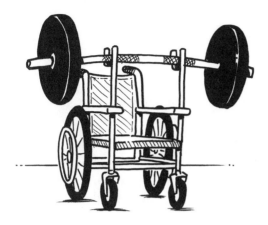

Chapter 30

Physically Challenged

In This Chapter

➤ Deciding that you can do it

➤ Using a wheelchair fitness regimen

➤ Finding clubs to get involved with

➤ Working out at home or in a gym

With its 30,000 runners, the New York City Marathon is one of the great parades in the United States. While it might sound like a line from a PR brochure, the theme that unites these highly mobile, scantily clad participants is ambition, will, and spirit.

Before the handful of world-class runners streak by, physically challenged athletes from the Achilles Track Club cruise the course with the same intensity and desire as anyone else in the race. Interspersed among the throngs of able-bodied runners are disabled athletes of every kind: the blind, amputees with prostheses, folks on crutches, and more. Perhaps these gutsy marathoners elicit the biggest cheers from the crowd because they remind us so graphically that it's not the body that holds us back, but the mind. Watch this race just once and you're likely to rethink any excuse you had about not working out because of that achy knee or stiff back.

In the 1980s when Joe worked as a reporter for *Newsday* newspaper, he was in the press tent in Central Park hours after nightfall collecting the results of the race. Still out on the course was a woman by the name of Zoe Koplowitz who was trying to finish the race before the next morning. Most runners can run six marathons in that time, but Koplowitz is afflicted with Multiple Sclerosis (MS), which causes balance impairment, spasticity, and fatigue. Despite her condition, she walks the course on crutches and for the last 10 years has been the final finisher of the race, including last year's 31-hour triumph. If you want a classic example of perseverance, know that the year before it had taken her nearly two days to finish the race. When she crossed the finish line late that night, there were more than a few jaded reporters shedding tears.

If anyone had an excuse not to complete a 26.2-mile marathon, it was that ambitious woman. What she and others have taught us is that, with few exceptions, there's no reason why the physically challenged shouldn't or can't run, hike, climb, swim, ski, and, of course, lift weights. In fact, the gains from strength training are probably greater for the disabled since they must work harder than the rest of us to do normal, everyday activities. And if you play wheelchair basketball, ski, or swim, strength training will help you perform at your chosen sport. Of course, the particular exercises one can do depends a great deal on the extent and type of disability.

Logistically Challenged

Improved technology and a change in attitude by the general public have enabled physically challenged folks to get out and participate. The Americans with Disabilities Act stipulates that all facilities must provide wheelchair accessibility for all buildings, and all buildings must provide a restroom stall that is large enough to allow a wheelchair access. However, even with those long-needed changes, people with disabilities often have significant logistics to overcome.

While there's no reason why virtually anyone can't strength train, it can often be a challenge to find a gym with the proper facilities. Consider the gym where Deidre and Joe work out. The entrance is clearly wide enough for a wheelchair to pass through and there are bathroom stalls available for wheelchair members. However, if you wanted to use the restroom, you'd have to negotiate two flights of stairs with no elevator to assist you. Even if you did negotiate the stairs, you won't be able to use the showers since the shower stalls are for a single occupant and have no place to sit. So, if you are wheelchair-bound you could get in the gym and work out, but using the facilities is not a practical option.

This is at least better than another gym where Deidre once worked out. It didn't even have an entrance wide enough to allow for wheelchair access. In addition, you had to pass through a *turnstile* in order to go *downstairs* to the gym. And forget about a wheelchair-accessible stall in the bathroom. (That would have added insult to injury.)

Before joining a gym, be sure to make a thorough visit first. Check on accessibility to the changing and shower facilities, as well as the equipment.

Benefits

Despite the particular obstacles one might encounter, the benefits of all forms of exercise are certainly worth the challenges. Although we've mentioned all these benefits before, it's worth repeating here. According to a report by the surgeon general, the benefits of exercise are:

➤ Reduces the risk of dying from coronary heart disease.

➤ Reduces the risk of developing high blood pressure, colon cancer, and diabetes.

➤ Helps people with chronic conditions improve stamina and muscle strength.

➤ Reduces symptoms of anxiety and depression.

➤ Helps control joint swelling and pain associated with arthritis.

➤ Helps reduce blood pressure for some people with hypertension.

While the above statements can be made with respect to anyone, a particular benefit of strength training for those who rely on a wheelchair is the reduction of shoulder and elbow injuries due to overuse. For people in wheelchairs who are always on the go, the possibility of developing rotator cuff or elbow tendinitis is greatly increased due to the constant flexion and extension that results from moving the wheels. With regular strengthening of the muscles in the shoulders and elbows, the likelihood of these injuries is greatly decreased. A strengthening program done two to three days per week would be extremely beneficial.

Similarly, people who rely on crutches for their mobility would profit from strengthening their lats, traps, shoulders, and triceps. Strength in these muscles provides the user with more control without muscular fatigue, especially when going up and down stairs or rushing after that impatient bus driver.

An outline of home and gym workouts is provided later in this chapter.

Safety

There's a fit, attractive woman Joe frequently sees working out. Like any other gym patron, she is fairly unremarkable in her attire and choice of exercises except that her arm has been amputated just below her elbow. In fact, what makes her exceptional is her ability to dress and work out just like everyone else. What Joe has never told her, for fear of sounding patronizing, is that her focused, consistent training and her refusal to accept her disability is inspirational. Each time Joe sees her he quickly realizes that the aches and pains that he's been complaining about are inconsequential (in fact they're welcomed) compared to the hardships of someone missing a limb.

For paraplegics or people with lower extremity amputations, strength training to maintain upperbody strength is extremely important. For wheelchair-bound athletes working out in a health club, there are numerous exercises that can be done without leaving the chair. Exercises like lateral raises, military presses, French presses, and seated biceps curls shouldn't present any major logistical problem, but be sure that your chair is stable when performing these exercises.

However, to get a more thorough workout, it's important to know that you'll be able to move safely and efficiently from the chair to the equipment. Practice working out with a spotter and/or trainer during off-hours so that you can make the transfer seamlessly. Have the trainer spot you several times to make sure that this transfer becomes second nature to you.

Except for exercises like biceps curls and triceps kickbacks, working out in the gym is safer and easier if you use machines instead of freeweights. Take the chest press, for example. Unless you have a buddy who will exercise with you at all times, setting up the bench can be time-consuming and even dangerous. Remember that for each body part, there is a machine equivalent for the freeweight exercise. So for safety's sake, use the machines.

This might be contradictory to just about everything we've already said, but since weight lifting requires a fair bit of motor control, people suffering from neuromuscular disorders like multiple sclerosis can injure themselves using either weights or machines. Why? If the neuromuscular system is disrupted, as it is with some disabilities, the strength that normally develops when you lift does not occur.

This isn't to say that you can't exercise if you're suffering from multiple sclerosis, just that some exercises should be abandoned. Those with neuromuscular disorders would be better suited doing the following:

➤ Stretching exercises to decrease *contractures* and maintain movement patterns that are as functional as possible

➤ Aerobic conditioning programs on a stationary bicycle

➤ Walking programs to maintain functional leg strength and aerobic conditioning

➤ Pool workouts such as organized water aerobic classes like those conducted at the YMCA

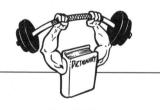

Bar Talk

A **contracture** is a condition where a joint (shoulder, elbow, wrist, finger, hip, knee, or ankle) is unable to be fully straightened or fully bent.

Guidelines

Some years ago, Dick Traum, the founder of the Achilles Club, who has worked tirelessly to help promote the club and its athletes, met Jonathan's father, Sy, who after a bout with cancer had his leg amputated below the knee. Mr. Traum pointed out that the reason most *disabled* people are unable to jog a few blocks is not because of their handicap but because of their sedentary lifestyle. In other words, missing a leg, being blind, or being wheelchair-bound often isn't as much of an impediment as being overweight and out of shape.

Mr. Traum would no doubt agree that the best medicine for a disabled person is some type of exercise done on a daily basis. The activities need not be strenuous, just consistent.

Whether you're able-bodied or not, if you've been sedentary you should see your physician before starting an exercise program. No matter how fit you think you are or what activity you choose, start slowly. Beginning with just 5 to 10 minutes of exercise is fine. Before you know it you'll be up to 20 to 30 minutes. Once you're working out for half an hour without looking for the closest lounge chair, you can do as much as you see fit.

For people who use a wheelchair to get around, the following aerobic activities can become part of a regular fitness regime:

➤ Try 30 to 40 minutes of wheeling around in your wheelchair. Refer to Chapter 26, "Mix It Up," for tips on calculating and monitoring your training heart rate. Keep in mind that 60 to 85 percent of your maximum heart rate is desirable.

➤ If you're a hoops fan, 20 minutes (or more) of wheelchair basketball is a fun way to get a good workout.

➤ Try a wheelchair road race if you're so inclined. There's no reason you can't compete.

➤ If your gym has an upperbody ergometer—described as a bicycle for the arms—this is a great aerobic conditioner. One of the best things about this machine is that you can increase the resistance as you get stronger.

➤ Try swimming. You can use flotation devices on your legs and do laps for cardiovascular fitness.

For those of you who are competitive, or for those who aspire to be, there is Mr. Traum's Achilles Track Club (ATC). This nonprofit organization was created to encourage people with all kinds of disabilities to participate in running events with the general public. They provide support, training, and technical expertise to runners at all levels. The club's credo states: "Achilles' athletes affirm their ability, not their disability, by competing alongside able-bodied runners."

When training in Central Park, Jonathan often sees wheelchair-bound Achilles athletes zipping around the park or blind runners holding tethers alongside a guide runner.

Another great organization that helps promote athletics among the physically challenged is The Challenged Athletes Foundation. Of all their many success stories, a young man by the name of Rudy Garcia-Tolson is perhaps the most inspiring.

Rudy Garcia-Tolson.

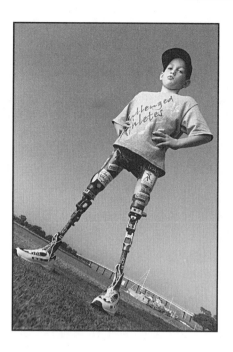

The next time one of us complains that our legs are too sore to train, we'll think of 10-year-old Rudy Garcia-Tolson. Rudy is truly an inspiration! Rudy was born with a condition known as Ptyregium Syndrome, one club foot, fingers of both hands webbed, and a cleft lip and palate. Faced with the decision between spending his life in a wheelchair or having his legs amputated, Rudy chose the latter. What he's done since then is nothing short of amazing.

Despite his condition, Rudy has completed triathlons and recently ran a mile in 8 minutes and 54 seconds. He has won awards in swimming and has competed on triathlon relay teams with teammates as diverse as comedian Robin Williams and pro triathlete Scott Tinley.

Let's Get Physical

As we've said many times, strength-training activities can be done at a health club or at home. Proper technique for the disabled is the same as for the able-bodied: Use a weight that you can only lift for 8 to 10 repetitions for three sets. Follow a count of three for the positive movement, one count pause and three for the negative movement.

If you work out at a gym, the following upper body routine offers a thorough workout.

Upper Body Routine—Gym

Body Part	Exercises
Chest	Machine pec deck, machine chest press
Back	Lat pull downs, machine rows
Shoulders	Machine shoulder press, dumbbell presses, dumbbell lateral raises, front raises, reverse flyes
Biceps	Dumbbell biceps curls
Triceps	Triceps kick backs, French curls
Forearms	Flexion and extension

As we mentioned earlier, there are several distinct advantages to working out in a gym:

➤ Space in your home is not an issue.

➤ There's usually a spotter at your disposal.

➤ There's camaraderie with fellow gym rats.

➤ Psychologically, you tend to work more consistently and harder when you go somewhere to work out.

Here are the disadvantages of working out in a gym:

➤ If the machines are spaced tightly together it may be a challenge to maneuver from station to station.

➤ If you don't have a workout partner, there are only certain exercises that you can do.

As we said in Chapter 5, "There's No Place Like Home," a working out at home routine affords you greater flexibility, assuming you have the space. After he was paralyzed in an automobile accident several years ago, Deidre's cousin Jerome purchased a bench, barbell, and dumbbells and began working out diligently to maintain upper-body strength. He is able to bench press, shoulder press, and do curls all in the comfort of his own home. Since he was known for his overall strength before his accident, his goal was to maintain upper body strength to assure his independence. He feared that weakness would make him dependent on others. Working out at home has allowed him to remain strong and to continue his pre-accident routine of exercise for fitness. Of course, if you're using freeweights, it's highly advisable to work out with a spotter.

If you don't have the space at home, you can rely on the old standbys: push-ups, chair dips, Dyna-Bands, and wrist or ankle weights.

If you want to go the home route, the following routine can be used.

Upper Body Routine—Home

Body Part	Exercises
Chest	Bench press, push-ups
Back	Dyna-Band rows
Shoulders	Dumbbell presses, lateral raises, front raises, reverse flyes
Biceps	Dumbbell curls
Triceps	French curls, kickbacks, chair dips
Elbow	Dumbbell curls, flexion, and extension

Whether you work out at home, in a gym, or in a cave, the most important thing is consistency, intensity, and desire. Perhaps the reason why most of us able-bodied athletes find the accomplishments of disabled athletes so inspiring is that they so graphically remind us that the struggle to get out there and exercise has more to do with matters of the heart and head than they do the body. As able-bodied athletes we worry—sometimes obsess—about the extra pounds we feel we need to lose, about our stiff lower back, or about setting a personal best in our next race. In short, we worry about so many meaningless concerns and tend to forget that the gift we've been given to run, jump, and lift weights can disappear suddenly and unexpectedly. Watching a Zoe Koplowitz or Rudy Garcia-Tolson reminds us of something Helen Keller once said: "Life is either a daring adventure or nothing at all."

The Least You Need to Know

➤ Disabled athletes make the most basic (and courageous) decision: to participate like anyone else.

➤ If you're confined to a wheelchair, make sure the gym you're considering has adequate facilities.

➤ No matter the disability, the Achilles Track Club has the event for you.

➤ Whether you strength train at home or in a gym, the most important things are consistency, intensity, and desire.

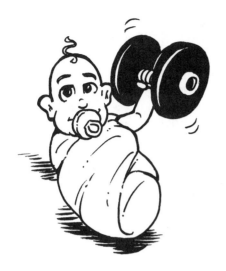

Chapter 31

Tots and Teens

In This Chapter

➤ Determining whether someone is too young

➤ Building bones 12 ways

➤ Hoisting your self-esteem

➤ Getting down to the nitty-gritty

Mention strength training and children in the same breath and people will threaten to call a child protection agency. Mention weights and teens together and more than a few eyebrows will be raised. However, in each case, strength training is not just possible: If it's done safely, it can provide many benefits.

The naysayers in the crowd may be thinking, "What do kids need to do this stuff for? They can't get strong and besides, they don't have the discipline or attention span to stick with a program over time!"

The fact is children and teens can make substantial strength gains just as adults and seniors can. The key, of course, is to be mindful of the do's and the don'ts, but the same could be said of strength training for adults. (In fact, that's exactly what we've been saying for the past few chapters.)

As for the attention span concern, children are more than able to focus on things that they enjoy—whether it be school, music, sports, or art. The key is making sure they are motivated and understand the benefits they can derive from the gym. They might not even know it, but working out regularly will not only improve their health and

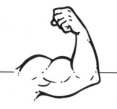

Flex Facts

More than four million kids between the ages of 10 and 17 are more than 20 pounds overweight. Since weight lifting can help in weight control, teens are perfect candidates for a lifting program.

appearance, but it can improve their self-esteem and mental tenacity as well. The key, as we said, is creating a program that caters to a young adult.

Much like the misinformation about gains that senior citizens can (or cannot) make, there are many myths and misconceptions about the safety and productivity of lifting for teens. We'll help separate fact from fiction and point out the reasons why youngsters can and should be physically active.

Consider a few reasons why children and teens should participate in a structured weight-training program:

➤ It fosters discipline at a young age.

➤ It increases self-esteem from participating in an activity that reduces stress and builds muscle.

➤ It affords a good opportunity to work on self-reliance away from parental supervision.

➤ It provides the opportunity to meet and associate with other kids in a positive environment.

In the rest of this chapter we'll outline the benefits of a weight-training program for children and teens and make sure you understand how to put one into practice safely.

Benefits

For years Joe worked out at the same time as a very fit bike-riding, marathon-running 50-year-old who lifted weights like a young madman—always heavy and always hard. One day he started working out with a young man who lifted just as he did. Only later did Joe realize that this was his 16-year-old son. "He's getting strong," said the senior member of the duo, "and he really pushes me to work harder."

The point really isn't *how* they worked out but that they worked out together. Not only did they push each other to work harder, they enjoyed the time they spent together. While it seems so basic for a father and son to lift weights together—what could be more of a manly bond than pumping iron?—we seldom see father and son strength training together and have yet to see mother/daughter teams in action. Come to think of it, we've not seen father/daughter or mother/son, but you get the point.

Surely any parent would be wildly enthusiastic to be part of his or her teen's strength-training program. There are several very basic physical and emotional benefits that come from participation in a supervised weight-lifting program:

➤ Strong muscles, bones, and connective tissue during the years of growth and maturation.

➤ Reduced risk of injury from play and/or sports.

➤ The development of exercise skills, which can lead to the pursuit of a healthful lifestyle.

➤ Strength that can be used to enhance performance in other sports.

➤ The development of self-confidence and self-esteem. Considering that the teen years can be torturously awkward, this cannot be overemphasized.

➤ The ability to maintain proper bodyweight.

➤ The opportunity to learn from and interact with adults other than teachers and parents in a relaxed environment.

Perhaps the biggest reason to encourage teens to participate in organized sports as well as in solo athletic activities like strength training is it bodes well for their future. By establishing a pattern of activity in their formative years, teens are able to develop good habits that they can carry through to adulthood. As we've said often in this book, establishing an active lifestyle has significant impact like staving off heart disease, obesity, diabetes, lower back pain, and a myriad of other ailments that often accompany a sedentary lifestyle.

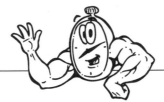

Weight a Minute

Always pay close attention to whether or not your child is enjoying their activity. Certainly don't force them just because it's what you want. This would probably have the opposite effect and push them farther and farther away from something that can be extremely beneficial to them later in life.

Safety

Of course, one of the reasons why many parents don't encourage or allow their teens to participate in organized sports is a concern over safety. With good reason. The National Youth Sports Safety Foundation (NYSSF), a nonprofit, educational organization whose mission is the reduction of injuries young people sustain in sports and fitness activities, provides the following facts:

➤ Sports participation has become a major cause of serious injury among youth.

➤ Sports activities are the second most frequent cause of injury for both male and female adolescents.

➤ Each year it is estimated that more than five million children seek treatment in hospital emergency rooms because of sports injuries.

➤ Most sports injuries are preventable. The NYSSF voices valid concerns about safety. By following the safety guidelines we'll present, most injuries can be prevented.

When we were kids, the general prevailing wisdom was that lifting weights could either stunt your growth or damage your skeleton. While we now know that this just isn't so, even incorrect pearls of wisdom are hard to shake. The primary reason that people worry about weight training with children is that their growth plates (the center of growth in the long bones of children) are still active and may be damaged with weight training. The fact is that in supervised weight-training programs, we know of no reported bone growth-plate injuries to preadolescent participants. As we've said, injuries come in unsupervised settings, where horseplay and bad form dominate—not where kids are taught proper form. However, before starting any program, have your child undergo a physical exam just to clear him or her of any problems that may exist that could be aggravated by a lifting program.

To ensure that preadolescents and adolescents remain injury-free in weight-training programs, you should follow these guidelines established by the ACSM:

➤ Remember that children are children; don't expect them to follow commands like adults do. Make the fun quotient high for them. The weight room isn't the place for playing around, but it need not be a silent, solemn place void of any pleasure.

➤ Teach proper weight-training techniques for all movements as well as proper breathing techniques.

➤ Make sure all exercises are performed slowly and smoothly.

➤ Do not use a weight that the lifter cannot use for at least eight repetitions. Overly heavy weight can cause damage to the bone growth plate.

➤ Don't allow any repetition to be done to the point of momentary muscle fatigue.

➤ As progress occurs, increase the number of repetitions, from 8 to 10 to 12, before you increase the amount of weight.

➤ Perform one to two sets of 8 to 10 different exercises (with 8 to 12 reps). Make sure that all major muscle groups are included.

➤ Limit sessions to twice per week and encourage other forms of exercise and play.

➤ Use multijoint exercises like pressing movements rather than one-joint exercises such as flyes.

➤ Always make sure that every training session is closely supervised by appropriately trained personnel.

➤ Machines may be preferable for the sake of safety. When using dumbbells or barbells, make sure that a spotter is always present.

➤ Never perform any maximal or competitive lifts. That's a sure way to court injury.

➤ Exercises that use body weight as resistance (such as push-ups, pull-ups, dips, and crunches) are excellent.

Here's a sample program for teenagers. As with other suggested programs, there's some flexibility built in, but remember to avoid exercises such as the bench press and military press, which can be dangerous unless a trustworthy spotter is available. In addition, because of the complexity and potential stress of the exercise, we do not recommend the use of deadlifts or squats for teens.

Body Part	Exercises
Legs	Lunges
	Leg extension
	Leg curl
Back	Pull-ups or lat pull downs
Chest	Push-ups or dumbbell bench press
Shoulders	Dumbbell military press
Biceps	Concentration curls
Triceps	Triceps push downs
Abs	Crunches
	Reverse crunches
	Oblique crunches

Here's another issue to consider: If the youngster is lifting to prepare for a particular sport, it may be appropriate to modify the program. Refer back to Chapter 25, "Lift Well, Play Hard," for suggestions on what exercises to include in sport-specific programs.

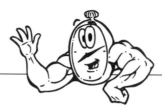

Weight a Minute

Strength training for teens and adolescents should never be competitive, and maxing out should never be part of one's program. Participants must understand that while lifting can be fun, safety needs to be taken seriously.

Walk, Don't Run

Although teens are full of restless energy and often have the attention span of, well, adolescents, they must be mindful of and adhere to the rules of the gym for their own protection. While you want the experience to be fun for them, they must understand that they can hurt themselves and/or others if the rules are not followed. When Joe was a mere lad of 16, he absent-mindedly removed a plate from a bar, which caused the bar to tilt like a seesaw when one of the players jumps off. This sent a 25-pound plate crashing down on his friend's large toe, which suddenly became much larger. The point is, safety in the gym is of the utmost importance, no matter what your age.

While strength training can benefit just about anyone, it's not for everyone. Children and teens must be emotionally mature enough to accept instruction and to follow guidelines. If not, he or she could get hurt and/or disrupt the session for other gym members. Knowing if your precocious youngster is up to the challenge can be difficult to discern. Because while your kid may not do what you ask without a fight—clean my room? I'd rather eat bugs!—he or she could listen to another adult without so much as a peep. Perhaps the best way to tell if this type of program is appropriate for your child is to discuss it with a teacher, especially a physical education teacher or coach your kid respects. This particular instructor may have insight into your child's physical and emotional makeup and direct them accordingly. Not surprisingly, if your child sees that you're excited and pleased with the results of your own fitness program, the odds are that they'll express interest in seeing what all this gym stuff is about.

The flip side of the coin is that sometimes teenagers are too eager to change their body image. According to the American Academy of Pediatrics, it is estimated that 6.6 percent of high school senior boys have used anabolic steroids. That's literally millions of youngsters who have tried potentially deadly drugs in an effort to improve their strength and appearance. Because of this staggering figure, it's very important that teens are made aware of the dangers of steroid abuse. Aside from the fact that steroid abuse can actually impair an adolescent's growth due to irreversible damage to the growth plates, side effects also include:

➤ Kidney disorders

➤ Liver disorders

➤ High blood pressure

➤ High cholesterol

➤ Reproductive system disorders (male and female)

➤ Acne

➤ Male pattern baldness (in boys and girls)

➤ Male breast enlargement

➤ Psychological disorders—mood swings ("roid rage") and sleep disturbances

➤ Connective tissue damage

➤ AIDS/hepatitis—steroid abusers often share needles

If that list doesn't sway your kid, then take him to a psychologist, since steroids are extremely toxic and highly hazardous to his health.

Guiding Light

Anyone participating for the first time in a new skill needs professional guidance. This is doubly true of newcomers like children, teens, and seniors, who may be more susceptible to injury. Many kids need to be reminded about what we've been telling you throughout this book—lifting should be fun but it must be taken seriously. The weight room is not the place for horseplay, competition, or carelessness.

We recommend that you seek out professionals who are certified in working with young people in this heavy metal environment. These experts should be knowledgeable in the ACSM's guidelines. We also recommend that you seek someone who has the temperament to work well with children. It's always wise to get references. You can contact the ACSM for referrals. Check Appendix B for ACSM's contact info.

It's hard to know if Joe's introduction to strength training in high school is typical of what many other teens may have to contend with, but we'll mention it because we think it might be. Joe's first taste of lifting came during gym class when the boys were let loose on a Universal Gym, an all-in-one unit with a dozen weight-lifting stations. Essentially, having that many adolescent boys in one room trying to demonstrate their strength is a very strange exercise in male superiority. The mooselike kids loaded up as much weight as they could and hoisted away, which intimidated the skinnier lads like Joe. Instead of inspiring him, it made him feel embarrassed since the amount of weight he could manage was so much less.

It was only when he lifted with his friend in the friend's basement (the same one whose toe he dropped the weight on) that any real progress was made. The larger point, however, is to try and communicate to your kid that the amount of weight they lift is utterly insignificant. What is important is that they're lifting safely and to the best of their ability. It's fine to lift weights with a vision of the body your budding Adonis (or Venus) wishes to build, but it's important to let your kid know that the body they have now is just fine. In fact, it's a wonderful gift from above.

The Least You Need to Know

➤ Common wisdom states that kids shouldn't lift weights. We're here to say that they can and should.

➤ The benefits of a safe strength-training program extend far beyond the physical.

➤ Check out a safe and successful strength-training program.

➤ Check your ego at the door. Lift because you want to, but don't get caught up in the numbers game.

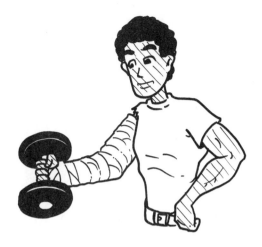

Injuries Nag

There's an old joke that perfectly captures how familiar we are with nagging injuries: A 92-year-old man wakes up in bed one morning and says to his wife, "I'm dead, I'm dead, I'm dead!" Ida replies, "Herman, what are ya talkin' about? You're lying next to me in bed." Herman says, "I'm telling you: I'm dead! I'm dead!" She asks, "How do you know?" and he says, "Nothing hurts!"

Injuries, injuries, injuries. What a strange and wonderful world it would be without them. First, what would we complain about? What would our grandparents discuss with their cronies? And finally, what would we do with all of the healthcare practitioners like Deidre whose livelihood depends on those very same injuries?

There are, of course, many reasons why we get injured. Let's take a look at the more common ways injuries occur.

Injuries occur from musculoskeletal imbalances—swimmers or gym rats who over-develop their pectoral muscles without regard for their traps, rhomboids, or rear delts, for example. The potential here for shoulder problems is great. There are also folks who have skeletal imbalances that can cause problems unless addressed—for example, scoliosis or leg length discrepancies.

Attempts to do more than the body is capable of doing can lead to injury. Take for example guys who try to impress their friends by bench pressing 300 pounds when they normally bench press 240. That extra 60 pounds can be enough to cause injury to the rotator cuff muscles that can last a long, long time.

Doing too much of one thing, with or without improper technique, is also a source of injuries. Even something as seemingly innocuous as typing can lead to a host of problems.

Regardless of the cause, we are here to assist you in the various ways to avoid injury. We'll also discuss ways to recognize what may cause an injury and finally what to do when you are ailing. Having said that, know that this chapter is not to be used as a diagnostic tool. If you are injured, the best thing to do is to go to a medical professional and get it checked out.

From our perspective, however, the most important thing to remember is to exercise according to the guidelines that we've laid out as well as to recognize what potential problems may befall you. (As far as we're concerned, preventive medicine is the best kind.) The most important thing to note is that exercise should not be painful. And don't make like a wounded war hero; never exercise with pain or through pain. Working out is supposed to be restorative—a sign of care—and not punishment for an imperfect body. While it's ironic, it should come as no surprise that our own worst enemy in the injury department is ourselves.

Back Attack

The most common complaint that plagues countless Americans is back pain. Although we hear a lot about *herniated disks*, relatively few people have herniations that cause them pain. Most people suffer pain brought on by poor posture and performing daily chores and/or working out with poor posture.

We cannot stress enough how important posture is to the health of your back. Eighty percent of the back patients that Deidre saw in private practice required instruction in proper posture. Most body alignment courses (Feldenkrais, Alexander Technique) are based on getting people to understand and improve upon faulty movement patterns caused by poor posture and mechanics.

For people who do have diagnosed herniations, we recommend that they get tips for exercises from their orthopedists or their physical therapists who are familiar with their conditions.

Bar Talk

A **herniated disk** is a protrusion of the disk material out of the vertebral canal onto a nerve. When the nerve is compressed, sharp pain or burning may be felt in various parts of the legs, depending on the amount of diskal protrusion there is.

Though many back pain sufferers resist the work of Dr. John Sarno, if you are afflicted with a chronically stiff or sore back, you should check out his eye-opening (or should we say, back-healing) *Healing Back Pain.* This simple book makes a convincing argument about how anxiety and repressed anger trigger muscle spasms and other debilitating back problems. Interestingly enough, many of Sarno's biggest converts were long-suffering back patients who had explored every avenue in conventional medicine.

Get Smart

The first and probably most important thing to get into the habit of is recognizing bad posture and integrating sound posture as part of your life. If your muscles are already weak, they're only going to get weaker if you spend a lot of time sitting, standing, or bending improperly. In fact, the domino effect of poor posture will create a litany of other ill effects like neck and upper back pain, which can lead to chronic headaches, shoulder pain, and middle and lower back pain.

For a refresher course on proper posture tips, refer to Chapter 11, "Safety First." In addition, pay careful attention to the photographs, and try to mimic the models. Study the way you stand in a mirror and/or in photographs of yourself and see how you stack up. Remember, breathing from your belly usually ensures that your posture is sound. So breathe well, and you're likely to stand well.

In fact, before you continue, take a deep breath right now. The restorative power of deep breathing is incalculable.

Solutions

Back pain from weak muscles requires strengthening of the muscles along the spine, scapula (shoulder blades), legs, and abdominals in addition to stretching of muscles that have been shortened from sitting in a slouched position for a prolonged period of time.

We recommend that in addition to improving your posture, you begin this regimen of stretching and strengthening exercises.

Body Part	Stretches
Pectorals	Pec stretch
Iliopsoas	Alternate iliopsoas stretch
Upper back, lower back, side of hips, rib cage	Spinal twist
Lower back and hip	Lower back and side of hip

Body Part	Exercises
Back	Lat pulls
	Reverse flyes
	Cable row
	Back extension machine
Abdominals	Crunches, reverse crunches,
	Obliques
Legs	Lunges
	Leg press machine
	Leg curl machine

For back pain resulting from a herniation, the exercises you need to do depend on the type of herniation. The most common herniation is a posteriolateral herniation where the symptoms increase when you bend forward. In this case, your exercises must emphasize backward bending. In acute cases or cases undergoing treatment, abdominal exercises are not recommended because of the forward bending required.

To develop sound muscular integrity, strengthening the middle and lower muscles in your back and legs is extremely important.

Body Part	Stretches
Iliopsoas	Alternate iliopsoas stretch
Hamstrings	Alternate hamstring stretch

Body Part	Exercises
Back	Lat pull downs
	Cable rows (from a neutral position, no forward bending)
	Back extension machine(from a neutral position, no forward bending)
Legs	Leg extension machine
	Leg curl machine
	Lunges (concentrate on holding the abdominals tight and keeping the back straight)

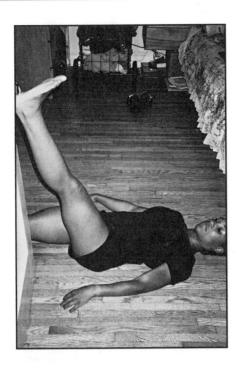

Alternate hamstring stretch.

Inflammation

The suffix *-itis* is short for inflammation. And as Herman, the man convinced that he was dead, could tell you, if there is a body part, there is an "-itis" for it: cellulitis, dermatitis, tenosynovitis, and so on. Our focus here, however, centers on the inflammation that involves tendons.

Elbow

Okay anatomy fans, which is the -itis that involves the elbow?

> Flexionitis
>
> Extensionitis
>
> Rotationitis
>
> Epicondylitis
>
> Punchitis

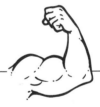

Flex Facts

Four out of five adults will experience some form of lower back pain sometime in their lives. In adults over 45, this condition is one of the most common causes of lost workdays. Common causes of lower back pain are sprains of ligaments and sprains of muscles as well as poor conditioning, improper mechanics, obesity, and smoking.

If you picked epicondylitis, you've been paying attention, and good things are in store for you. If you picked any of the others, return to the beginning of the book and give it another go.

Epicondylitis is an inflammation of the tendons that attach to the bony prominence at the elbow and its surrounding tissues. Typically, it results from a strain or overuse.

If you begin to feel pain in the area on either side of your elbow while turning a doorknob, opening a jar, or squeezing an object, and if it is tender to touch, this may be the -itis you have. Until you see a health professional, you should refrain from any activity that causes such pain. (Again, pain is a very wise guide. Respect it!) Ice the tender area for 10 minutes several times a day and consider taking a recommended dose of anti-inflammatories.

Once the pain subsides with normal activities, you can begin strengthening.

Body Part	Stretches
Wrist Flexors	Flexion stretch
Wrist Extensors	Extension stretch

Wrist flexion stretch.

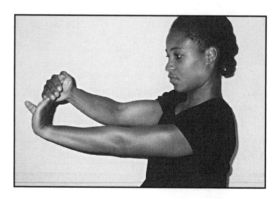

Wrist extension stretch.

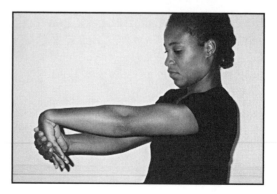

Body Part	Exercises
Wrist flexors	Dumbbell flexion
Wrist extensors	Dumbbell extension
Wrist flexors	Gripping exercises, with a ball or a sock

Knee

There's an old adage that the human knee is so fragile (dare we say flawed) that it's conclusive proof that God doesn't exist. Theology aside, of all the joints, the knee is the most problematic—probably because it bares so much of your weight and is called on to do so many diverse tasks. (For this reason alone, artificial turf should be outlawed from all sports arenas.)

Although this section will cover the -itis conditions that affect the knee, there are other knee problems you can be afflicted with which we will review here.

Patellar Tendinitis

The most common knee injury is patellar tendinitis. This condition is a result of overuse during jumping activities such as basketball, volleyball, and tennis. In fact, name an NBA star from Julius "Dr. J" Erving to Patrick Ewing to Michael Jordan and patellar tendinitis is all too familiar.

Symptoms:

➤ Tenderness just below the patella (kneecap)

➤ Swelling

➤ Pain that intensifies by jumping

➤ Pain with a full squat

➤ Area below patella tender to touch

If you find that you have some of these symptoms, stop the offending activities. (This is like the old joke where the man goes to the doctor and says he has a sharp stabbing pain in his elbow when he plays the violin and the doctor tells him to stop playing immediately.)

Again, your automatic response should be rest, ice, and anti-inflammatories until you can get to an orthopedist or physical therapist. If the symptoms normalize, begin the stretches and exercises below. If the symptoms return, stop and get to a health professional. Common-sense stuff, but you'd be surprised how often people, especially highly motivated athletic types like us, try to push through the pain.

Body Part	Stretches
Quadriceps	Quadriceps stretch
Hamstrings	Hamstring stretch
Calves	Gastroc/soleus stretch

Body Part	Exercises
Legs	Leg press machine
	Lunges
	Leg curl machine

As we stated earlier, some injuries are not a result of improper form or technique, but are from a weakness that stems from asking the body to do more than it's capable of.

To illustrate: Deidre had a patient in physical therapy who, a year before she came to her, had an anterior cruciate ligament reconstruction. On discharge from her outpatient clinic, she returned to running three miles, three days per week. About a month afterward, she felt knee pain while running. Not long after that, she experienced swelling just below her kneecap. On evaluation, she was found to have reduced quadriceps strength. She also lacked full range of motion in her knee, meaning she did not have enough strength to straighten (extend) the leg fully (this is to say that instead of having full extension at 0°, she had less than full extension at 2°).

By being zealous and doing too much too soon—noble aim, bad result—she developed patellar tendinitis. In short, before you can return to your normal workout routine, you've got to recover fully.

Patellofemoral Syndrome

Patellofemoral syndrome is an overuse condition of the knee joint that afflicts runners, cyclists, tennis players, and swimmers. Loretta Robertson, orthopedic clinical specialist and advanced clinician at the outpatient department in New York City's Columbia Presbyterian Medical Center, related the story of a patient who developed patellofemoral syndrome while training for the marathon. She increased her mileage too quickly and ignored the pain and swelling that ensued. Consequently, the condition worsened, and she was unable to compete. By the time she saw a doctor and physical therapist, she had significant swelling, muscle atrophy, and very tight hamstrings. She was in rehab for two to three months before she was able to return to running.

Symptoms:

➤ Diffuse ache in the front of the knee.

➤ Pain increases with walking up and down stairs.

➤ Pain when sitting for prolonged periods of time with the knee bent. This is called the "movie sign."

➤ Sometimes a feeling of the knee "giving way" or buckling with walking or climbing stairs.

➤ Sometimes you'll feel a "catching" sensation in the knee.

➤ Mild swelling occurs occasionally

Causes:

➤ Muscle tightness of the hamstrings, calves and iliotibial band.

➤ Muscle imbalance that would need evaluation by an orthopedist or physical therapist.

➤ Overtraining caused by a runner's or cyclist's sudden increase in mileage, increase in hill work, stairs, or change of training surface or shoes

➤ Biomechanical abnormalities that would require evaluation by an orthopedist or physical therapist.

Again, if you begin to feel any of these symptoms, stop the offending activity. Rest, ice, and use a recommended course of anti-inflammatories. And don't forget your secret weapon—stretching. Again, if the pain resolves with day-to-day activities, begin to do the exercises listed below. If the pain returns with these exercises, stop at once and get thee to a physician or physical therapist.

Body Part	Stretches
Quadriceps	Standing quadriceps
Hamstrings	Hamstring
Gastrocnemius	Standing gastroc
Iliotibial band	Lower back and side of hip

Body Part	Exercises
Legs	Leg press machine
	Leg curl machine
	Standing/sitting calf raises

Iliotibial Band Syndrome

The iliotibial band or ITB is a tough, fibrous band that is found on the outside of the thigh from the hip to the knee. It can be extremely tight in athletes, particularly endurance jocks like runners, skiers, and cyclists.

Causes:

➤ Overtraining

➤ Variations in training like increased mileage, different surface, changed footwear

➤ Muscle imbalances that need to be evaluated by a professional

➤ Faulty biomechanics that need to be evaluated by a professional

Symptoms:

➤ Pain over the lateral (outside) aspect of the knee

Body Part	Stretches
Iliotibial band	Lower back and side of hip
Quadriceps	Standing quadriceps

Body Part	Exercises
Legs	Machine adduction
	Leg press machine
	Leg curl machine

What to do:

Sure we've been telling you this over and over in this chapter, but it can't be stressed enough: Only after you've rested, iced, taken anti-inflammatories, and stretched should you begin the exercises—assuming you're pain-free. If pain accompanies these exercises—that's pain, not discomfort—or if day-to-day pain returns after exercise, stop and see a health professional.

Rotator Cuffs

Unless you hurl a baseball for a living—or injured one of these itty-bitty muscles that virtually no one thinks about until they demand attention—you've probably not spent much time worrying about your rotator cuffs. Well, you should because they're quite valuable when you have to reach into your back pocket or put on your jacket.

The following is a list of the most common rotator cuff injuries, symptoms, causes, stretches, and exercises.

Impingement Syndrome

An impingement syndrome is a condition whereby the soft tissues in the shoulder—the rotator cuff tendons; bursa or biceps tendon—are squeezed by a structure called the coracoaromial arch. (Don't fret about all of these names, just take our word for it.)

Causes:

➤ Tightness within the shoulder joint

➤ Weak rotator cuff

➤ Development of bony spurs

Symptoms:

➤ A pain when raising your arm upward or outward

Afriqiyah Woods, a prominent New York City physical therapist, had a patient, a young male, who regularly lifted weights at least three days per week. He began to experience pain when doing overhead lifting activities like the shoulder press and lat pull downs. First he followed doctor's orders and rested, iced the injured area, and took anti-inflammatories for two weeks. When he returned to the gym, the pain was back. What she discovered was that his rotator cuff and scapular muscles were weak and the muscles surrounding his shoulders were tight. Once all of this was addressed, Ms. Woods found that the amount of weight that he was lifting was too heavy, too soon.

Rotator Cuff Tendinitis

Rotator cuff tendinitis is most commonly an inflammation of the following tendons of the rotator cuff: the supraspinatus and infraspinatus.

Causes:

➤ Overuse during racket sports or any repetitive overhead activity (for example, any job that involves hoisting heavy objects up onto or off of a shelf).

Symptoms:

➤ Sharp pain felt on various movements such as bringing the arm out to the side, or putting on a jacket or putting a hand in a back pocket.

Rotator cuff.

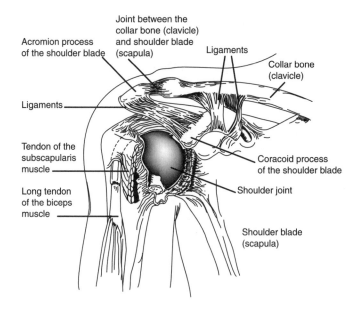

Joint between the
collar bone (clavicle)
and shoulder blade
Acromion process   (scapula)
of the shoulder blade   Ligaments

Collar bone
(clavicle)

Ligaments

Coracoid process
of the shoulder blade

Tendon of the
subscapularis
muscle

Shoulder joint

Long tendon
of the biceps
muscle

Shoulder blade
(scapula)

Exercises:

The rotator cuff depresses the head of the long arm bone during overhead activities like reaching up toward your kitchen cupboard or up into your closet. With weakness (decreased muscle tone), the long arm bone is not depressed with elevation and compresses soft tissues, which causes pain. Therefore, it is important to improve the strength in and around your rotator cuff prior to introducing shoulder movement beyond 90°.

Stretching:

A classic test for rotator cuff tendinitis is to stretch the two rotator cuff muscles—the supraspinatus and the infraspinatus—that are most commonly involved. This stretching will elicit pain in the tendons of the respective muscles if tendinitis is present. During rehab, the key is to stretch after the pain has subsided. Your aim is to ensure that the muscles remain sufficiently separated to allow a free range of motion. Don't stretch before the muscles are warmed up. It's wise to do all of your exercises first, then stretch three times for 30 seconds each time.

Body Part	Stretches
Infraspinatus	Infraspinatus stretch
Supraspinatus	Supraspinatus stretch

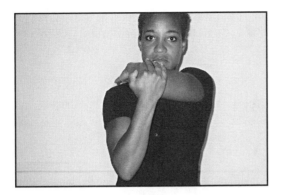

Infraspinatus stretch.

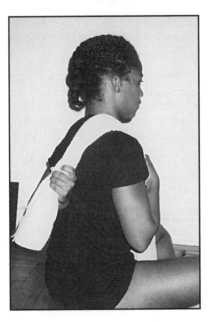

Supraspinatus stretch.

Body Part	Exercises
Anterior deltoids	Front raises
Serratus	Push-ups with arms out at 90°
Medial deltoids	Lateral raises
Rhomboids/middle traps	Cable rows
Upper traps	Shrugs
Subscapularis	Internal rotation
Infraspinatus/supraspinatus	External rotation

All of the exercises listed previously should be performed in a limited range without pain. Before increasing the range, always perform the movements first without any weight. If this feels fine, you can then use two pounds, three pounds, and so on.

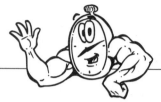

Weight a Minute

Lateral raises during rehab should be done with the palms facing forward, thumbs toward the ceiling. If your palms are facing downward (the way it's most commonly performed), impingement will occur, and the irritation will only get worse.

As we have stated previously, the first response to pain is to stop the aggravating activity. The second course of action is to use ice several times per day for 10 to 20 minutes. The third is to use the recommended dosage of anti-inflammatories.

Once you no longer have pain on a daily basis, you can begin stretching (make sure that you are stretching without pain—if there is pain, stop). Add exercises once you are able to stretch without pain. If these exercises result in a recurrence of symptoms, go to an orthopedist or physical therapist for an evaluation.

The Least You Need to Know

➤ Injuries are part of life, but you can prevent most and treat the rest.

➤ The key to a sound back is good posture.

➤ Being informed will help you avoid overuse injuries, which head the list of sports injuries.

➤ Once the pain is gone, there are stretches and exercises you can do to return to full strength.

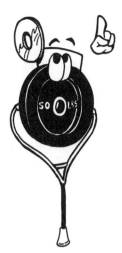

Chapter 33

What's Up, Doc?

In This Chapter

➤ Exercise and AIDS

➤ Combating cancer

➤ Diabetes need not be debilitating

➤ Maintaining a healthy heart and lungs

➤ Living longer with Lupus

Here's a late-breaking news flash: Exercise is good for you. Research shows us that exercise can reduce your risk for more than just heart disease. According to the *Physician and Sports Medicine* journal, exercise will help reduce the incidence of the following:

➤ Heart disease

➤ Stroke

➤ High blood pressure

➤ Diabetes

➤ Arthritis

➤ Osteoporosis

➤ Excess body weight

> ➤ Depression

> ➤ Cancer

> ➤ Chronic obstructive pulmonary disease. (This is a category of disease processes that prevent the lungs from properly ventilating.)

Again, moderation is essential. Moderate intensity of an aerobic activity performed for 30 minutes every day—combined with healthy eating habits and rest—is more than enough to produce significant benefits. (In fact, research shows that one of the biggest contributors to disease is chronic stress.)

A six-week study comparing 16 patients in a control group with no exercise to a group of 16 patients who participated in a supervised program of gradually increasing aerobic activity revealed that those who participated in the supervised exercise program regained their strength and energy levels faster. As a result, activities like climbing up stairs and carrying groceries were easier.

Despite a serious illness or condition that you may be afflicted with, a combination of aerobic exercise and strength training will help you deal with it. That's not to say that exercise is a cure-all; however, it is a terrific way to get better, and, if the disability is permanent, it will help you live a more "normal" life.

In fact, the more we researched this chapter, the more amazed we were to find some of the incredible stories of people with seemingly incurable diseases refusing to yield to conventional medical wisdom and give up the ghost. One man with AIDS ran, biked, and swam across the United States. Another who is paralyzed below the waist climbed Yosemite's El Capitan, one of the great big wall climbs in the world. And the list goes on.

In this chapter, we'll discuss weight training for folks with a variety of conditions that many people might assume would prevent them from lifting weights. While weight training can offer benefits to just about anyone, it's important to note some of the specific precautions that must be taken in terms of intensity and rest periods.

HIV/AIDS

The inevitable question that comes to mind when people think about HIV and exercise is, "How will it affect the immune system?" Good question. As we've said before, and emphatically repeat here, for someone with a serious illness exercising for the first time, make sure you consult your physician.

However, research shows that exercise will boost your immune system. In a recent 12-week study of people with HIV, 45 participants (at various stages of infection) did aerobic conditioning and resistance training for an hour per day, three times per week. While the strength and conditioning of the participants improved (no surprise there), the immune system was not significantly affected.

In an article on exercise and HIV written by Melanie Walgren, RD, research shows that people with HIV often have a moderate to severe depression of the male hormone testosterone, a contributing factor of AIDS wasting syndrome. Testosterone, as we mentioned earlier, is responsible for lean body mass. Strength-training exercises can increase testosterone levels in the blood, which will increase lean body mass.

Aerobic exercise can also help boost the immune system. Some studies show that people who do 45 minutes of brisk walking five days a week may reduce the number of colds they get by 50 percent compared to people who do no exercise at all. It appears that moderate amounts of exercise may even boost the body's natural killer cells without decreasing the number of CD4 cells, which are the immune cells, attacked by HIV.

For most HIV positive people, the key word is *moderate*. While moderate exercise can boost the immune system, too much can suppress it. Why? It is thought that excessive exercise can stimulate an increase in free radicals, which are chemicals formed in the body when oxygen is burned. Some studies have found that the levels of immune cells found in the blood are lower after extreme amounts of exercise. The theory is that these immune cells temporally leave the blood and go to the muscle to repair damaged muscle fibers. The suggestion is that risk of infection may increase immediately after high-level activity because these immune cells are not available to fight. (Although it is thought that the immune system does return to normal approximately 9 to 24 hours later.)

For people who train to race, or just train a lot because they love to eat banana splits, the balancing act between "enough" and "too much" can be like walking on a precarious ledge.

Jonathan, who cycles, runs, and lifts weights from March through September, often gets ill a month after his cycling season ends around November. When Deidre was competing, she often suffered from a low-grade fever when she stepped up her powerlifting training in preparation for the nationals. Don't let this alarm you. Exercise is like drinking red wine; it's good for you as long as you do it in moderation.

Whether you have HIV/AIDS or not, here are some do's and don'ts to help you to remain healthy in your exercise pursuits.

The following is a list of do's:

➤ Spend 30 minutes on some type of moderate activity at least three or four days a week, but never seven days a week. Cycling, brisk walking, or swimming are three excellent ways to go.

➤ If you run, your goal should be 10 to 15 miles per week. Once you log more than that, you're doing it more for your head than for your body.

➤ To maintain muscle mass and bone density, lift weights three times per week.

➤ For cardiovascular conditioning, your target heart rate should be about 60 to 85 percent of your maximum heart rate for 20 to 30 minutes.

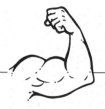

Flex Facts

In 1989, Jim Howley was diagnosed with AIDS and told that he had 12 to 18 months to live. Then he began competing in triathlons. Through new medications and daily exercise he is now healthy and symptom-free. Howley's T-cell count has risen from a low of 2 cells to 260, a remarkable increase, though still lower than that of healthy adults. In 1997, Howley competed in the "Polar Transcontinental Triathlon for Life" in which he ran, cycled, and swam 3,375 miles from Los Angeles to New York City in 52 days.

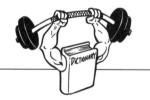

Bar Talk

T cells are responsible for enhancing antibody production and for killing foreign cells in the body.

➤ Eat a balanced diet. Include lots of fruits and vegetables.

➤ Get plenty of rest.

➤ If you exercise heavily, some nutritionists recommend antioxidant supplements, including 1,000 milligrams of vitamin C, 400 IC of vitamin E, and 25,000 IU of beta-carotene.

➤ If you have a cold, make sure the symptoms are above the neck (primarily nasal) before you work out.

The following is a list of don'ts:

➤ Don't exercise if you have symptoms below the neck like a bad cough, fever, or muscle aches. If you have bronchitis, exercise may trigger asthma.

➤ Unless you are a trained athlete who has competed for more than a season, avoid intense exercise for more than 90 minutes at a time. Working out more than that often sponsors the release of cortisol, which is a stress hormone and immune suppressant.

➤ If you are already under stress in other areas of your life, make sure you don't overtrain.

➤ Don't lose weight too fast. More than two pounds per week may compromise *T cells*.

For individuals living with HIV, weight training and aerobic conditioning can help to maintain and increase strength as well as decrease fatigue and depression.

Cancer

Consistent exercise has been shown to reduce the risk of breast, colon, and prostate cancer. Exercise has also been shown to help people who have undergone chemotherapy minimize the debilitating side effects.

Men and woman have their own particular concerns when it comes to cancer. For men, there is an avoidable but predictable pattern that we see again and again. The combination of aging, being sedentary, and an increase in the percentage of body fat (along with a decrease in lean body mass) alters hormone levels and leads to an increase in the risk of prostate cancer.

For women, research has shown that women who exercise regularly have a 37 percent lower risk of developing breast cancer than sedentary women. Women whose jobs involved walking, lifting, or heavy manual labor also showed reduced risks of breast cancer as compared to sedentary women. In fact, the women who participated in the most strenuous work had the lowest risk. Studies show that the effect was greater in premenopausal women than in postmenopausal women. The speculation is that exercise may alter levels of naturally circulating hormones.

The effects of exercise for both men and women regarding the decreased risk of colon cancer may have a lot to do with the fact that people who exercise regularly watch their diets more carefully than those who do not. Studies that compare incidents of colon cancer in America versus colon cancer in Japan reveal that the Japanese suffer less colon cancer primarily because their diets are low in fried, fatty foods and high in complex carbohydrates and alternate protein sources. The *typical* American diet, rich with an assortment of fatty fast-fried food, is a breeding ground for health problems.

We can hear the cynics citing the examples of world-class athletes like Olympic figure skating champion Scott Hamilton and 1999 Tour de France winner Lance Armstrong, who were both diagnosed with testicular cancer. (When Jim Fixx, an avid runner and author, died of heart failure some people said, "Why bother?") True, exceptions abound; we all know an uncle who drank a pint of whiskey and smoked two packs of cigarettes a day who died dancing with his 23-year-old girlfriend at the age of 103. But the irrefutable bottom line is that exercise combined with a healthy diet will lower your risks of getting cancer.

It's also safe to say that athletes like Hamilton and Armstrong, who continued working out as part of their recovery, return to their previous levels of activity much sooner than those who do not exercise regularly. We would dare to speculate that their drive to survive was in some way linked to their extremely active lifestyles.

Diabetes

There are two types of diabetes, type I (juvenile diabetes), which usually requires insulin injection, and type II (adult-onset diabetes), which can usually be controlled by diet or oral medication. Regardless of the type of diabetes you have, you can benefit from an aerobic and weight-training program.

One of the most important things for people with diabetes to pay attention to is their diet—especially before a workout. Your preexercise meal—a high-carbohydrate, low-fiber, low-sodium, low-sugar, low-fat, and moderate-protein meal—should take place at least three hours before exercise. This is important so that your blood has sufficient levels of circulating glucose.

Now let's take a look at the aerobic side of the equation. Cardiovascular exercise improves blood glucose control, improves circulation, and is just plain good for your heart. Again, don't go bounding up the steepest hill you can find until you're about to drop. Work out for 20 to 40 minutes at a time. The intensity should be 55 to 75 percent of your maximum heart rate at least three to five times per week.

At the beginning of your weight-training program, perform one to three sets of a weight that you can lift no more than 8 to 12 times. Make sure you exercise all major muscle groups using 8 to 10 exercises that we've described in Chapters 15 through 20.

For individuals taking insulin, exercise can influence how insulin is used. In fact, exercise can cause hypoglycemia (low blood sugar) or hyperglycemia (high blood sugar). Consider the following are tips from www.mylifepath.com for insulin-dependent individuals:

➤ Avoid injecting insulin into a part of the body that will be used during exercise. Injecting into a muscle that will be active can accelerate the insulin's effect and cause hypoglycemia.

➤ Don't exercise at the peak of insulin activity. Different types of insulin reach their peak at different times. Check with your doctor or pharmacist about yours.

➤ Avoid alcohol and beta-blocker drugs around the time of exercise because they promote hypoglycemia.

➤ Eat a healthy snack just before and during exercise.

➤ Keep simple carbohydrates like fruit or hard candy handy at all times.

➤ Always carry emergency cash and identification listing your medial conditions and medications.

➤ If you experience pain in your chest, nausea, heart palpitations, or severe short-ness of breath during exercise, stop and call your doctor.

➤ Test blood glucose before, during, and after exercise.

➤ Watch for postexercise hypoglycemia up to 15 hours after activity

➤ If blood glucose levels are above 240 mg/dL, or below 60 mg/dL, don't exercise. If you have low blood sugar, ingest simple carbohydrates prior to exercise. This will raise your blood sugar to a normal level (90-110 mg/dL).

While hydration is important for everyone, it's even more so for diabetics. Drink two cups of water two hours before exercise, one to two cups 30 minutes before exercise, and ½ cup every 15 minutes during exercise as well as enough afterward to replenish whatever was lost during your workout.

Cardiovascular Disease

When it comes to minimizing heart disease (and all diseases in general), nothing seems to be as effective as a sound diet, regular exercise, and proper rest.

The following cardiovascular diseases are greatly decreased with regular exercise:

➤ *Heart disease.* Cardiovascular exercise (CV) helps to reverse established disease and control the risk factors for heart disease, including high blood pressure, high cholesterol, and obesity. It also lowers LDL (bad fat) and raises HDL (good fat).

➤ *Stroke.* Cardiovascular exercise helps to decrease the risk of stroke and helps to restore the ability to function after a stroke.

➤ *High blood pressure.* Cardiovascular exercise promotes a lower blood pressure for mild to moderate hypertensives without the use of drugs.

It goes without saying that if you've had a heart attack, you'll need to work carefully with your physician to get back on the bandwagon. Generally, cardiac patients are referred to an in-patient cardiac rehabilitation program.

According to American College of Sports Medicine guidelines, following the first 48 hours of a heart attack or cardiac surgery, the only activities should be self-care activities (bathing, dressing, grooming), and very low-resistance activities done progressively from supine (lying face up) to sitting to standing. For uncomplicated cases, the use of a treadmill three to five days afterwards is indicated as a good barometer of exercise tolerance. Upon hospital discharge, patients may be referred to an outpatient cardiac rehabilitation program. At that time, various goals are laid out and closely followed by exercise physiologists, nurses, and physicians.

While resistance exercise is important in improving muscular strength and endurance, it is not suitable for all cardiac patients. People suffering from congestive heart failure should not participate in strength-training activities.

In fact, all cardiac patients should defer resistance training until after four to six weeks of cardiorespiratory endurance exercise has been completed. Every precaution should be taken to ensure that proper breathing techniques are used throughout each and every repetition for each and every set to make sure you don't hold your breath, which can send your blood pressure through the roof. Strength training should incorporate all major muscle groups: legs, calves, back, chest, shoulders, and arms. The following exercises are appropriate for cardiac patients beginning a resistance program.

Exercises for Cardiac Patients Beginning a Resistance Program

Body Part	Exercises
Legs	Leg extensions, leg curls, leg presses, standing calf raises, sitting calf raises
Chest	Pec deck, machine chest press
Back	Lat pull downs, cable rows, back extensions
Shoulders	Machine lateral raises, machine shoulder press
Biceps	Machine curls
Triceps	Triceps extensions
Abs	Crunches, oblique crunches

Note that all of the above exercises require machines. Machines are much less strenuous and require less skill and balance than freeweights. As a result, the patient is free to concentrate on proper breath control while performing the exercises. Again, to state the obvious, if you feel any adverse reactions during or after your strength-training routine, please contact your physician immediately.

Sadly, with all of the benefits available for people who have suffered a heart attack, research shows that those who need it the most are least likely to eat right and go to the gym. (Which may explain why they had a heart attack in the first place.) While it may sound preachy, get smart, work out before your heart tells you that you must, and avoid becoming a statistic.

Asthma

Asthma is a treatable lung disease that can strike at any age; however, about half of all patients are under the age of 10, with twice as many girls affected as boys. Asthma has three main characteristics associated with it:

➤ Airway obstructions

➤ Airway inflammation

➤ Airway hyperresponsiveness to a variety of stimuli

Symptoms associated with asthma are wheezing, coughing, shortness of breath, and chest tightness.

EIA and *EIB* are terms used interchangeably to describe asthma symptons that are brought on by exercise. EIA stands for exercise-induced asthma and EIB stands for exercise-induced bronchiospasm. Symptoms of both include shortness of breath, a tight feeling in the chest, and coughing. EIA usually occurs within three to eight minutes of exercise with the aforementioned symptoms.

Following are factors that may determine whether you have exercise-induced asthma. This is by no means an absolute diagnostic tool, just a guideline.

➤ Coughing, wheezing, difficulty breathing, or chest discomfort when you exercise

➤ Symptoms that vary by season or outdoor temperature

➤ Discontinued, decreased, or altered exercise regimen

➤ Complaints of decreased or limited endurance

➤ "Out of shape" label used to describe a well-conditioned athlete by his or her coach

➤ Minimal problems with swimming because of the warm, humid environments

If you experience any of the above, see your physician for further assessment.

For those of you diagnosed with EIA, the following are factors that may contribute to the severity of the affliction:

➤ Ambient air conditions (cold air, low humidity, and/or pollutants)

➤ Duration, type, and intensity of exercise

➤ Exposure to allergens in sensitive individuals

➤ Poor physical conditioning

➤ Respiratory infections

➤ The amount of time since the last episode of exercise-induced asthma

➤ Underlying bronchial hyperactivity

Asthma is not a sentence to a sedentary lifestyle; as a matter of fact, it can be brought under control with proper precaution during exercise. As any athlete can tell you, having asthma is merely a hindrance, not a reason to stand on the sidelines. Just ask Jackie Joyner-Kersee, the Olympic long jumper and hepthatlete considered the best female athlete ever. (Our own fitness maven Jonathan Cane has asthma.)

Several sports that are recommended for asthma sufferers are baseball, softball, and volleyball—all sports that involve brief rest periods. However, more strenuous sports like swimming, cycling, running, or soccer are fine as well, although the asthmatic athlete may require inhalation of his or her bronchodilator before participation.

Weight training is far less problematic to asthmatics than cardiovascular activities. However, since symptoms can be triggered by allergens in the air, it's possible that symptoms like wheezing and coughing can kick in if you're allergic to something in the gym. Since environmental factors such as cold, dry air, pollens, dust mites, and air pollutants can exacerbate EIA, it's a good idea to have your bronchodilator nearby.

For those of you who do have asthma, weight training would be no different for you than it would be for anyone else. Good form, technique, and proper breath control should be your mantra. A basic beginner's routine incorporating all major muscle groups with a base of three sets of 10 to 12 reps is fine.

For those who run, cycle, and do the mambo, the following precautions should be taken to avoid triggering symptoms:

➤ Warm up before you run a 10K or swim the English Channel. In other words, before any intense endurance effort.

➤ Wear a face mask during activities that take place in cold, dry conditions.

➤ Breathe in through your nose as opposed to your mouth to warm and humidify inspired air.

Lupus

Lupus is an autoimmune disorder, which means that for reasons no one seems to know, the body turns against itself. Right now there is no known cause for Lupus and no known cure. The best way to manage the disorder is through medication and a healthy lifestyle—good nutrition, proper hydration, exercise, and rest.

There are three types of lupus. Discoid lupus erythematosus (DLE) attacks the skin and scalp. Lesions are round, scaly red patches that are not itchy or painful, but when it attacks the scalp, hair loss can occur. People with this variety of Lupus are usually very sensitive to the sun.

The second type, Systemic lupus erythematosus (SLE) is called "The disease of a thousand faces" because no two people with this form have the same symptoms. It can affect any organ of the body and is more severe than discoid lupus.

The third type is drug-induced, and it usually occurs after the ingestion of certain prescription drugs. The symptoms are similar to SLE; however, once the drugs are stopped the symptoms disappear, and the illness does not progress to a chronic stage.

While Lupus can affect any part of the body, the most common symptoms involve the skin, joints, kidneys, heart, and lungs. The objective in treatment is to try to prevent flare-ups. Patients must take an active role in their day-to-day physical health and take note of their responses to physical activity, diet, and sleep. Because some of the medications used to treat Lupus can cause muscle weakness, it's extremely important to make weight training a part of your life as you deal with the disease.

Before beginning any exercise, it's important to gently stretch all of your major muscle groups—with an emphasis on gentle since the muscles weakened by medication have a tendency to tear. Warm up with easy aerobic exercise until you're perspiring lightly. Then go through a gentle stretching routine for your legs, chest, and back. Once you've stretched, begin your weight-training routine.

It is important to exercise at a moderate pace. We recommend that you begin with one set of each exercise using a weight that you can handle for 8 to 10 reps. Afterwards, take stock of how you're feeling. Are you extremely fatigued compared to prior workouts? If so, decrease the amount of weight that you selected and have at it.

Once you've found a weight that is appropriate, experiment with increasing the number of sets: first two sets, then three sets. Don't increase the weight. Once you've adapted and have not noted any adverse reactions, you can slowly increase the amount of weight you're using, but only by 2.5 to 5 pounds at a time.

On the Bright Side

While disease is often unavoidable and death is a certainty, there is one thing that we can control—our attitude to the adversity that visits us. People who state that they're going to "beat" a particular ailment often do, in part because they refuse to give in to the depression that often accompanies the affliction. As one coach we know likes to say, "Postitive thinking is a healthy tonic." His logic is simple but profound: Think well of yourself, and you'll think yourself well.

The Least You Need to Know

➤ Strength training and aerobic exercise for HIV/AIDS patients will make their bodies stronger without weakening their immune systems.

➤ Studies have shown that exercise dramatically reduces some of the most common types of cancer for men and women.

➤ Diabetics can work out normally, assuming they take special precautions.

➤ Heart disease is often directly related to poor eating habits and a sedentary lifestyle.

➤ Asthmatics have won Olympic gold medals. Asthma is not a sentence to a sedentary lifestyle; as a matter of fact, it can be brought under control with proper precautions during exercise.

➤ Lupus has no known cure, but strength training is one of the best ways to combat the medication that weakens your muscles.

Glossary

Abdominals (abs)   muscles of the midsection.

Abduction   sideways movement away from the body.

Abductors   muscles that move your leg away from the body.

Adduction   sideways movement in the direction toward the body.

Adductors   muscles that draw your leg in toward your body from an outward position.

Aerobic   exercise that requires a significant and sustained supply of oxygen. Literally means in the presence of oxygen.

Alternating grip (reverse grip)   a grip where you hold the bar with the fingers of one hand facing your body (pronated) and the fingers of the other hand facing away from your body (supinated).

Amino acids   the structural material or "building blocks" of protein.

Anaerobic   exercise that can take place in the absence of oxygen.

Anterior   refers to the front of the body.

Assisted reps   repetitions performed with the help of a spotter.

Atrophy   the loss of size of a muscle. The opposite of hypertrophy.

Barbell   a straight freeweight, on which plates can be added for increased resistance.

Bench press   a power-lifting exercise that involves lying on your back and pushing a weight from your chest.

Biceps   the muscle in the front of the upper arm, responsible for bending (flexing) the elbow.

Breakdowns   a technique in which once you fatigue, you decrease the weight being used and do a few extra reps.

Bursa   a padlike sac that acts to reduce friction between tendon and bone or tendon and ligament.

Bursitis   inflammation of the bursa.

Cardiovascular exercise   any activity that improves your cardiovascular system. Your body's cardiovascular system includes your heart, lungs, and circulatory system.

Carpal tunnel syndrome   a condition that is often caused by repetitive activities done with improper body mechanics, such as typing with your wrists in an extended position, or repetitive squeezing activities. The median nerve swells and is unable to pass comfortably through the small bones in your wrist (carpals). Symptoms of carpal tunnel syndrome are numbness, tingling, or a sharp, shooting pain into your hand.

Clean and jerk   an Olympic weight-lifting exercise in which the lifter hoists the weight from the platform to the shoulders in one motion (clean) and then thrusts the bar from his/her shoulders to a position over head in one motion while splitting his/her legs (jerk).

Collar   a safety device that helps secure plates on a barbell.

Compound movement   an exercise, such as the bench press, squat, or lat pull down, that involves the movement of more than one joint at a time.

Concentric contraction   the shortening of a muscle as it exerts force.

Contract   literally speaking, to draw together or shorten. When contracted, a muscle shortens and produces movement.

Contracture   a condition where a joint (shoulder, elbow, wrist, finger, hip, knee, or ankle) is unable to be fully straightened or fully bent.

Deadlift   a powerlifting maneuver in which the weighted bar is on the floor, and the lifter bends his or her knees and hips to reach the bar. The bar is then lifted to midthigh.

Delayed onset muscle soreness (DOMS)   the temporary pain you feel in your muscles after a workout, usually within 24 hours of your workout, which peaks after 48 hours.

Deltoid   major muscle of the shoulder. Divided into medial, posterior, and anterior sections.

Diaphragm   a muscle used in respiration.

Dumbbell   handheld freeweights.

Eccentric contraction   a lengthening of the muscle as it exerts force but is overcome by the resistance.

Erector spinae   muscles of the back that run along the spine.

Ergogenic aid   any product that improves athletic or physical performance.

Extend   to increase the angle between body parts, as in straightening the elbow or knee.

Fast-twitch muscle fiber   a powerful, easily fatigued muscle fiber.

Female athletic triad   a phenomenon common among competitive female athletes, that consists of eating disorders, amenorrhea (absence of the menstrual flow), and osteoporosis.

Flex   to decrease the angle between body parts, as in bending the elbow or knee. (Commonly, but incorrectly, used to refer to contracting a muscle.)

Freeweights   handheld weights such as barbells and dumbbells.

Gastrocnemius   a muscle in the back of the lower leg, responsible for raising the heel over the toe, especially when the knee is straight.

Gluteus (glutes)   generally refers to the gluteus maximus (the gluteus medius and gluteus minimus are much smaller and weaker), responsible for extension of the hip.

Hamstrings   muscles of the back of the upper leg, responsible for bending the knee and extending the hip. Made up of the biceps femoris, semitendinosus, and semimembranosus muscles.

Hyperextend   to extend a joint beyond straight.

Hyperplasia   an increase in the amount of muscle fibers. Does not appear to occur in humans.

Hypertrophy   the growth of a muscle and the individual fibers that make it up. This growth usually occurs as a result of an external stimulus like weight lifting.

Impingement   the pinching or squeezing of the internal structures of the shoulder (tendons of the rotator cuff, bursa, ligaments, and nerves). This pinching causes pain on elevation of the arm.

Isolation exercise   a lift that uses only one joint and therefore focuses on one muscle.

Isometric contraction   a muscle action that results in no movement because the muscle force and the resistance are equal.

411

Lactic acid by-product of anaerobic work that causes fatigue and a burning sensation.

Latissimus dorsi (lats) the large, fan-shaped muscles of the middle and upper back.

Ligaments the connective tissue between bones.

Lordosis the natural inward curve of the lumbar or lower spine.

Muscle pull See *muscle strain*.

Muscle strain a trauma to the muscle or tendon caused by excessive contraction or stretching.

Negatives an advanced technique in which you stress the eccentric phase of an exercise.

Olympic weight lifting a competitive sport that includes the snatch and the clean and jerk.

Overtraining a phenomenon that occurs when you exercise excessively without allowing sufficient recovery between workouts.

Palpitations an abnormally rapid throbbing or fluttering of the heart.

Pectorals (pecs) the large muscles in the chest.

Phlebitis an inflammation of a vein.

Plates weighted disks that are added to a bar to increase its weight. Plates most often come in denominations of 2½, 5, 10, 25, 35, and 45 pounds.

Plyometrics controversial exercises that use bounding techniques to build "explosive" power.

Posing a facet of bodybuilding where the competitor demonstrates his or her physical assets by assuming various positions that show off his or her muscularity and proportion.

Posterior refers to the rear of the body.

Powerlifting a competitive sport that includes the squat, bench press, and deadlift.

Pronation turning the hand so that the palm faces downward. Opposite of *supination*.

Quadriceps muscles of the front of the upper leg, responsible for straightening the knee. Made up of the rectus femoris, vastus lateralis, vastus intermedius, and vastus medialis muscles.

Range of motion (ROM)   the movement from the beginning to the finishing point of an exercise. Moving a joint from complete extension to complete flexion is considered a full range of motion.

Recovery   the rest period between two sets or workouts.

Repetition (rep)   the execution of an exercise one time. Consecutive repetitions are grouped into a set.

Rotator cuff   group of muscles (supraspinatus, infraspinatus, teres minor, and subscapularis) located under the deltoid.

Set   a series of repetitions performed consecutively.

Slow-twitch muscle fiber   a muscle fiber that has great endurance but relatively low power.

Snatch   an Olympic weight-lifting exercise in which the lifter pulls the bar up from the platform. Then he or she leaps into a squat position under the bar, securing it overhead with arms held straight.

Soleus   a muscle in the back of the lower leg, responsible for raising the heel over the toe, especially when the knee is bent.

Specificity of training   a physiological theory that suggests that adaptations made during training depend on the type of training used.

Split routine   a workout scheme in which the body is divided into different parts that are exercised on different days.

Spotter   someone who stands by to help the lifter if and when he or she can't finish a repetition. The spotter is responsible for the safety of the lifter.

Sprain   damage due to overstretching of ligaments.

Squat   a power-lifting maneuver that involves performing a deep knee bend with a barbell across your back.

Sticking point   a particular position during your range of motion where you have difficulty completing the repetition without assistance.

Supersets   an advanced strength-training method that involves doing two exercises with no rest.

SuperSlow   a protocol that involves extremely slow movement—10 seconds for the positive phase and 5 seconds for the negative.

Supination   turning the hand so that the palm faces upward. Opposite of *pronation.*

T cells   the cells responsible for enhancing antibody production and for killing foreign cells in the body.

Target heart rate (training zone)   the desired heart rate range to elicit a training effect while performing cardiovascular exercise.

Tendinitis   a condition characterized by inflammation of a tendon.

Tendon   connective tissue that attaches muscle to bone.

Trapezius (traps)   the muscle that covers the rear of the neck and shoulders.

Triceps   the muscle in the back of the upper arm, responsible for straightening (extending) the elbow.

Valsalva maneuver   holding the breath while lifting. May lead to excessive increase in blood pressure and decrease in blood returning to the heart.

VO$_2$ max   a measure of an individual's capacity for aerobic work. It is generally considered to be one of the most important factors in predicting an athlete's ability to perform in activities of more than three to five minutes.

Weight belt   a thick, wide, dense leather belt used for added support for the lower back when lifting.

Working in   the practice of alternating sets on a particular bench or machine with another person.

Resources

Achilles Track Club
    42 West 38th Street
    New York, NY 10018
    (212) 354-0300
    www.achillestrackclub.org

Aerobics and Fitness Association of America (AFAA)
    15250 Ventura Boulevard
    Sherman Oaks, CA 91403
    (800) 225-AFAA
    www.afaa.com

American College of Sports Medicine (ACSM)
    P.O. Box 1440
    Indianapolis, IN 46206-1440
    (317) 637-9200
    www.acsm.org

American Council on Exercise (ACE)
    5820 Oberlin Drive
    Suite 102
    San Diego, CA 92121-3787
    (800) 825-3636
    www.acefitness.org

AquaBells
    115 Marin Valley Drive
    Novato, CA 94949
    (800) 987-6892
    www.metro.net/aquabells

Bowflex
2200 NE 65th Avenue
Vancouver, WA 98661
(800) 269-3539
www.bowflex.com

Challenged Athletes Foundation
2148-B Jimmy Durante Boulevard
Del Mar, CA 92104
(619) 793-9293
www.challengedathletes.org

Concept II
105 Industrial Park Drive
Morrisville, VT 05661-9727
(800) 245-5676
www.concept2.com

Cyberpump
www.cyberpump.com

Cybex
2100 Smithtown Avenue
Ronkonkoma, NY 11779-9003
(516) 585-9000

DynaBand
Fitness Wholesale
895-A Hampshire Road
Stow, OH 44224
(800) 537-5512

Fitness World
www.fitnessworld.com

Gatorade Sports Science Institute
617 W. Main Street
Barrington, IL 60010
(800) 616-GSSI (4774)
www.gssiweb.com

Hammer Strength
2245 Gilbert Avenue
Cincinnati, Ohio 45206
(513) 221-2600
www.hammerstrength.com

Healthclubs.com Guide to Health and Fitness
www.healthclubs.com

Healthfinder
U.S. Department of Health and Human Services
www.healthfinder.gov

Icarian
12660 Branford Street
Sun Valley, CA 91352
(800) 883-2421

International Health, Racquet & Sportsclub Association (IHRSA)
263 Summer Street
Boston, MA 02210
(800) 228-4772
www.ihrsa.org

LifeFitness
10601 West Belmont Avenue
Franklin Park, IL 60131
(800) 735-3867
www.lifefitness.com

Nancy Clark Sports Nutrition
www.nancyclarkrd.com

National Sports Performance Association (NSPA)
700 Russell Avenue
Gaithersburg, MD 20877
(800) 494-6772
www.nspainc.com

National Strength and Conditioning Association (NSCA)
1640 L Street, Suite G
Lincoln, Nebraska 68508
(888) 746-CERT (2378)
www.nsca-cc.org

Natural Strength
www.naturalstrength.com

Nautilus
709 Powerhouse Road
Independence, VA 24348-0708
(800) NAUTILUS
www.nautilus.com

Polar
370 Crossways Park Drive
Woodbury, NY 11797
(800) 227-1314
www.polarusa.com

Power Blocks
Intellbell
1819 South Cedar Avenue
Owatonna, MN 55060
(800) 446-5215
www.powerblock.com

Powerlifting USA
P.O. Box 467
Camarillo, CA 93011
(800) 448-7693

Quinton
3303 Monte Villa Parkway
Bothell, WA 98021-8906
(800) 426-0337
www.quinton.com

Soloflex
Hawthorn Farm Industrial Park
570 NE 53rd Avenue
Hillsboro, OR 97124-6494
(800) 547-8802
www.soloflex.com

StairMaster Sports
12421 Willows Road NE
Suite 100
Kirkland, WA 98034
(800) 635-2936
www.stairmaster.com

Star Trac
14410 Myford Road
Irvine, CA 92606
(877) STAR-TRAC
www.startrac.com

SuperSlow Exercise Guild
P.O. Box 180154
Casselberry, FL 32718-0154
(407) 862-2552
www.superslow.com

Trotter
10 Trotter Way
Medway, MA 02053
(800) 677-6544

Total Gym
(800) 541-4900
www.totalgym.com

U.S. Food and Drug Administration (FDA)
5600 Fishers Lane
Rockville, MD 20857
(888) INFO-FDA 463-6332
www.fda.gov

USA Powerlifting
124 West Van Buren Street
Columbia City, IN 46725
(219) 248-4889
www.usapowerlifting.com

USA Weightlifting
One Olympic Plaza
Colorado Springs, CO 80909
(719) 578-4508
www.usaweightlifting.org

VersaClimber
Heart Rate, Inc.
3188-E Airway Avenue
Costa Mesa, CA 92626-2771
(800) 237-2271
www.versaclimber.com

Women's Sports Foundation
Eisenhower Park
East Meadow, NY 11554
(800) 227-3988
www.lifetimetv.com/WoSport/index.html

Index